# Research for Physiotherapists

*For Laura*

*For Churchill Livingstone:*

*Commissioning Editor:* Mary Law
*Project Editor:* Dinah Thom
*Project Manager:* Neil A. Dickson
*Project Controller:* Nicola S. Haig
*Copy Editor:* Teresa Brady
*Sales Promotion Executive:* Maria O'Connor

# Research for Physiotherapists

## Project Design and Analysis

**Carolyn M. Hicks** BA MA PhD PGCE CPsychol
Senior Lecturer in Psychology, School of Continuing Studies,
University of Birmingham, UK

SECOND EDITION

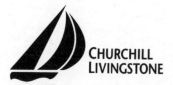

CHURCHILL LIVINGSTONE
EDINBURGH HONG KONG LONDON MADRID MELBOURNE NEW YORK AND TOKYO 1995

CHURCHILL LIVINGSTONE
Medical Division of Pearson Professional Ltd

Distributed in the United States of America by Churchill
Livingstone Inc., 650 Avenue of the Americas, New York,
N.Y. 10011, and by associated companies, branches and
representatives throughout the world.

First edition 1988
Second edition 1995
    Reprinted 1995
    Reprinted 1997

ISBN 0-443-04999-8

**British Library Cataloguing in Publication Data**
A catalogue record for this book is available from the
British Library.

**Library of Congress Cataloging in Publication Data**
Hicks, Carolyn.
    Research for physiotherapists : project design and
analysis /
    Carolyn M. Hicks. -- 2nd ed.
        p.    cm.
    Rev. ed. of: Practical research methods for
physiotherapists. 1988.
    Includes bibliographical references and index.
    1. Physical therapy--Research--Statistical
methods.    I. Hicks, Carolyn. Practical research methods
for physiotherapists.
    II. Title.
    [DNLM: 1. Psysical Therapy.    2. Research
Design.   3. Statistics.
    WB 460 H631r 1995]
    RM708.H53 1995
    615.8'2'072 -- dc20
    DNLM/DLC
    for Library of Congress                     94-25780

**Note**
Medical knowledge is constantly changing. As new information
becomes available, changes in treatment, procedures, equipment
and the use of drugs become necessary. The authors and the
publishers have, as far as it is possible, taken care to ensure that
the information given in this text is accurate and up-to-date.
However, readers are strongly advised to confirm that the
information, especially with regard to drug usage, complies with
latest legislation and standards of practice.

The
publisher's
policy is to use
**paper manufactured
from sustainable forests**

Produced by Longman Singapore Publishers Pte Ltd.
Printed in Singapore

# Contents

# Preface

There have been many changes in the health care system since the first edition of this book was written. Managerial and organisational structures, policy-making, training and service delivery are now all quite different, and this inevitably means that the whole health care culture has shifted immeasurably.

One of the most significant changes to have taken place recently is the Government's commitment to the role of research in health care provision. It is no longer considered acceptable to base paramedical clinical practice on time-honoured ritual; instead, clinical practice must be properly and integrally related to research findings in order to increase its public accountability. At a time when the British National Health Service is experiencing a diminution in resources with a simultaneous need for enhanced efficiency, economy and effectiveness in its provision, research is seen to be one important way in which these aims can be achieved. Consequently, health care practitioners from every branch of the service are being urged to use research to justify their practice.

In parallel with these directives are the changes taking place in paramedical training, with the professions complementary to medicine increasingly seeking academic accreditation, by universities, polytechnics and colleges, for their pre- and post-registration training courses. Inherent to many of these courses, as a result of such developments, is an emphasis on research skills and awareness. Thus, both existing clinical practitioners as well as new trainees are being encour-aged to develop research projects, and a general research-mindedness, as routine parts of their job.

This book is an attempt to support these changes. There are, undoubtedly, numerous excellent texts on research currently on the market, but methodology research is a dry topic, which usually holds little interest for the intending researcher. If individuals are to be enticed into the research arena, it is important that the essential, but turgid concepts of research methodologies are made meaningful to them. Consequently, a text on physiotherapy research should translate the theoretical ideas into situations and terms which make sense to a physiotherapist. I have, over the years, taught numerous research methods courses to a wide range of health care professionals, and all my experience suggests that the most effective way of engaging the participants' interest and enhancing their understanding is to 'customise' the essential concepts, using examples relevant to their own experience. In this respect, I believe that this text differs from many others presently available.

A side-effect of the movement in health care provision towards scientific accountability of clinical practice, is the diffidence felt by many health carers under the pressure to undertake research, at whatever level. The traditions of the paramedical professions have been vocational rather than academic, and the shift towards research, with its connotations of intellectual exclusivity and scientific rigour, has concerned many practitioners who, despite being clinically qualified and very experienced, have not had the opportunity to develop research skills.

An elitist attitude has undoubtedly been fostered by many academics who perceive research to be solely within their domain, and who consequently resist the notion that research expertise should be the right of any interested professional. One technique used by people who wish to retain rather than share their particular knowledge is the use of excessive and unnecessary jargon. Consequently, many research methods and statistics books are stuffed full of complex and incomprehensible words, and their message, inevitably, will remain inaccessible to all but the most intrepid and determined of readers.

I hope that this text will not fall into the same trap. I am not a statistician but rather a psychologist who often has a mental block when confronted with new statistical formulae and concepts. This, I trust, will mean that I am perhaps more aware of the anxieties and problems many new researchers and non-statisticians experience when confronted with formulae and figures; as a result I have attempted, as far as possible, to demystify the text and remove the jargon.

Similarly, I have included as little statistical theory as one can get away with. Many books on research methods and statistics incorporate detailed theoretical derivations of esoteric concepts and formulae. While a full understanding of the principles of research design and analysis are crucial to sound research, such information overload can have a demoralising effect on students, who then feel deterred rather than fully equipped to undertake a research project. This book is intended to help physiotherapists to understand the most important aspects of how to design, undertake and analyse a relevant piece of research, without submerging them in too much jargon and theory.

That having been said, there is, of necessity, some research-specific terminology, and this raises a note of caution. Terminology within research and statistics is notoriously inconsistent, and consequently cross-referencing with other books may be confusing. To minimise confusion I have tried to give common alternatives to some of the terms as and where relevant.

Finally, the emphasis in this text is primarily on experimental research in physiotherapy. A full explanation of what this means in practice will be given later, but it is important to justify, at this point, why this particular approach has been chosen. Experimental research is important in all the paramedical professions because it allows them to compare procedures, treatments and patient groups. In the context of physiotherapy, this means that the relative effectiveness of different interventions for a given medical problem can be evaluated, allowing the physiotherapist to rationalise his/her practices; it allows the comparison of different patient groups, so that it can be ascertained whether one type of person is more likely to benefit from a given procedure than another, and it allows the evaluation of the efficiency or reliability of various makes of equipment. In short, the experimental approach is critical in the development of physiotherapy as a research-based profession. It should, however, be noted that it is not the only valid approach to research and nor is it the most valid; but it is a particularly worthwhile way of investigating many problems which arise in physiotherapy practice. While other methodologies will be referred to in the text, it is the experimental approach and the statistical analyses which go with it that will receive most attention.

In these ways, this second edition is similar to the first. However, there is some new material which has been incorporated, largely on the recommendations of many of the physiotherapists who were kind enough to provide feedback on the first text.

While there are numerous minor changes and updatings, all of which will, I hope, serve to clarify the essential points, the most significant modifications to this edition have been the inclusion of additional material.

First, a broader overview of the different approaches to research has been included in the Introduction, in order that the reader may gain a wider perspective of other methodologies relevant to physiotherapy research.

Secondly, sections on surveys and questionnaire design have been included in Chapter 3. Both topics are of considerable use in health care research, enabling the physiotherapist to undertake studies which provide an overview of the health, sickness or take-up of care in any given community.

Thirdly, a new chapter on estimation and confidence intervals has been included. These techniques are particularly useful in care planning and resource allocation, both of which are familiar tasks to any physiotherapist who has a management responsibility.

There is also a chapter on how to read research critically. Many physiotherapists, for a variety of reasons, may not wish to embark on any research of their own. However, it is still essential that they are able to evaluate the work of others prior to implementing research findings into their own practice, since without this, it is conceivable that patient well-being could be compromised. Chapter 12 provides guidance on how to make informed judgements on published research.

Finally, there is a glossary of terms, providing a quick reference for any readers who wish to check or confirm their understanding of essential concepts and terminology.

In conclusion, I would like to acknowledge the many people who helped and supported me in writing this book.

I am indebted to Doreen Caney, retired Principal of the Queen Elizabeth School of Physiotherapy in Birmingham, who furnished me with numerous ideas, guidance, information and help; without her, the book would not have been started in the first place, and nor would it have been completed. If inaccurate statements about physiotherapy remain in the text, it is because I misused her advice. Sincerest thanks are due to her. Secondly, I wish to thank my excellent secretaries; Janet Francis, who ploughed her way through the manuscript of the first edition with consummate skill and good humour, and Christine Corbett, who took on the equally awful task of interpreting my revisions for this second edition with similar goodwill and expertise. Thanks are also due to Christine O'Donoghue and Christine Marshall who were prime movers and facilitators in getting the initial project off the ground. I am also indebted to Christine Greatbatch who read the revised manuscript with great thoroughness. Her suggestions and comments have been invaluable. And lastly, I owe a great deal to my husband, Professor Peter Spurgeon, for his comments on the theoretical content of the book and the lucidity of its presentation, and to my children, Tom and Laura. When they stopped helping me, I started to make some progress.

Birmingham 1994                    C. H.

# Acknowledgements

I am indebted to the following sources for granting permission to reproduce the statistical tables in Appendix 2 of this book:

*Tables A2.1, A2.5 and A2.6* from Lindley D V, Scott W F 1984 New Cambridge Elementary Statistical Tables, 10th edn. Cambridge University Press, Cambridge

*Table A2.2* from Wilcoxon F, Wilcox R A 1949 Some Rapid Approximate Statistical Procedures. American Cyanamid Company. Reproduced with the permission of the American Cyanamid Company

*Table A2.3* from Friedman M 1937 The use of ranks to avoid the assumptions of normality implicit in the analysis of variance. Reprinted with permission from the Journal of the American Statistical Association. Copyright (1937) by the American Statistical Association. All rights reserved

*Table A2.4* from Page E E 1963. Reprinted with permission from the Journal of the American Statistical Association. Copyright (1963) by the American Statistical Association. All rights reserved

*Table A2.7* from Runyon R P, Haber A 1991 Fundamentals of Behavioral Statistics 7th edn. McGraw-Hill, New York

*Table A2.8* from Kruskal W H, Wallis W A 1952 The use of ranks in one-criterion variance analysis. Reprinted with permission from the Journal of the American Statistical Association. Copyright (1952) by the American Statistical Association. All rights reserved

*Table A2.9* from Jonckheere A R 1954 A distribution-free k-sample test against ordered alternatives. Biometrika 14 (Biometrika Trustees)

*Table A2.10* from Olds E G 1949 The 5% significance levels for sums of squares of rank differences and a correction. Annals of Mathematical Statistics 20 (The Institute of Mathematical Statistics)

*Table A2.11* from Table VII (p. 63) of Fisher R A, Yates F 1974 Statistical Tables for Biological, Agricultural and Medical Research, Longman Group Ltd, London (previously published by Oliver and Boyd Ltd, Edinburgh). I am grateful to the Literary Executor of the late Sir Ronald Fisher, FRS, to Dr Frank Yates and to Longman Group Ltd, London for permission to reprint Table VII from their book, Statistical Tables for Biological, Agriculture and Medical Research, 6th edn. 1974

*Table A2.12* adapted from Friedman M 1940 A comparison of alternative tests of significance for the problem of m rankings. Annals of Mathematical Statistics

# Basic principles of research

# 1

# Introduction

## THE NEED FOR RESEARCH IN PHYSIOTHERAPY

Why carry out research in physiotherapy? Surely the profession is sufficiently well-established to make such activities irrelevant – after all, many of the therapeutic techniques currently in practice have been developed over the years and consequently are tried and tested. Is there really any need to start introducing experiments and statistical analysis?

I have heard these arguments on a number of occasions and have some sympathy with this point of view. However, as I have written this book on experimental design and statistics for physiotherapy, it must be apparent that my opinion differs from this. While this is no place to enter the debate, I would like to outline briefly why I feel that research is fundamental to the profession.

My first argument is a general one. There is an increasing trend towards physiotherapy becoming an all-graduate profession, and the current degree courses all have a substantial science component. Nor is this inappropriate, since physiotherapy is clearly scientific in content. However, all sciences have at their root, a reliance on experimentation, data collection and statistical analysis. If physiotherapy is to submit to the scientific rigour inherent in a degree course, it must incorporate research methodology and statistics. Such a component lends credibility, not only academically, but professionally.

A second point relates to the need for physiotherapists to understand research methods and statistics in order to evaluate other professionals' research activities and reports. In a climate of increasing accountability, particularly in the public service sector, it is becoming imperative for professionals to justify their actions and to increase their effectiveness and efficiency. Clearly, one way to achieve these aims is to make clinical practice more firmly informed by proper empirical evidence rather than based on more traditional modes of operating. As a result, physiotherapists and other paramedical professionals are turning more and more to published research, in order to rationalise and streamline their own service delivery. Consequently, it is essential that health carers are able to understand and evaluate the quality of published research prior to any decision to implement the conclusions in their own practice. Therefore, an additional, equally important reason for physiotherapists to develop their research competencies is the need to be able to make properly informed judgements concerning other people's research work. Without this, it is highly likely that patients' well-being, both physical and psychological, might be adversely affected in a direct or indirect way, through the implementation of findings from poorly conducted research.

The third argument in favour of research in physiotherapy relates to much more specific problem-driven issues. There are many physiotherapists who, at the risk of disagreement from their colleagues, would admit that many of the therapeutic procedures they use are selected on the basis of intuition, personal preference and familiarity, rather than on the basis of empirically established information. To illustrate this point, consider the following problem issues:

1. You are about to treat a recent injury where pain is the predominant symptom. Do you select ice or ultrasound? Why? When I asked these questions of a group of highly trained physiotherapists, their opinions were divided. While this could suggest that both methods are equally effective, in this instance I do not think this was the case. Every member of the group put forward an argument for one treatment or the other, based on his/her own experience and not on any research evidence. In other words, their views were divided because treatment selection was a matter of opinion and not of hard factual evidence deriving from scientific research. Research in areas like this might compare the outcomes of different types of treatment, thus removing the subjective element and making the decision process clearer, less ambiguous and hopefully more effective.

2. The uniform/no uniform issue continues to be contentious in some quarters. There are sound arguments on both sides, with the pro-uniform lobby claiming that the uniform inspires greater confidence and trust in the patient, while the anti-uniform contingent argues that it decreases rapport. So how can the issue be resolved? The answer lies in the use of experimental method and statistical analysis – if the effects of wearing uniform vs. wearing 'civvies' are measured and analysed using scientific techniques, the debate can be settled.

3. You are presented with a new piece of apparatus for treating frozen shoulders. Do you try it on the first patient who comes along and then, if the outcome appears to be favourable, order half a dozen more? Or do you set up a controlled experiment whereby you systematically compare the effectiveness of the new apparatus with that of the standard treatment procedure? If you opt for the latter you will need a sound knowledge of scientific methodology and data analysis.

I hope that you can see from these examples of problem-driven issues that experimentation and statistical analysis are essential if physiotherapeutic procedures are to be appropriately and effectively used.

In the current era of increasing pressure on resources, hit-and-miss policies of treatment, based on opinion and preference rather than hard evidence, are too wasteful of time and money to be justified. Therefore it is crucial for physiotherapists to evaluate their procedures systematically to make the profession even more efficient, cost-effective and successful. To do this, a knowledge of experimental design, research methods and statistical analysis is essential.

## APPROACHES TO RESEARCH

It will be clear from the foregoing arguments that

the main emphasis of this book is on *experimental* research. This doesn't mean that physiotherapists are expected to sit in laboratories surrounded by chemicals and Bunsen burners, but rather that they apply the basic principles of experimental methods to their own clinical practice. In this context, an experiment simply means that different groups of people – patients, colleagues or whoever – are treated in certain ways, to see if there are any differences in the groups' outcomes which could be attributed to the intervention they received. In this way, treatments can be compared for effectiveness, along objective scientific lines, in order to try to optimise procedures. The whole issue of designing an experiment will be dealt with in more detail in the course of the book.

However, the experimental approach is not the only way of conducting physiotherapy research, and nor is it necessarily the most valid. It should be remembered that research is about asking questions and finding answers to those questions in a systematic and logical way. There are many ways of asking and answering questions and these variations constitute the different methodologies in research. Experimental research techniques deal with research problems in a way which has enormous value to physiotherapy, as I hope you will discover as you read this text. However, there are alternative approaches which are more appropriate under certain circumstances. To include all the possible variations on the research theme would be impossible in a single text, but it may be useful to refer to some of them briefly here.

## SINGLE-CASE DESIGNS

Like all person-oriented professions, physiotherapy is involved in treating individuals, with their own particular medical problems, personality, motivations etc. Consequently, it may be appropriate on occasions, not to establish whether groups of patients do better on a given intervention than another group, but rather to ask whether a single *individual* patient is benefiting from the treatment given. This has given rise to a research approach known as the **single-case design**.

Let us imagine you are dealing with a 73-year-old lady who has just had a stroke and has lost the use of her left arm which now has very weak muscle contraction. You decide to try to increase the strength of contraction by the use of sensory facilitation. After five treatments, you check her movement control and note that it has improved. This would appear to confirm your choice of treatment for her.

The phases is such a procedure are given labels. The period prior to beginning treatment is called the baseline phase or A. The period during which the patient received the facilitation is called the treatment phase or B. Hence this design is known as an AB design.

However, the approach is not quite as conclusive as might appear at first, since it is possible that the patient's movement control would have improved over time anyway, just as a result of the natural recovery process. The AB design, then, by itself, cannot prove definitively that an improvement occurred as a function of treatment, because that improvement might have happened irrespective of any physiotherapy. One way of getting over this problem is the ABAB design.

In this single-case ABAB approach, our patient would have the sensory facilitation treatment stopped, and consequently would enter another no-treatment phase (a second A stage). If the facilitation had been responsible for the improvement previously observed, we would anticipate that during the second A phase there would be some deterioration in movement control. Then another treatment phase (the second B phase) would be introduced into the study, to find out whether movement control improved again, as a result of sensory facilitation. These phases are outlined in Figure 1.1.

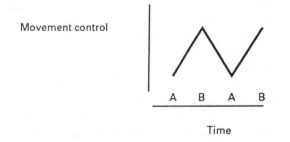

**Figure 1.1** Graph of patient's movement control whilst being treated by sensory facilitation on an ABAB design.

Whilst this design might be useful for looking at individual case histories, it is clearly inappropriate in some situations. For example, it is quite likely that the improvement in movement control noted during the first treatment phase is irreversible and would not, therefore, deteriorate. There are also serious ethical objections, too, to withholding treatment and this must, of necessity, be a cause for serious deliberation prior to the use of an ABAB design. And finally, these single-case designs have little predictive power for other comparable situations. Our stroke patient in this study might have improved, but we have no basis for expecting other stroke patients to derive benefit from the same treatment. Where quick decisions have to be made it is often more useful to be able to rely on findings derived from groups of people rather than from individuals.

## QUALITATIVE RESEARCH

All research involves the collection of facts about an individual or a group of people. Where this information is numerical in nature (such as percentage range of movement, distance walked, blood pressure and temperature readings), the research is classified as **quantitative**. However, how do you quantify a patient's feelings about their condition, or their thoughts on their progress? While numbers can be applied to many fairly objective events, a person's thoughts, feelings and beliefs cannot adequately be subjected to this type of numerical assessment. What is often more appropriate in these circumstances is a description, such as a verbal or pictorial recording, of the individual's responses. Information collection which avoids numerical approaches is called **qualitative** research, and is a means by which the researcher can gain insights into another person's views, opinions, feelings and beliefs, in their own natural settings.

Techniques of qualitative research rely heavily on accurate reporting in a natural environment, without control or restriction being imposed by the investigator. Moreover, unlike quantitative research where small aspects of an individual's behaviour are selected for study, in qualitative research, the individual as a whole and in relation to their social setting, is described. Thus, qualitative research can be thought of as **holistic**. Furthermore, qualitative approaches usually focus on specific individuals, rather than on groups, or types, of individuals.

Another important aspect of qualitative research is the role of the investigator who, rather than being detached and objective as s/he would be in quantitative research, must become enmeshed and integral with the people being studied. This subjectivity, while bringing bias to the research environment, allows for a measure of sensitivity and intuition in the assessment and this can have a considerable benefit in some subject areas. Nonetheless, it should be pointed out that unless the information collection process in qualitative approaches is carefully structured, there is enormous potential for researcher bias. This problem is made worse by the involvement the investigator typically has with the people being studied, since when we know we are being watched or monitored our behaviour changes, often in quite fundamental ways.

Such qualitative approaches can be of great importance to paramedical research. However, it should be pointed out that academic and professional regard for quantitative techniques tends to be higher, rather unjustifiably, which may mean that qualitative research is disregarded and trivialised (see Hunt 1987). However, qualitative techniques can be very usefully employed to describe phenomena such as hospital or unit cultures, or patient experiences, particularly where these are likely to be unusual. My own feeling is that qualitative and quantitative research should be seen not in superior/inferior terms, but rather as complementary techniques, each bringing their own insights to a given problem.

## OBSERVATIONAL TECHNIQUES

One research technique which is inherent to both qualitative and quantitative approaches is observation. Observation in research simply means that a researcher can collect information on a given topic through direct recording and perception of the relevant events.

Observational techniques may involve self- or other evaluations. Self-evaluations are simply reports of subjective responses to certain situations. Pain measurement is a classic example of self-observation, where a patient is required to make a subjective evaluation, of either a numerical or qualitative kind, of how much pain they are experiencing. Other-evaluation involves the use of a third party to observe and record events. Many clinical assessments of student physiotherapists rely on observations of aspects of their clinical expertise, such as the ability to establish rapport with the patient, and as such, these assessments constitute an observational technique.

Observations may be carried out either in natural settings, such as outpatients' clinics, or in more controlled environments, such as laboratories. Both have advantages and disadvantages; for example, while a natural setting cannot be adequately controlled in terms of external or biasing influences, it does have the advantage of realism, so that events can be observed in the way in which they normally occur. Laboratory settings on the other hand can control extraneous influences, but the results so obtained may not translate into more natural surroundings.

There are, inevitably, problems with observational techniques, just as there are in all research methodologies. The reliability of an observation may be a problem, and consequently, some research topics may require a number of different independent observers, or the use of video monitoring systems. Nonetheless, observational information gathering can be an invaluable approach either on its own or in conjunction with other data collection techniques.

These topics re covered in more detail in Polgar & Thomas (1991) and the reader is referred to this book for a fuller explanation of the range of approaches to research.

## SURVEYS, QUESTIONNAIRES AND OTHER DESCRIPTIVE TECHNIQUES

These approaches to research are essential tools for the physiotherapy researcher and will be covered separately in Chapter 3. These techniques are useful for establishing an overview or picture of a given problem within a specified group of people. For example, the researcher might wish to follow up a group of leg fracture patients to establish whether or not they have had any further physical problems, such as residual pain or restricted movement; whether or not they have complied with their exercise plan; attended their outpatient's appointment, or whatever. The survey technique, using a specially devised questionnaire, would be a highly appropriate way of conducting such a study. An introduction to these approaches will be described in more detail in Chapter 3.

## USING STATISTICS

Statistics are a crucial part of quantitative research. Whenever someone carries out an experiment it is essential that the results are analysed and presented in a way that can be understood by other interested parties. Statistics are one means by which this is achieved. For example, if an experiment had been carried out to compare ultrasound with passing accessory movements in treating arthritic toe joints, it is insufficient just to present a table of figures showing the range of movement for each patient following treatment, and expect the reader to make sense of it. The data has to be analysed, described and interpreted using statistical methods, so that an objective conclusion can be reached about the study's outcomes.

The main type of data analysis covered in this book is a technique known as **inferential statistics**, which is the most common way of analysing results derived from experiments. The concepts and procedures relating to this approach are described in Chapters 6–9 and 13–18.

However, data can also be analysed using techniques of **descriptive statistics**. This method allows the researcher to describe the findings in terms of their most interesting features. Descriptive statistics are often used to analyse survey data and for this reason, will be referred to in more detail in Chapters 3–5.

However, many people are put off research because of the statistical procedures that are required. They see a page of formulae and figures, panic and slam the book shut. This suggests the first and most important rule of statistics – **don't panic!** Inability to understand statistics is rarely an intellectual problem, but an emotional one, and anyone who feels diffident in the face of figures should remember this. As long as you approach the statistical analysis systematically and in a step-by-step manner, there should be few problems.

Another point should be raised here. Do not imagine that the object of statistical analysis is to test your long multiplication and division – it isn't. Statistics are no more than a tool for analysing data. So, always use a calculator, as it is faster and usually more reliable than even the quickest mind.

And lastly, remember that you don't need to memorise formulae: as long as you know where to look them up and how to use them, there is no need to commit them to memory. Further, at the risk of being hammered by purists, I would also add that there is no need to understand how the formulae were derived from statistical theory. While many statisticians would vehemently disagree with that rather bald statement, I would liken statistical analysis to any other tool or piece of apparatus; you don't need to understand the workings of a car or television in order to use it. If that were the case, only garage mechanics would be allowed to drive cars. Many would argue, of course, that if you do understand the mechanism, then you are able to put it right if the apparatus goes wrong. However, if you know when, why and how to use a statistical method, and if you follow the procedure step-by-step, then the statistical tool will not break down. It is the when, why and how of statistics that this book aims to explain.

## STRUCTURE OF THE BOOK

The book has been divided into two sections, the first of which is devoted to the design of research projects and the second to statistical procedures. I would recommend that anyone who feels unsure of themselves mathematically should read Appendix 1 at the end of the book. The rest of you may only want to refresh your memories on some basic rules of mathematics. These are presented briefly in the next section. Once you have read as far as Chapter 10 you should have a sound idea of how to design research studies and which

analysis to use on any data resulting from them. After that point, the chapters are devoted to outlining the procedures involved in particular statistical tests. You should read the relevant chapter as and when required. For this reason, these chapters are independent of each other and so may contain common material. I make no apologies for this repetition, since I find nothing more irritating than to open a statistics book at the appropriate chapter only to discover that certain essential elements have been covered earlier, necessitating the reading of additional chapters in which I have little immediate interest. For this reason, the chapters on statistical tests are virtually self-contained.

Throughout the book, too, there are exercises to test your understanding of a particular principle. If you decide to do these, you will find the answers at the back of the book. Also, within each chapter, at appropriate intervals, there are 'Key Concept' boxes, which summarise the most important points. These can be used to refresh your memory without having to plough through several pages to find what you want.

Finally, there aren't a lot of laughs in statistics. Many students find the topic dry, so I've tried to make the style as chatty as possible. Nonetheless, jokes are hard to come by, but do persevere – statistics are an essential part of research life.

So, I hope you will find that this book equips you with the basic elements you need for your research. Happy experimenting!

P.S. All the experiments and data in the book are entirely fictitious!

P.P.S. Please note that all the calculations in the examples and activities have been worked to three decimal places throughout.

P.P.P.S. A final caveat: I am not a physiotherapist, a point which will undoubtedly become clear to you as you read this book. As a result, I have a tendency to make up physiotherapy as I go along, so if there are examples which strike you as ludicrous, naive or just impossible, please forgive me.

And a final word from a student: 'If I had only one day to live, I would spend it in my statistics class. It would seem so much longer.'

Sanders, Eng & Murph 1985

## SOME BASIC MATHS

Most of us have forgotten many of the basic mathematical concepts we learnt for 'O'-level or GCSE, simply because we don't use them very often. Even though you are advised to use a calculator for the statistical tests in this book, it is still essential that you are familiar with the basic mathematical principles, for two main reasons. Firstly, even though a calculator will do all the most complex multiplying, dividing and square-rooting for you, you will need to know the order in which these processes are carried out, because, as you will no doubt remember, some types of computation must be done before others. This will be clarified later. Secondly, even though you will be using a calculator, it is still quite possible to come up with some odd results, either because some information has been entered wrongly, or simply because on occasions, calculators have been known to go haywire. So you need to be able to 'eyeball' the results of your calculations to see if they look right. If you have any doubts or reservations about any of this, read on.

This section is just a brief reminder of some of the basic principles you will need. These principles are discussed in greater detail in Appendix 1, so if you are unsure of any of them, turn to page 205.

## Basic rules

1. If the formula contains brackets, you must carry out all the calculations inside them first.
2. If the formula contains brackets within brackets, you must do the calculations in the innermost brackets first.
3. If the formula contains no brackets, do the multiplications and divisions first.
4. If the formula contains only additions and subtractions, work from left to right.
5. Adding two negative numbers results in a negative answer.
6. Adding a plus number to a minus number is the same as taking the minus number from the plus number.

7. Multiplying two positive numbers gives a positive answer.
8. Multiplying a positive number and a negative number together gives a negative answer.
9. Multiplying two negative numbers gives a positive answer.
10. Dividing a positive number by a negative number (or vice versa) gives a negative answer.
11. Dividing two negative numbers gives a positive answer.
12. The square of a number is that number multiplied by itself. It is expressed as $^2$.
13. The square root of a given number is a number which when multiplied by itself gives the number you already have. It is expressed as $\sqrt{\phantom{x}}$ .
14. To round up decimal points, start at the extreme right-hand number. If it is 5 or more, increase the number to its left by 1. If it is less than 5, the number to its left remains the same.

You might like to do the following exercises just to satisfy yourself that you're happy with these rules.

**Activity 1.1** (Answers on page 227)

Calculate the following:

1. $14 + 8 + 27 - 3$
2. $14 + 8 - (27 - 3)$
3. $17 + (30 - 4)$
4. $11(19 + 4)$
5. $19 \times 3 + 8$
6. $12 + (14 \times 3) - 5$
7. $6[(4 + 8) - 3]$
8. $15 - 4 \times 4 + 12$
9. $(49 - 1) + 7 \times 8$
10. $36 - (12 - 6) + 17$
11. $-18 + 22 - 10$
12. $24 + 16$
13. $12 \times +4$
14. $-18 - 26$
15. $14 \times -3$
16. $-51 + 3$
17. $51 - (+3 \times +2)$
18. $+17 - 4 - 26$
19. $-19 + 11 + 15$
20. $-5(4 \times 12)$

## SYMBOLS IN STATISTICS

You will find the following symbols appearing in formulae throughout the book. Although they will be explained when they appear, this page can serve as a quick reference point.

$\Sigma$ = sum or total of all the calculations to the right of the symbol e.g.
$$\Sigma\, 3^2 + 6^2 + 4^2 = 61$$

$x$ = an individual score

$\bar{x}$ = the average score

$\sqrt{\phantom{x}}$ = the square root of a figure or calculations, e.g.

$$\sqrt{89} = 9.434$$

$$\sqrt{17 + 15 + 86} = 10.863$$

$$\sqrt{51 \times 3} + 4 = 12.369 + 4$$

$$= 16.369$$

$N$ = the total number of scores in an experiment

$^2$ = the number times itself,
e.g. $8^2 = 8 \times 8$
$= 64$

$<$ = less than,
e.g. $5 < 7$ (5 is less than 7)

$>$ = more than,
e.g. $10 > 2$ (10 is more than 2)

$C$ = the number of conditions in the experiment

$n$ = the number of scores in a subgroup or condition.

# 2

# Research design and statistics: some basic concepts

When you engage in research, you will almost always end up measuring something – muscle tone, recovery rate, vital capacity, numbers of patients, etc. These measurements are called **data**. In order for the research to have some value, the meaning of this data has to be presented in ways that other research workers can understand. For example, there is no point in carrying out a well-designed experiment to compare the effectiveness of two bladder control techniques in multiple sclerosis sufferers, if the data on this is left as a jumbled mass of figures. In other words, the researcher has to make sense of the results.

There are various ways of making sense of the results, but for the physiotherapist two methods are of major importance. The first approach is called **descriptive statistics**, where the researcher collects a set of data, usually from a form of survey and then describes it in terms of its most important features, e.g. average scores, range of scores etc. The second approach is called **inferential statistics** in which the data, which has usually been collected from an experiment, is subjected to statistical analysis, using tests which allow the researcher to make inferences beyond the actual data in front of him/her. The differences between these approaches will be discussed briefly now, and then later in more detail in later chapters.

## DESCRIPTIVE STATISTICS

As has already been mentioned, descriptive statistics are often used in conjunction with survey methods. A survey is a research approach which involves collecting information from a large number of people using interviews or questionnaires, in order that an overall picture of that group can be described in terms of any characteristics which are of interest to the researcher. Examples are take-up of community physiotherapy services, use of antenatal clinics, health states, vaccination rates etc. The information that is collected can be analysed using techniques of descriptive statistics in order to highlight some of the most interesting findings.

The way in which a survey is carried out will be described in more detail in the next chapter. However, some general introductory points about survey methods and descriptive statistics will be described here so that the reader can get an overview of how descriptive and inferential statistics differ.

Let's take an example. Supposing you are interested in the general topic of community physiotherapy. You could easily gather a vast quantity of data on this topic, for example:

1. The number of community physiotherapists currently employed in a particular district and their specialities.
2. The number of calls made on average per week within the district over the last year.
3. The types of patients seen (their ages, ethnic origin, social class, sex, etc.) over the last year.
4. The average amount of time spent treating a particular category of patient.
5. Any changes in the execution of community physiotherapy over the previous 10-year period could be noted, e.g. any increase in provision to a particular patient group.

From all this survey data, you could gain the following sorts of information:

- what is going on in a particular area (type and extent of community physiotherapy service provision)
- identification of areas of existing or potential problems (e.g. less provision in some geographical areas or for some categories of patient)
- measurement of the extent of these problems
- the generation of possible explanations for them.

In addition to all this, the survey could identify past trends and so could be used to predict future patterns. (For example, with the population growth in the over-75 age group and the increasing trend towards community-based care, the need for greater provision of community physiotherapists with a special interest in the problems of the older person might be highlighted).

The outcome of such surveys can radically influence major, as well as minor, policy decisions. And if such policy changes are implemented, survey techniques may be used to evaluate the impact these changes have. (For further information on survey methods see Cartwright (1983).) It might be useful at this point to look at some of the ways in which descriptive statistics might be useful to the physiotherapist, by means of a more specific illustration.

### Descriptive statistics: an example

Suppose that you are the head of a school of physiotherapy. Obviously, in this role you will be concerned about the standards of student performance, both clinical and theoretical, in your school. In particular, you may want to find out: (a) whether these standards are dropping or rising from year to year, and (b) how they compare with other schools throughout the country. To do this you need to employ some common mathematical techniques in order to highlight certain features of the data, in other words, descriptive statistics. Let's take the first example. To find out whether the standards are changing from year to year, you could take the average mark in both final theory and clinical exams over, say, the last 10 years. From this you can draw a graph to get the general picture of the standards of performance. You might end up with something like Figure 2.1.

From such a graph of average marks, you can get the general picture of the trend of performance and also the comparative performance on clinical and theory exams.

To solve your second problem of how your school compares with others, you can collect the average marks from all the other schools for 1984, and compare yours with these. You might obtain the data in Table 2.1.

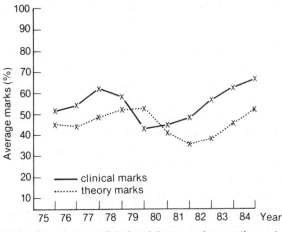

**Figure 2.1**  Average clinical and theory marks over the past 10 years in a school of physiotherapy.

Your own averages for 1984 (66% for theory, 52% for clinical, see Fig. 2.1) can be compared with the other schools to find out how well your school does. It can be seen, then, from this information that your school comes 3rd in the theory exams, but only 7th in the clinical exams. From this information, too, you can see that although school E has the best marks on theory, they have the biggest discrepancy between theory and practice, while school H appears to be the most consistent. In other words, you can glean a considerable amount of information from such data.

It should be pointed out that there are many ways of describing your data besides the methods illustrated above. However the three most commonly used forms of descriptive statistics are **graphs**; **measures of central tendency**, which present data in terms of the most typical scores

**Table 2.1**  Average exam marks from all the schools of physiotherapy in 1984

| School | Average theory mark (%) | Average clinical mark (%) |
|--------|-------------------------|---------------------------|
| A | 63 | 58 |
| B | 45 | 55 |
| C | 48 | 59 |
| D | 57 | 45 |
| E | 70 | 50 |
| F | 52 | 60 |
| G | 54 | 61 |
| H | 67 | 66 |

and results, and **measures of dispersion**, which present data in terms of the variation in the scores. Each of these will be discussed, in Chapter 5, 'Techniques of descriptive statistics'.

Descriptive statistics, then, are used when the researcher has collected a large quantity of data, usually from a survey of some sort, and wishes to extract certain sorts of information from it in order to provide a description of the data.

It is important to recognise that descriptive statistics allow you to make statements about features of your data that are of interest, but they do not allow you to infer anything beyond the results you have in front of you. In other words, if you were measuring the muscle power of a group of 20 muscular dystrophy patients, you could use descriptive statistics to make statements about the muscle power data of that particular group of patients in terms of average power, range of power, speed of contractions etc. What you could not do would be to infer anything about the muscle power of muscular dystrophy patients as a whole, simply on the basis of the data from your particular group. To be able to do that you have to use the techniques of inferential statistics.

## INFERENTIAL STATISTICS

Prior to every election, we are bombarded with the results of opinion polls which tell us how well one political party is likely to do compared with the others. In order to obtain this sort of information, a sample of the general public is questioned, since it would be impossible to ask the opinions of every member of the electorate. From the responses given by this sample, the attitudes of the rest of the voters are predicted, or inferred. However, we all know that these opinion polls may be quite incorrect. For example, if the opinion pollsters only went to a polo match in Surrey and asked the views of the spectators, they would be likely to get a very different picture of the prevailing political opinion than if they only went to a rugby match in South Wales. In other words, if the opinion poll is to have any value in predicting the outcome of an election, the sample of potential voters selected for the poll must be representative of the population as a whole and not representative of just one section of it.

The usual method of selecting a sample which is representative of the population from which it is drawn is a technique called **random sampling**. For a sample to be random, it must have been selected in such a way that every member of the relevant population had an equal chance of being chosen. For example, if 6 playing cards are to be randomly selected from a pack, the pack is first shuffled and any 6 cards are chosen. Assuming the dealer did not hide any or keep his thumb on some, then these 6 cards will be a random sample because every one of the 52 cards had an equal chance of selection.

Now, there are two important points here. Firstly, if these cards are not replaced and a second random sample is drawn from the same population, it will not be the same; so, if another set of 6 cards is selected from the pack, they will be different from the first set because there is only one ace of clubs, seven of hearts etc. in a pack. Similarly, any two groups of hysterectomy patients, if randomly drawn from a population of hysterectomy patients, will not be identical in their characteristics (age, height, fitness, etc.) Secondly, the larger the random sample drawn, the more likely it is that it will be fairly representative of the population from which it comes. So, a random sample of 3 hysterectomy patients out of a total population of 60 will stand less chance of being representative than a random sample of 35. More information about the ways in which the researcher can select a random sample in practice and other ways of selecting a sample are provided in Chapter 3.

Returning to the opinion poll, even if the sample is representative of the whole population, there will still be an element of error in the predictions about the election (because some voters subsequently change their views, fail to vote, or misunderstand the questions etc.).

Nonetheless, if the voters selected for the poll have been chosen randomly, according to certain statistical principles, then this degree of error can be calculated using a branch of statistics known as inferential statistics. Essentially what this approach enables the researcher to do is to select a small sample of people for study, and from the results of that study to make inferences about the larger group from which that sample was drawn. In other words, techniques of inferential statistics allow the researcher to move from what they *know* to be the case, as indicated by the data they have collected, to what they *predict* will be the case in other similar situations.

In case this sounds a rather complex procedure, it should be stated that these inferential techniques are used by everyone on a daily basis. For example, your children, for as long as you can remember, have had cereal for breakfast. This is your data, the facts that you know are true. On this basis, then, you anticipate that this morning they will again want cereal so you put the packets out for them on the assumption that this is what they will want. This is your **inference**, based on the information collected from previous mornings and generalised to another similar situation. There are doubtless numerous examples that you can think of, where your knowledge about one situation leads you to make assumptions about other comparable situations. The actual techniques of inferential statistics are rather more complex than this, but the basic idea is the same.

The proper scientific procedure for making these inferences involves formulating an hypothesis; setting up an experiment to test the hypothesis, and using inferential statistics to analyse the results of your experiment to see if your hypothesis has been supported. Thus, inferential statistics are used in testing hypotheses. It should be pointed out at this stage, that there are two main types of research design which are used to test hypotheses: **experimental designs** and **correlational designs**. They will be described in detail in Chapter 6.

### Using inferential statistics: an example

A classic way in which the physiotherapist might use this approach is in the comparison of different treatment techniques with patients. Let's suppose you were interested in trying to establish bladder control among middle-aged women suffering from stress incontinence. You have two techniques, A and B, and you want to find out which is more effective.

For a host of practical reasons, you cannot test every middle-aged women with stress incontinence, and so you select a random sample of, say, 20 women and assign them to treatment A and a further random sample of 20 women and assign them to treatment B. Both groups are managed in exactly the same way except for the nature of their treatment, and at the end of a given period, you compare the groups in terms of bladder control.

Suppose you find that the incidence of stress incontinence is less (i.e. improved) for the treatment A group than for the treatment B group. Now you would expect that there would be some differences between the groups anyway, simply because of chance factors, like the mood swings of the patients, personality factors, current state of health, fatigue etc., but the question is whether the difference between the two groups in terms of the incidence of stress incontinence can be accounted for by these chance factors, or whether the difference is due to the relative effectiveness of the treatments.

If the experiment has been carried out properly and in accordance with certain prerequisite conditions (see Chapters 7 and 8 for details on this), then statistical tests can be used to analyse the data and to conclude whether or not the difference between the groups is, in fact, attributable to the type of treatment. If it is found to be due to the treatment procedure, then you would conclude that treatment A is more effective with this group. If you have selected your sample of patients randomly from the whole group of middle-aged women with stress incontinence as a whole, then you could reasonably infer that treatment A is likely to be more effective than treatment B with other sufferers, and hence you would recommend it to other physiotherapists.

In other words, you have selected a small sample for study and from the results of this study, you can make inferences about the whole population from which the sample was drawn. This is the basis of inferential statistics.

---

**KEY CONCEPTS**

Data from research must be presented in a way that can be understood by the reader. There are two main ways of doing this:

- Descriptive statistics, which summarise the main features of the results from a survey by describing the average scores etc.
- Inferential statistics which are used to test hypotheses and which involve selecting a small sample of people for study and from the results of this, allowing the researcher to make inferences about the population from which the sample was drawn.

In other words, descriptive statistics allow the researcher to make statements only about the results obtained, but do not permit any assumptions to be made beyond the data collected, whereas inferential statistics allow the researcher to make assumptions beyond the set of data in front of her/him.

# 3

# Questionnaires, surveys and sampling

It was noted in the previous chapter that surveys often used questionnaires as a means of collecting information about a group of people. However, while questionnaires are commonly used in this way, they can also be used in experimental or single-case designs, and as such are an invaluable method of data collection. This chapter will look at the basic principles of questionnaire design, as well as providing more details on carrying out surveys.

## QUESTIONNAIRE DESIGN

Designing a good questionnaire is a skilled business and does not involve simply jotting a few questions down on paper. The design and use of a good questionnaire should follow six steps:

1. Identifying the general topics to be covered by the questionnaire, which will reflect the objectives the researcher has in mind.

2. Initial draft of the questions covering all these topics.

3. Piloting the questionnaire; i.e. giving out the questionnaire to a number of people (who do not necessarily come from the population at whom the questionnaire is targeted) in order to collect feedback on unclear or insensitive questions, ambiguous instructions etc.

4. Modification of the questionnaire using the information collected from the pilot trial.

5. A second pilot trial to establish whether or not the earlier problems have been ironed out.

6. Final administration of the questionnaire in the actual study or survey. The completed questionnaire can then be analysed in a variety of different ways.

## ASKING THE QUESTIONS

Questions come in two main forms: open-ended and closed. Open-ended questions are those which allow respondents free range when supplying their answers. They are questions which do not provide boundaries or constraints on the answers. Closed questions, on the other hand, do just that: they allow the respondent only a limited choice of how to answer the question.

To illustrate the difference between the two, let us take a simple enquiry that any physiotherapist might make about a patient's health. He or she might ask the patient:

'How do you feel today?'

or alternatively

'Are you feeling any better today?'

The first is an open-ended question since the patient is being given the opportunity to make statements about their pain levels, appetite, anxiety level or whatever. The second example is a closed question, since the patient can really only answer 'yes' or 'no'. This example is a simplistic one, but it does illustrate the different ways in which questions can be used to elicit information.

As with every other aspect of research, both types of question have their pros and cons. Open-ended questions allow the respondent more flexibility and consequently much more information can be derived, often of a type the researcher hadn't thought of. On the debit side, though, such answers are difficult to analyse objectively which means that it can be difficult to compare one person's answer with another's. In consequence, the analysis may be much wider, less informative and more unsophisticated. Also, open-ended questions are more time-consuming to complete, and without answer guidelines many respondents may miss the point completely and provide responses which are neither relevant nor useful.

Closed questions overcome a lot of these difficulties, since the structured response format means that answers can be completed quickly, analysed easily and direct comparisons between people can be made. The level of analysis can also be more sophisticated and useful. (This point will be discussed in more detail later in this chapter as well as in Chapter 4.) However, the value of such questions is largely governed by the skill of the question-setter, who needs both to ask sound questions, devoid of ambiguities and bias and to provide a comprehensive and appropriate answer structure. Too often respondents get irritated by answer formats which don't meet their needs and consequently they refuse to fill in their replies.

These points raise two particularly important issues in questionnaire design: how to word the questions and how to structure a response format for closed questions.

### Wording the questions

Asking the right questions is a skilled science and is not a topic which can be covered adequately here. I would therefore refer the reader to Oppenheim's (1966) seminal text *Questionnaire Design and Attitude Measurement* which remains a leader in the field.

However, some guidelines can be given here, as a start. Good question design is dictated by a list of do's and don'ts, each of which will be illustrated in turn:

1. *Don't* use complex sentence structures.
   *Do* keep your sentences clear and simple.
   For example, ask:

   'Do you think that cystic fibrosis is a sufficiently serious condition to merit top priority for Government funding for genetic engineering?'

   and not:

   'Do you think that cystic fibrosis, which is a life-threatening and frightening disease and one which causes untold anxiety, misery and pain to sufferers and families alike, should be given top priority in terms of Government funding for genetic engineering projects?'

2. *Don't* use medical or professional jargon.
   *Do* use words and phrases that the respondents will understand.
   For example, ask:

   'When did you have your gallbladder operation?'

   and not:

   'When did you have your cholecystectomy?'

3. *Don't* confuse the respondent by asking about more than one thing at a time.
   *Do* keep to one idea per sentence.
   For example, ask:

   'Do you experience any pain after eating?'

   and 'Do you experience any pain after walking?'

   and not:

   'Do you experience any pain after eating or walking?'

4. *Don't* assume everyone will know what you mean.
   *Do* keep your questions unambiguous.
   For example, ask:

   'Do you do your exercises for at least 20 minutes every day?'

   and not:

   'Do you do your exercises regularly?'

5. *Don't* use double negatives.
   *Do* ask questions positively.
   For example, ask:

   'Have you ever wanted anything to eat after doing your exercises?'

   and not:

   'Have you ever not wanted to have nothing to eat after doing your exercises?'

6. *Don't* ask leading questions.
   *Do* ask questions in an unbiased, unemotional way.
   For example, ask:

   'Do you think that smoking should be banned throughout the hospital?'

   and not:

   'Do you agree that the filthy habit of smoking should be banned throughout the hospital?'

Instructions on how to complete the questionnaire should also be clear and unambiguous. In addition, it may be necessary to enclose a definition of what the essential terms are to avoid misunderstanding for example:

'Doing your exercises' should be taken to mean 'Doing all the exercises you have been shown in the way they were demonstrated and for the time suggested'.

Remember that if the questionnaire is piloted in the way suggested earlier, then many of these potential problems can be ironed out.

## Response formats for closed-ended questions

The way in which the response options are structured is important in questionnaire design, since it can dictate how honestly the respondent answers as well as the value and amount of information that can be derived from the questionnaires. These response formats can be thought of as ways of measuring a person's reply to your question and these measurements range from simple through to sophisticated scales. The whole area of **scales** or **levels of measurement** is a crucial one in all sorts of research and is dealt with in Chapter 4 in much more detail. However, a brief introduction will be given here.

Let's imagine you have been treating a group of prostatectomy patients for postoperative incontinence, and you wish to send them a follow-up questionnaire, 6 months after the operation, to find out how they are progressing. One question you want to ask is: Do you still suffer any incontinence?

You can structure the possible answers to this in a number of ways, for example:

(a) Do you still suffer any incontinence?
    Yes □    No □
(b) Do you still suffer any incontinence?

    |⎯⎯⎯⎯|⎯⎯⎯⎯|⎯⎯⎯⎯|⎯⎯⎯⎯|
    1         2         3         4         5
    never  infrequently  often  very often  all the time

(c) Do you still suffer any incontinence?
    Never                          □
    Once a day                     □
    Twice a day                    □
    Three times a day              □
    Four times a day               □
    Five times a day               □

The first response format is a simple one and gives us only basic information. For instance, a respondent who ticks the 'Yes' box might suffer urinary incontinence once a month or once an hour, but this sort of answer format doesn't provide that level of detail.

The second answer format is somewhat more sophisticated, since it allows us to collect a range of information on the overall frequency of incontinence. However, the descriptions 'infrequently', 'often' etc. are open to subjective interpretation, and while they provide more information about the patient's level of incontinence than the previous format, are still lacking in objectivity and precision.

The last response format is the most sophisticated of the three, since it gives us detailed and accurate information about how often the patient is incontinent, in absolute terms.

These different types of response need different techniques to analyse them and this point is referred to in some detail later. As a rule of thumb, it is better, where possible, to use the most sophisticated and objective response formats as they supply a lot more information about our respondents.

It is also important to note, too, that respondents are not always honest in their answers, not necessarily because they deliberately wish to deceive the researcher, but simply because they want to present themselves in the best possible light. This tendency is known as a social-desirability response set and topics which are sensitive or emotive are particularly vulnerable to this type of bias.

Finally, do treat your respondents with respect. Don't ask embarrassing or intrusive questions, don't use their replies to compromise them, don't mislead them in any way and if you tell them their responses are anonymous or confidential, mean it.

## ADVANTAGES AND DISADVANTAGES OF QUESTIONNAIRES

The main advantage of questionnaires is that they can be designed and customised for any purpose or group of people.

In addition, because a questionnaire does not have to be administered by the researcher in person, it means that a large sample of people can be included in the study by posting the questionnaire to them. This has added advantages. Firstly, posting a questionnaire is considerably cheaper

than the time and travel expenses which would be incurred either by transporting the individual participants into the project centre, or by the researcher travelling to meet the participants. Secondly, if questionnaires are to be posted, the possibility of the researcher influencing the respondent's answers either unwittingly or deliberately is reduced considerably.

However, questionnaires have their disadvantages too. If the questionnaires are sent by post there is a very high chance that a lot of recipients will not return them. While this non-return rate can be reduced somewhat by the inclusion of stamped addressed envelopes, it does, nonetheless, mean that the researcher usually has to send out considerably more questionnaires than are actually needed in order to compensate for the non-returners, and this, of course, adds to the cost. However, it has been found that sending out reminders to respondents can increase the response rate (e.g. Cartwright, 1983).

Furthermore, whether a questionnaire is administered in person or by post there is still a high probability that some questions will be ignored, or incorrectly completed, instructions may be misinterpreted and some answers will be inadequately detailed.

Also, while it seems an unbelievably obvious thing to say, it is still a point which is commonly overlooked by a lot of researchers: the respondent should be able to read the questions. This means that issues of visual impairment, non-English speakers and illiteracy must be considered.

This having been said, questionnaires are still a very popular and very useful technique of data collection within the health care area.

---

**KEY CONCEPTS**

1. Questionnaires are a very useful way of collecting data in the health care area.
2. Asking the appropriate questions is a very skilled task and requires consideration of a number of issues.
3. Questions can be **open-ended** or **closed-ended**, both of which have advantages and disadvantages.
4. Closed-ended questions require structured answers, and the way in which the questioner sets out the answer structures is an important consideration.

## SURVEYS

In the previous chapter a survey was described as a research technique which involved collecting data from a large number of people, so that a general overview of the group could be obtained. Surveys usually use questionnaires or interviews as a means by which information is gathered, but since a key characteristic of the survey is the large number of people who take part, it is often quicker and much cheaper to use questionnaires rather than interviews. Indeed, so costly is it to interview hundreds of people that it is often outside the scope of most researchers. Consequently, this section will not cover issues concerning interviews. If you would like to find more about interview techniques, Polgar & Thomas (1991) and Cartwright (1983) both provide useful overviews.

## GENERAL PRINCIPLES OF SURVEYS

The first stage in designing a survey is to establish its aims. In other words: what questions do you want answered? So, for example, you may want to describe the services of a back pain clinic, and consequently might want to ask:

1. How many people use it in the course of a year?
2. Where do they come from?
3. How many men use the clinic?
4. How many women use the clinic?
5. What are the ethnic origins of the users?
6. What are the ages of the users?
7. What are the occupations of the users?
8. What were the presenting medical problems?
9. For how long do users come to the clinic per session?
10. How do the users rate the quality of physiotherapy care they receive at the clinic?

etc.

You then have to decide the best ways of finding answers to these questions; in other words you have to design your survey.

## THE DESIGN OF THE SURVEY

Two commonly used survey designs are **prospec-**

**tive designs** and **retrospective designs.**

Prospective designs involve identifying the group of people you want to study and then collecting the information you require when they use the particular service. So, for example, you might want to focus on patients using a back pain clinic who have no clearly identifiable trauma to the back. As soon as such patients enter the clinic the researcher would collect the relevant information from them.

However, by far the most common survey approach is the retrospective design which focuses particularly on past events. For example, you might identify, from the medical records department in the back pain clinic, patients who had been given different treatments for their condition. You would then contact these patients to collect the information you require, such as their subsequent problems, perceptions of care, etc. The main problem with this approach is the fact that when people are asked to recall events their memory may be selective and consequently this might bias the data you collect.

Once you have decided on the design, you then have to identify the people who will take part in your survey.

## SELECTING THE PEOPLE TO TAKE PART

Finding the appropriate number and type of people to take part in your study is called **sampling**. This is an essential part of good research design of any sort, whether it be surveys or experimental approaches. While some reference has already been made to sampling in the earlier section on inferential statistics (Chapter 2) it is sufficiently important to merit a section on its own.

### Sampling

When you carry out a piece of research it is impossible to involve every person who might be of interest to you, both for practical and financial reasons. For example, you might want to conduct some research on women with osteoporosis, but as there must be many thousands of these women within the UK it would be completely impossible to study them all. Consequently, you would select just some of them to take part in your study. These women would be your **sample**.

However, if the data collected from the sample is to be of any value, the sample must be representative of female osteoporosis sufferers as a whole. This entire group of all the osteoporosis patients is called the **population**. The population can be defined as all those people (or even events) who possess the characteristic(s) in which the researcher is interested. Thus, the sample of osteoporosis sufferers is a subset of the population of osteoporosis sufferers as a whole. To take another example, you may wish to look at the treatment procedures for meniscectomy patients in a regional health authority. All the meniscectomy patients in that authority would constitute the population and you might select a sample of 50 of them for your study.

However, if you are to collect any useful information from your sample, you have got to try to ensure that the sample is pretty well representative of the population from which they are drawn. If it is not, then the conclusions you reach from your study cannot readily be generalised to the rest of the population and might lead you to make invalid assumptions about that population.

Let's illustrate this idea with an example. Supposing you wanted to conduct a survey looking at the incidence of asthma in the under-fives, perhaps with a view to planning future physiotherapy provision more carefully. You devise your questionnaire and send it out to every family within two postal districts. When you get the returns and analyse the data, you find to your amazement that 70% of the respondents' under-five children suffer from asthma. You then assume that 70% of all under-fives in your region have asthma and you set about recruiting four specialist physiotherapists to meet the anticipated demand for services. Two years later, you find that two of these specially recruited physiotherapists have insufficient work to do and you have to terminate their contracts. What could have gone wrong with your planning?

One possible reason might be the way in which you selected your survey sample. When you go back to check this, you realise that the two postal areas you chose were both inner city areas lying close to a network of motorway junctions. Consequently, atmospheric pollution was likely to be extremely high in the areas. Moreover, you then read a new report which claims that smoking is more prevalent in inner city areas. Therefore, the children in your sample were also likely to have been subjected to high levels of atmospheric pollution in their home as well. Small wonder, then, that your survey results suggested an incredibly high incidence of early childhood asthma. It also becomes clear why your specialist physiotherapists were underemployed – your resource planning was based on findings from a very biased sample which could not be generalised to the rest of the region's population.

Consequently, it is imperative that the sampling techniques employed in any study, be it survey or experimental, must be sound if you are to draw valid conclusions from your data. The most commonly used sampling methods in scientific and health research are **incidental sampling** and **random sampling**.

## Incidental sampling

Incidental sampling involves selecting the most easily accessible people from your population and consequently it is relatively easy to do. Let's imagine you're interested in doing a survey of cystic fibrosis children, and you ask a community physiotherapist to give your questionnaire to all the cystic fibrosis patients she sees in her area.

This is undoubtedly an easy way of accessing a sample but it may not give you a representative selection of patients. For example, the community physiotherapist may only see those patients who have very severe problems associated with the cystic fibrosis, or alternatively he or she may only see the least affected patients, because the others are in hospital. In other words, this incidental sample may or may not be representative of the population and, unless you had a lot more information about the population of cystic fibrosis patients, you wouldn't know whether the sample was biased or representative.

One way round this is to use a variation of incidental sampling called **quota sampling**.

## Quota sampling

Suppose you know that 40% of all cystic fibrosis sufferers between the ages of 10 and 15 are hospitalised at least once a month, and 60% are hospitalised less than 5 times per year, while 70% of those between 5 and 9 years are hospitalised at least once a month and 30% are hospitalised less than 5 times per year (Table 3.1).

**Table 3.1** Age and frequency of hospitalisation for cystic fibrosis sufferers

| Age (years) | Frequency of hospitalisation | |
| --- | --- | --- |
| | Once per month | Less than 5 times per year |
| 5–9 | 70% | 30% |
| 10–15 | 40% | 60% |

Having this information you would then collect your cystic fibrosis sample by quota, ensuring that:

1. 70% of the 5–9 year olds in your sample were hospitalised at least once a month.
2. 30% of the 5–9 year olds in your sample were hospitalised less than 5 times per year.
3. 40% of the 10–15 year olds in your sample were hospitalised at least once a month.
4. 60% of the 10–15 years in your sample were hospitalised less than 5 times per year.

However, this approach means that you must know what particular characteristics are likely to be important in your study (in the above example, these were assumed to be age and frequency of hospitalisation) and secondly, you have to know what proportions of the cystic fibrosis population come into these categories. Both pieces of information may be difficult or even impossible to obtain, and this makes proper quota sampling problematic.

## Random sampling

This is perhaps the most commonly used and best way of selecting a sample. The basic concepts were referred to in the section 'Inferential statistics' in the previous chapter (pages 13–15) and consequently only a review will be presented here. The fundamental principle underpinning random sampling is that every member of the target population should have an equal chance of being selected for study. There are a number of ways in which this can be achieved. For instance, you can put the names of all members of the population into a hat and then draw out the number you need for your sample, just like a raffle. Alternatively you can use **random number tables**. This involves giving a number to every member of the population and then using a set of random number tables to select the sample size you need. (Random number tables can be found in a number of research texts, e.g. Robson 1974.) Essentially, the process works like this. Random number tables consist of the numbers 0–99 occurring with the same probability at any point in the table. If you wanted to select 25 paraplegic patients from a population of 100 such patients then you would assign each one of the numbers from 0–99 to a patient, shut your eyes and stick a pin into the random number table. From that number you work in any direction you like, making a note of the first 25 different numbers you encounter. You then tally these up with the corresponding numbers assigned to your patients and you have your random sample. Remember not to change direction once you have started; also, if you need to select another random sample then you should enter the table at a different point and move in another direction.

Random samples have an important advantage over other sampling techniques in that the sample, because it is more representative of the population, does not have to be a large one. (Sample size will be dealt with later in this chapter.) However, there are major disadvantages. The researcher must know the names of all the population members before a random sample can be selected. If we think about the prospect of doing this with the topic of diabetes or cardiovascular disease, the task becomes impossible. Allied to this is the cost; it is much cheaper to use an incidental sample simply because they are by definition, easily accessible.

Two variations of random sampling are worth a brief mention: **stratified random sampling** and **systematic sampling**.

## Stratified random sampling

This is akin to quota sampling in that it involves

the researcher defining relevant subgroups of the population. A random sample, using either the 'raffle' or the random number technique, would then be drawn from each subgroup. This approach ensures that all the important subsets of a population are represented in the sample but like random sampling it requires the names of all members of the population and is therefore costly, difficult and time-consuming.

### Systematic sampling

This involves choosing every third, seventh, thirteenth or whatever, member of the population. While this is not a truly random technique, it usually provides a sample which is adequately representative of the population.

## Sample size

When you have chosen an appropriate method for selecting your sample you then have to decide how many people you want to survey.

Many would-be researchers are deterred from undertaking research because they believe they need hundreds of people to participate. This is not necessarily so and indeed in many situations it may be inadvisable to have crowds of people taking part, particularly if painful procedures or ethical issues are involved. There is no easy way of establishing the best size of sample since this decision depends very largely on the research which is being undertaken. However, as a general rule of thumb, a larger sample is more likely to be representative of the population than a smaller one and secondly, where techniques of inferential statistics are being used, small sample sizes are corrected by an increase in the stringency with which the analysis is conducted. In crude terms, then, if you have only a small

sample, then your results have to be 'better' before you can draw any conclusions from them. This will be discussed in more detail later.

Once you have collected your results you then have to make sense of them. Some ways in which this can be done are described in the next chapter.

It may be worth pointing out that decisions concerning surveys or any other type of research approach can never be perfect; because of the practical difficulties and complexities of field and applied research, compromises in design always have to be made. However, it is important that the researcher knows the pros, cons and implications of any decision before implementing it, and this text is an attempt to provide some of this basic information.

If you are interested in finding out more about health surveys, Cartwright's (1983) book may be useful.

---

**KEY CONCEPTS**

1. Surveys are a research approach which involves collecting data from a large number of people, either by questionnaires or interviews, so that an overview of that group can be obtained.
2. Surveys can be **prospective** in design or **retrospective**. Retrospective surveys are more commonly used but, as they rely on people's recall of events, they may be flawed by selective or inadequate memory.
3. Deciding on who takes part in your study is called **sampling**. The general idea behind sampling is that you can generalise the results from your sample to the rest of the population from which they were drawn.
4. There are a number of different sampling methods, each of which has its own advantages and disadvantages.
5. The appropriate size for the sample is not easy to determine, since it depends very much on the subject being studied, as well as on the researcher's knowledge of the relevant population's characteristics.

# 4

# The nature of the data

## LEVELS OF MEASUREMENT

Whatever sort of research you're interested in, whether it's a survey or an experiment, you will probably be involved in measuring something, e.g. exam performance, distance walked, vital capacity, range of movement and so on. These measurements form your data or results. If we look at the above examples a bit more carefully, we can see that each of them involves a different sort of measurement:

- exam performance may be measured as marks out of 20 or 100, say
- distance walked may be measured in yards or metres
- vital capacity may be measured in litres
- range of movement may be measured in degrees.

You can doubtless think of other sorts of measures that might be involved in physiotherapy research and it might be useful to make a list of these.

However, any measurement you use belongs to one of four main **categories of measurement.** It is important to be able to distinguish which category your data belongs to because it will affect the way in which you analyse your results, since some analyses can only be used with particular categories of measurement.

### KEY CONCEPT

When you carry out research you will be involved in measuring something. These measurements form your **data** or results and fall into one of four main **categories of measurement.** You need to be able to identify which category your own measurements come into, because this will affect the way in which you analyse your data, since some statistical tests can only be used with certain categories of measurement.

The four categories are called 'levels of measurement' and each category gives us a different amount of information:

1. **N**ominal level: the most basic level which gives us least information.
2. **O**rdinal level: the next level which provides all the information of the nominal scale plus some additional information.
3. **I**nterval level: a higher level of measurement which provides all the information of the nominal and ordinal scales but which offers additional information.
4. **R**atio level: the highest level of all which provides all the information of the nominal, ordinal and interval scales but which offers further information still.

For the purposes of statistical analysis, the interval and ratio scales are combined to form a single category, and this is how we will be dealing with them in this book.

Before we go on to look at what these levels actually mean, you may find it useful to remember the mnemonic **NOIR** (as understanding which category is which becomes a 'bête **noir**e' for many students) to help you with the order of the different levels.

## NOMINAL LEVEL

Let's take the nominal level first of all. As you may have guessed, this is simply a 'naming', category, in that it only gives names or labels to your data without implying any order, quality or dimension. So, for example, you might want to ascertain how many of the applicants for places at a school of physiotherapy come from particular areas. You call one region Area A, another Area B, and another Area C and count up how many applicants fall into each category. This is a **nominal level** of measurement, because it has simply allowed you to allocate your data into one of three named categories.

Two important points are worth noting here. I have just said that this level of measurement has no implication for degree, order or quality of the data, which means that we could very easily alter the headings of the categories in any way, without affecting the results. So, for instance,

Area A could just as easily have been called Area C or D, or X, Y or Z or Banana or Apple, since it will not affect the number of applicants who have come from that region.

Secondly, the categories are mutually exclusive, in that an applicant can only come from one area. Thus, once we have allocated a subject to one particular category, they cannot be allocated to any other category.

Let's take an example. If you were looking at the final exam success of two different schools of physiotherapy, you might take School A and School B and count up the number of passes and fails at each.

What you are measuring here is exam success, but all you have done is to use two labels – 'pass' and 'fail' – and have counted up how many students in each school achieved more than 50% (pass category) and how many achieved less (fail category). You might end up with the data in Table 4.1.

**Table 4.1**

|  | Pass | Fail |
|---|---|---|
| School A | 29 | 11 |
| School B | 33 | 7 |

A student who comes into the pass category cannot also come into the fail category and so this level of measurement involves mutually exclusive categories.

Measurement at this level gives us very little information about our data. You don't know how well the students have passed; all School A's pass students may have achieved 90 + %, while all School B's passes may have been between 50–55%. You also don't know how bad the fails are, e.g. 0% or 43%. All you know is that a certain number of students can be labelled 'pass' and a certain number 'fail'. Therefore, this is a nominal level of measurement, and as you can see, it doesn't tell us a great deal. For example, if you had to recommend one of these schools on the basis of nominal data, you would probably suggest School B because it achieved 33 passes to School A's 29. But if School A had pass marks of 90 + % as opposed to School B's 50–55%, you might want to change your recommendation. However, you wouldn't know this from nominal data alone, since all this category allows you to do is to classify your data under the broad headings of 'pass' and 'fail'.

Political opinion polls which simply categorise people into Conservative, Labour, Liberal Democrats and Don't Knows are nominal scales. Voting on a particular issue in a meeting categorises people into 'For', 'Against' and 'Abstain' and so is a nominal scale. We don't know how Conservative a respondent in a poll is, or how 'against' a voter in a meeting is; we just know that they can be allocated to a particular category.

The following are also examples of the nominal level of measurement:

• The number of male vs. female applicants for physiotherapy places at School A may be 39 males to 123 females. You don't know how old applicants are, how good their 'A'-level results are, or how suitable they are, all you know is that you have 39 male applicants and 123 females.

• You send a questionnaire to all the clinical physiotherapists in a district asking them to indicate:

Do you smoke?   Yes _____   No _____

You get a set of replies, which suggests that 42 people smoke, and 101 do not. But you do not know how many cigarettes the smokers get through; it may be 5 per day or 65. All you know is that 42 physiotherapists in a particular district smoke and 101 do not.

It may be worth noting that the nominal level of measurement is referred to as 'categorical' data in some text books.

---

**Activity 4.1**   (Answers on page 227)

Look at the following measures you might use in a piece of research, and indicate how these might be converted into a nominal category of measurement:

1 improvement in incontinence following therapy
2 reduced incidence of chest infections following breathing exercises
3 increased range of movement in a leg, following manipulation
4 keeping appointments at an outpatients' clinic
5 perceptions of the quality of physiotherapy.

---

## ORDINAL LEVEL

The next category of measurement is the **ordinal**

scale which tells us a bit more about our data. The ordinal scale allows us to **rank order** our data according to the dimension we are interested in, for example:

most preferred — least preferred
most improved — least improved
most competent — least competent.

Suppose you asked a clinical supervisor to rank order a set of students on their competence during a placement, because you wanted to see if clinical performance was related to 'A'-level grades. The supervisor may come up with the list in Table 4.2.

**Table 4.2**   Students arranged in order of competence

| Competence position | | Student |
|---|---|---|
| 1 | (Most competent) | Catherine A. |
| 2 | | Jane C. |
| 3 | | Jackie S. |
| 4 | | Carol R. |
| 5 | (Least competent) | Susan D. |

What we have is a rank ordering of these students in terms of the dimension we're interested in: their competence. We still don't have a great deal of information about them, however, because we don't know how much better Catherine A. is than Jane C., or how much worse Susan D. is from the rest (or in fact, whether any of them are competent at all). All we know is that Catherine A. is better than Jane C. who in turn is better than Jackie S.; but we don't know how much better. In other words, we have a *relative* and not an *absolute* measure of competence. It is also important to note that the differences between each pair of ordinal positions is not necessarily the same, i.e. the difference in competence between Catherine A. and Jane C. may not be the same as the difference between Jane C. and Jackie S.

## Point scales

Another example of an ordinal scale of measurement is the use of a point scale. For example, in the previous study with another set of students, you might alternatively have asked the clinical supervisor to indicate on the following scale how competent each student was:

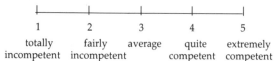

Here we have a dimension of most competent to least competent on a 5-point scale, (although we could use fewer or more than 5 points) and on which each student may be rated. Therefore, had we asked the clinical supervisor to assess students using this scale, we might have found the results shown in Table 4.3.

**Table 4.3**

| Competence score | Students |
|---|---|
| 5 | Laura B. |
| 4 | Julie N, Mark S. |
| 3 | Chris D. |
| 2 | Jill F., Liz H. |
| 1 | Sally C. |

Again, the difference between each pair of scores must not be assumed to be the same. The difference in competence between:

5 (extremely competent)
and
4 (quite competent)

may not be the same as between:

1 (totally incompetent)
and
2 (fairly incompetent)

In our earlier example on the smoking questionnaire, you could modify your question from:

Do you smoke? Yes _____ No _____

to:

What sort of smoker would you classify yourself as:

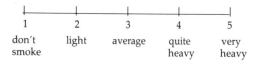

Again, we don't know whether the physiotherapist who selects 'very heavy' smokes 60 or 100 cigarettes a day, but we do know that she smokes more than the light smoker. Similarly, someone who scores 4 may not smoke twice the number of cigarettes as someone who scores 2. All we know is that someone with a score of 4 does smoke more than someone with a score of 2.

We can see particularly clearly from this example how the ordinal scale gives us more information than the nominal scale. If we use this rank ordering technique, we can count up the number of non-smokers (anyone who scores 1) and the number of smokers (those who score 2, 3, 4 and 5) and this gives us the information provided by the nominal scale. However, the ordinal scale adds a *dimension* to the label of 'smoker', in that it allows us to measure people according to whether they are heavy, average or light smokers. In other words, it gives us a bit more information than the nominal level.

It should be noted, though, that the ordinal scale is a rather imprecise measurement. It is commonly used to assess things like pain, attitudes, levels of agreement etc; consequently it relies on very subjective interpretations and so cannot be assumed to have any absolute meaning.

**Activity 4.2** (Answers on pages 227–228)

Look back at the examples given on page 27, and convert each of these to an ordinal level of measurement.

## INTERVAL/RATIO LEVEL

The interval level or scale of measurement is like the ordinal scale, except that it does assume *equal intervals* in its measurement. Interval scales are measures such as percentage in an exam, temperature etc. Interval and ratio measurements have two things in common.

Firstly, they assume equal intervals, such that it is possible to say that the difference between scores of 30 and 60% (i.e. 30%) is half the difference of that between scores of 30 and 90% (i.e. 60%). Similarly, the difference between marks of 40 and 50% on an exam is exactly the same as the difference between 80 and 90% (i.e.

10%). If we look back to the ordinal scale of measurement, we cannot make these statements, because we simply don't know whether the difference between scores of 1 and 3 on a 5-point scale is the same as the difference between 3 and 5. In order words the gap between 'no smoker' and 'average smoker' is not necessarily identical to the gap between 'average smoker' and 'very heavy' smoker (see above).

The second point to note is that the interval scale does not have an absolute zero point although sometimes one is arbitrarily imposed. This means that a zero score on an interval scale does not necessarily mean an absence of the quality being measured. A good example of this is temperature on the Centigrade scale, where zero temperature does not mean an absence of temperature, but rather that the temperature is at freezing point.

The ratio level of measurement is like the interval level except that it does have an absolute zero. It includes measures such as distance, height, weight, time, etc. Do not worry about this point, because for the purposes of statistical tests, interval and ratio scales are treated as the same. From now on, these two levels of measurement will be collapsed to form one category, which will be referred to as the interval/ratio level.

If, then, we look back at the example of students' competence on clinical placement, our clinical supervisor could have given the students a test (marks out of 50, say), rather than rank ordering them. The results might have looked like Table 4.4.

**Table 4.4**  Test marks of students

| Mark | Student |
| --- | --- |
| 44 | Laura B. |
| 39 | Julie N. |
| 36 | Paul S. |
| 30 | Chris D. |
| 22 | Liz H. |
| 20 | Jill F. |
| 11 | Sally C. |

From this data, we can see that the difference between Laura B. and Liz H. is twice the difference between Liz H. and Sally C. In addition,

from this data we could rank order the scores to find each student's position in the group (ordinal level of measurement), and also we could classify the students into pass/fail (nominal level of measurement). Therefore, the interval/ratio level of measurement gives us more information than the ordinal scale, which in turn tells us more than the nominal scale.

Again, if we look at our smoking example, we could modify our questionnaire again and simply ask 'How many cigarettes do you smoke per day?' We might get a range of answers from 0 to 60, and from this, we can say that someone who smokes 60 daily, smokes twice the amount of the person who smokes 30, three times the amount of the person who smokes 20, four times the amount of the person who smokes 15, and so on. We could also:

- rank order the replies from heaviest smoker to lightest (ordinal scale)
- classify the replies into smokers and non-smokers (nominal scale)

As a result, it can be seen that the interval/ratio level of measurement gives us all the information of the nominal and ordinal levels, plus a bit more. Other examples of interval/ratio data include temperature, blood pressure, time measures, length, weight, volume and heart rate.

### Point-scales: ordinal or interval?

It should be mentioned here that sometimes researchers treat point-scales as though they were interval rather than ordinal scales, because when constructing the point-scale they have *assumed* equal intervals between the points. Sometimes this is entirely legitimate, for example, when analysing questionnaire data. As a broad rule-of-thumb, if you construct a point-scale with at least 7 points on it, and are assuming that the distances between the points are comparable, then you may wish to classify this as an interval scale for the purposes of analysis.

This point is highlighted by the visual analogue method of measuring pain. This commonly used technique involves presenting patients with an unmarked line of length exactly 10 cm, with 0 cm representing no pain and 10 cm representing excruciating pain:

---

no pain                                        excruciating pain

The patient is then asked to mark on this line how much pain they're experiencing. The line up to the mark is then measured. In this way, one patient may report 54 mms of pain, and another 19 mms and so on. The problem then emerges of how to classify the data. Pain is subjective, so should this be called an ordinal scale? However, length measurement in centimetres, millimetres, or whatever is an interval/ratio scale so how can the issue be resolved? There is no right answer here and it must be left to the researcher. However, as a general rule of data collection, it is usually advisable to use the most sophisticated level of measurement you can, since more detailed analyses can be performed. Therefore, it may be preferable to treat visual analogue data as interval/ratio.

---

**Activity 4.3**   (Answers on page 228)

1–5  Look back at the five examples given on page 27 and convert the measures to interval/ratio scores.

6    Suppose that you wanted to look at the incidence of low back pain among welders at the local car factory, you could measure:

(i)  How many had experienced low back pain and how many had not experienced low back pain over the last 2 years (nominal).

(ii) Frequency of back pain, using a 5-point scale, by asking the question:
How often have you experienced back pain over the last 2 years? (ordinal):

| 1 | 2 | 3 | 4 | 5 |
|---|---|---|---|---|
| never | rarely | sometimes | quite often | very often |

(iii) Frequency of back pain using absolute number of incidents (interval/ratio) by asking: How many times have you experienced back pain over the last 2 years? Using the same format, construct nominal, ordinal and interval/ratio levels of measurement for the following:

(i)  accuracy of shooting an arrow at a target
(ii) improvement in mobility after a hip replacement operation
(iii) relief of neck and arm pain following use of a cervical collar.

7  Look at the following measurements and say whether they are nominal, ordinal or interval/ratio:

(i)  Number of attenders vs. non-attenders at an outpatients' clinic.

(ii) Patients' ratings of the degree of confidence they have in their physiotherapist, on a 7-point scale.
(iii) Number of work hours lost through low back pain in physiotherapists on a neurological ward.
(iv) Percentage of knee movement regained following physiotherapy for leg fractures.
(v) Recovery time in days following physiotherapy for cardiothoracic surgery patients.

Remember that you need to be able to distinguish between nominal, ordinal and interval/ratio levels of measurement, because the level of measurement will affect how you analyse your data. More information about this will be given throughout the text.

Finally, it is generally advisable to use the highest levels of measurement you can (i.e. interval/ratio rather than ordinal, ordinal rather than nominal) because not only do the higher levels provide you with more information than the lower levels, but also the type of analysis that can be carried out with the higher levels is more detailed and sophisticated. Clearly, there will be occasions when you have no choice but to use nominal or ordinal levels of measurement. For instance, if you're collecting information about the number of left hip replacements vs. right hip replacements, you would have to use the simple nominal categories of 'left hip' and 'right hip', since nothing else would be appropriate. However, as a general rule-of-thumb, use the higher levels of measurement whenever you can.

---

**KEY CONCEPTS**

There are four levels of measurement, each of which gives us a different amount of information about our data.

• **Nominal scales** give us least information and simply allow our data to be labelled or categorised, e.g. pass/ fail, male/female, over-60/under-60, improvement/no improvement.
• **Ordinal scales** give us a bit more information in that they allow us to put our data into a rank order, according to the dimension we are interested in, e.g. most competent to least, heaviest smoker to lightest, greatest movement to least etc.
• **Interval/ratio** scales give us more information, in that they deal with actual numerical scores, e.g. weight, height, time, percentage, pressure, capacity, etc., which allow direct mathematical comparisons to be made.
• The interval and ratio levels are combined to form a single category for the purposes of data analysis.

# 5

# Techniques of descriptive statistics

The information or data collected from your project has got to be interpreted, in order to make sense of it. It was noted in Chapter 2 that there are two main techniques you can use to interpret your data: inferential statistics which are used to check whether your results support your hypothesis, and descriptive statistics which are methods of describing your results in terms of their most interesting features. Techniques of descriptive statistics are commonly used to make sense of survey data, where large quantities of information are collected. Once this data has been organised and presented in a more accessible way, it is then possible for the researcher to formulate hypotheses from it. These can then be tested using the appropriate inferential statistics. In this way, descriptive statistics are sometimes thought of as the first stage in analysing results from surveys or whatever, and inferential statistics the second stage. This chapter is concerned with some frequently used techniques of descriptive statistics.

## ORGANISING DATA INTO A TABLE

It is very difficult to make any sense out of a large amount of information simply by looking at the raw data. However, if this data is organised into a table, then it is much easier to understand.

Let's imagine you have been conducting a survey of your sports injuries service and you have a mass of information concerning the nature of the injuries, the pain levels, type of treatment and progress rates. This information can be tabulated to make the key points clearer. To focus, for example, on leg fractures, the first set of information you have concerns the causes of injury, which are mainly football, rugby, ski-ing, motorcycle racing and athletics, i.e. nominal data. This information can be represented as in Table 5.1.

**Table 5.1** Frequency of causes of leg fractures seen at a sports injuries clinic over a period of 1 year

| Cause of injury | Frequency |
| --- | --- |
| Football | 52 |
| Rugby | 21 |
| Ski–ing | 11 |
| Motorcycle racing | 14 |
| Athletics | 19 |
| Other | 9 |
| Total | 126 |

From Table 5.1 you can see at a glance the most common, as well as the least common, source of injury. In order to construct this sort of table, then, you must group the data into the important nominal categories, which here were the sources of the injury. The number of patients falling into each category is counted up and this information is then represented in a table.

You then decide to look at the reported pain levels of the leg fracture patients. In order to collect this data you have asked every patient on admission, to rate how much pain they experienced, using a 5–point ordinal scale:

| 1 | 2 | 3 | 4 | 5 |
| --- | --- | --- | --- | --- |
| no pain | mild pain | moderate pain | severe pain | excruciating pain |

You tabulate this data as in Table 5.2.

**Table 5.2** Frequency of pain levels among leg fracture patients at a sports injuries clinic over a period of 1 year

| Pain level (score) | Frequency |
| --- | --- |
| No pain (1) | 0 |
| Mild pain (2) | 5 |
| Moderate pain (3) | 29 |
| Severe pain (4) | 76 |
| Excruciating pain (5) | 16 |
| Total | 126 |

Therefore, you needed to count up all the patients in each ordinal pain category before presenting the figures in table form.

The next set of data you need to interpret is the distance each patient could walk unaided immediately the plaster cast had been removed. The raw data ranges from less than a yard to 15 yards. You may recall from the previous chapter that length measurements are of an interval/ratio type. The data is organised as in Table 5.3.

**Table 5.3** Frequency of distance walked by leg fracture patients at a sports injuries clinic immediately upon removal of plaster cast

| Distance (yards) | Frequency |
| --- | --- |
| less than 1 | 1 |
| 2 | 3 |
| 3 | 5 |
| 4 | 8 |
| 5 | 13 |
| 6 | 16 |
| 7 | 16 |
| 8 | 12 |
| 9 | 15 |
| 10 | 11 |
| 11 | 15 |
| 12 | 5 |
| 13 | 3 |
| 14 | 1 |
| 15 | 2 |
| TOTAL | 126 |

Again, to arrive at this table, you would need to count up the total number of patients falling into each distance interval; these intervals should be arranged *in order* from lowest to highest and then set out accordingly.

However, if there are a lot of intervals, as there are in Table 5.3, then the table can be large and unwieldy and rather difficult to interpret. Consequently, it may be better in such cases to group the intervals (Table 5.4).

While Table 5.4 may be neater table, it should be noted that a lot of detailed information is lost by collapsing the intervals in this way. If you decide to combine your data intervals like this, you should ensure that the grouped intervals are of an equal size.

**Table 5.4** Frequency of distances walked by leg fracture patients at a sports injuries clinic, immediately upon removal of the plaster cast

| Distance (yards) | Frequency |
| --- | --- |
| 0–3 | 9 |
| 4–7 | 53 |
| 8–11 | 53 |
| 12–15 | 11 |
| Total | 126 |

It can be seen by looking at Tables 5.1–4, that they provide at-a-glance information about your patients, and consequently they are a valuable technique for describing your results. Remember, though, that all tables should be clearly labelled and self-explanatory.

## GRAPHS

Sometimes it is easier to make sense of a set of data if it is presented as a graph rather than as a table of results. While a graph tells you no more than a table of figures, it often shows trends and other features of the data more clearly. Since we have all drawn graphs in school and elsewhere, the principles pertaining to graph-drawing will be outlined only briefly here.

For the purpose of physiotherapy research the frequency distribution graph is probably the most important. A frequency distribution refers to how often a particular event occurs, for instance, how many coronary patients in a particular age group have heart rates of the order of

60–65 beats per minute,
66–70 beats per minute, or
71–75 beats per minute.

The most common forms of frequency distribution graph are the **histogram** and related **bar graphs, pie charts** and the **frequency polygon**. The features of each will be outlined shortly, and some general rules for drawing graphs will be presented at the end of this section.

### Histograms and bar graphs

These two graphical techniques are very similar, though many people feel the bar graph is clearer.

Bar graphs are typically used to present nominal and ordinal data, and histograms for interval/ratio data. Each technique presents the data in a series of vertical rectangles, with each rectangle representing the number of scores in a particular category. However with the histogram, the vertical bars are directly adjacent to one another, whereas with the bar graph there are spaces between them.

These techniques can best be demonstrated by illustrations. Suppose you want to find out what the distribution of multiple sclerosis (MS) sufferers is within districts in your particular health region, you might come up with the figures in Table 5.5.

**Table 5.5** Geographical distribution of multiple sclerosis (MS) patients

| Geographical district | No. of MS patients |
| --- | --- |
| Bridgetown | 15 |
| Henley-by-the-Sea | 32 |
| North Downs | 26 |
| Wallsend | 10 |
| Brick Lane | 6 |

The frequencies for the nominal categories in Table 5.5 can be represented in a bar graph as in Figure 5.1. Note that the categories of event go

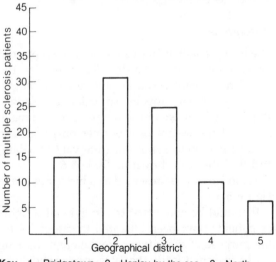

**Key** 1 = Bridgetown  2 = Henley-by-the-sea  3 = North Downs  4 = Wallsend  5 = Brick Lane

**Figure 5.1** Bar graph showing distribution of MS sufferers by district within a health region.

along the horizontal or X-axis and the frequency with which they occur go along the vertical or Y-axis.

If the categories along the horizontal axis have no natural order, then they may be arranged in order of size, with the greatest frequency on the left and the smallest on the right. Figure 5.2, showing the 'A'-level subjects of physiotherapy students, is an example of this.

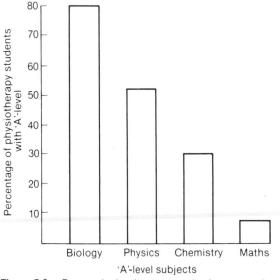

**Figure 5.2** Bar graph showing comparative frequency of 'A'-level subjects among physiotherapy students.

### Histograms

The histogram, which is usually used to represent interval/ratio data, can be illustrated by the following example. You are interested in carpal tunnel syndrome, and in particular its relationship to the body weight of the patient. You make a note of the weight of every person presenting with carpal tunnel syndrome (interval/ratio data) and find the data shown in Table 5.6.

Table 5.6 can be presented as a histogram, as in Figure 5.3.

It should be noted that the individual weights of patients have been allocated to categories for the purpose of simplifying the data and drawing the histogram. Clearly the category size should be appropriate for the range of data available; a small number of categories will lose much of the detailed information of the data, while too many

**Table 5.6** Body weight of patients with carpal tunnel syndrome

| No. of patients | Body weight |
| --- | --- |
| 0 | 10% or more underweight |
| 3 | 5–9% underweight |
| 7 | 0.9–4% underweight |
| 9 | 0–4% overweight |
| 15 | 5–9% overweight |
| 23 | 10–14% overweight |
| 38 | 15–19% overweight |
| 47 | 20% or more overweight |

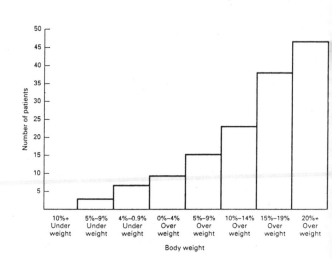

**Figure 5.3** Histogram showing the weights of patients presenting with carpal tunnel syndrome.

will complicate the table or graph. No more than nine categories are used as a rule.

## Pie charts

Nominal data can also be represented graphically using pie charts. A pie chart is a circle which is divided into sections, each section representing proportionately the number in each category or event. In order to do this, the figures in each category must be converted to percentages of the total number first.

Let's imagine you wish to represent Table 5.5 as a pie chart rather than as a bar graph. You would need to convert the figures for each district into a percentage of the total number of MS sufferers in the region (Table 5.7).

**Table 5.7** Percentage of total MS sufferers in each district

| District | No. of MS sufferers | Percentage |
|---|---|---|
| Bridgetown | 15 | 16.85 |
| Henley-by-the-Sea | 32 | 35.96 |
| North Downs | 26 | 29.21 |
| Wallsend | 10 | 11.24 |
| Brick Lane | 6 | 6.74 |
| Total | 89 | 100.00 |

The pie chart would look like Figure 5.4. To construct the pie chart, the percentages for each district must be converted to degrees. Each 1% equals 3.6° since 100% is the equivalent of 360°.

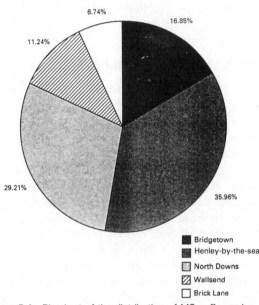

**Figure 5.4** Pie chart of the distribution of MS sufferers by district.

The value of a pie chart lies in its immediate visual appeal and the ease with which proportions can be compared. However, if there are a lot of categories pie charts can be confusing and difficult to construct and interpret accurately.

## Frequency polygons

Data of an interval/ratio type can also be plotted as a frequency polygon, in which the frequency of occurrence of each unit or event on the horizontal axis is plotted at the midpoint of the unit, and these points are then joined by a continuous straight line.

Imagine that your survey of MS sufferers has also included the age of onset of the disease (interval/ratio data), as in Table 5.8.

**Table 5.8** Age of disease onset for MS patients within the regional health authority

| Age of onset (years) | No. of MS patients |
|---|---|
| 15–24 | 21 |
| 25–34 | 30 |
| 35–44 | 17 |
| 45–54 | 10 |
| 55 + | 11 |
| Total | 89 |

This can be represented by a frequency polygon as in Figure 5.5.

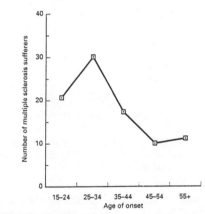

**Figure 5.5** Frequency polygon showing age of onset of MS within a particular region.

In the above example the graph does not touch the horizontal axis. Some people are of the opinion that this gives a rather odd appearance to the graph, and so, in cases where it is appropriate, you can add a class to either end of the units with scores on the horizontal axis.

To give an example, you might wish to plot the frequency of average final examination marks across a number of schools of physiotherapy for 1985. The results you obtain are shown in Table 5.9. Your graph might look like Figure 5.6.

**Table 5.9** Average final exam marks in schools of physiotherapy

| Average final exam mark | No. of schools attaining mark |
| --- | --- |
| 31–40 | 0 |
| 41–50 | 1 |
| 51–60 | 3 |
| 61–70 | 4 |
| 71–80 | 1 |
| 81–90 | 1 |
| 91–100 | 0 |

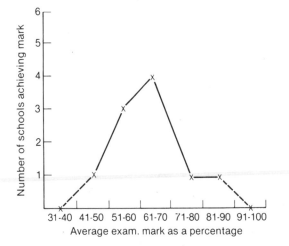

**Figure 5.6** Frequency polygon showing distribution of average final examination marks, in 1985, across a number of schools of physiotherapy.

There are no schools who achieve an average mark of 31–40% or of 91–100%. Therefore, to give this graph a more complete appearance, the line can be extended to the values for the categories 31–40% and 91–100% (dotted line in Figure 5.6).

Obviously, more than one set of data can be plotted on a frequency polygon, so that direct comparisons can be made. In the above example, you might want to plot the average marks for the year 1984 as well, so that you can compare performance.

## Which type of graph should you use?

Whether you decide to use a histogram, bar graph, pie chart or a frequency polygon depends on the nature of the data you wish to present. Nominal data, for instance, should not be plotted as a frequency polygon, but rather as a bar or pie chart.

Generally, the frequency polygon is more suitable if two or more sets of frequencies are to be compared, since a number of lines can be represented in different colours or styles on the same graph. A similar comparison using bar graphs or histograms is very confusing, since it will involve overlapping rectangles. However, that being said, lay people often find histograms and bar graphs easier to interpret, when they are not familiar with the subject area.

In short, which technique you use will depend on what your objectives are, and the nature of your data.

## Producing a smoother graph

There is one further point of interest when plotting frequency distributions. Generally, the larger the amount of data to be plotted, the smoother the resulting frequency distribution curve and conversely, the fewer the scores plotted, the more irregular and uneven the resulting graph. If you are concerned to identify trends, patterns and regularities in your data, you will obviously be keen to produce a smooth frequency distribution. If you cannot achieve this because you have only a limited number of scores to plot, you can obtain greater regularity by reducing the number of categories along the horizontal axis.

Let's suppose, for example, you were interested in the recovery rates of patients following hysterectomy operations. Having looked at some patient records over a 6-month period, you find that:

    4 patients were discharged after 4 days
    6 patients were discharged after 5 days
  10 patients were discharged after 6 days
  13 patients were discharged after 7 days
  10 patients were discharged after 8 days
    9 patients were discharged after 9 days
  15 patients were discharged after 10 days
    3 patients were discharged after 11 days
    5 patients were discharged after 12 days
    2 patients were discharged after 13 days

If this data is plotted as presented, we get the graph shown in Figure 5.7.

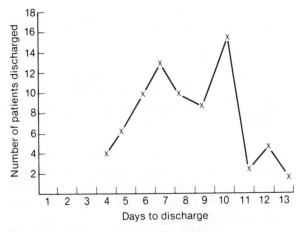

**Figure 5.7** Frequency polygon showing frequency distribution of recovery period following hysterectomy.

However, if we collapse the categories along the horizontal axis, as shown in Figure 5.8, we achieve a rather smoother graph:

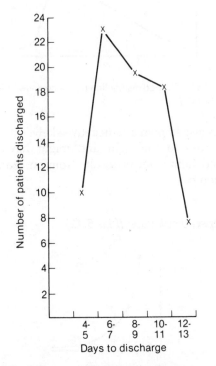

**Figure 5.8** Frequency polygon showing frequency distribution of recovery period following hysterectomy. The categories in Figure 5.7 have been collapsed.

You can see from the above illustration that reducing the categories along the horizontal axis makes the graph appear more regular, and in so doing allows you to get a clearer idea of the trends in the data. (A word of caution, though! Reducing the categories in this way may also distort your data, and obscure important features.)

## Ten rules for drawing graphs of frequency distributions

1. The horizontal axis, also known as the X-axis, must be used to represent the categories or events.

2. The vertical axis, also known as the Y-axis, must be used to represent the frequencies with which each event occurs.

3. The intervals along the axes must be of a suitable size, so that the graph may be drawn and interpreted accurately.

4. The intersection point of the axes conventionally should be zero. If this does not suit your purposes, ensure you make a note of this so that it is clear to the reader.

5. All graphs should be clearly labelled and self-explanatory. Both axes should also be labelled.

6. Nominal and ordinal data are usually described in bar graphs or pie charts.

7. Interval ratio data are usually described in histograms and frequency polygons.

8. Interval ratio data can be combined so that the graph can be inspected for *trends*.

9. If the categories are to be combined to form larger subgroups you should not use too many groups, otherwise the graph may be difficult to interpret. Similarly, you should not use too few subgroups, otherwise a lot of information will be lost.

10. If you subgroup your data, the subgroups should be of equal size, otherwise you will distort the information.

## Shapes of frequency distribution curves

If you plot a large number of graphs over a period of time, you will notice that some shapes of frequency distribution tend to occur time and again. It may be useful to outline some of these briefly.

*Normal distribution (Fig. 5.9)*

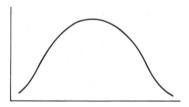

**Figure 5.9** Normal distribution.

This is probably the most important frequency distribution shape of all and has numerous implications for statistics. So important is it that the next section will be devoted entirely to a more detailed description of it. For the time being, suffice it to say that it is typically a symmetrical bell-shaped curve, and were we to plot heights or heart rates of a population as a frequency distribution, we would find that both are normally distributed.

*Skewed distribution (Fig. 5.10)*

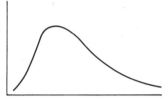

**Figure 5.10** Skewed distribution (1). This is also known as a positive skew.

This is also known as a positive skew. It is skewed to the left and is the sort of graph that might result from an overly difficult exam, i.e. too many students achieved marks near the bottom end of the score range.

*Skewed distribution (Fig. 5.11)*

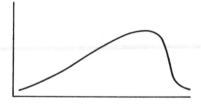

**Figure 5.11** Skewed distribution (2) – also known as negative skew.

This is also known as a negative skew. The graph is skewed to the right and might have been derived from a set of results from an exam that was too easy.

*J-shaped distribution (Fig. 5.12)*

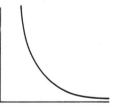

**Figure 5.12** J-shaped distribution.

This is the sort of frequency distribution which might result from monitoring the number of gastric contractions in a group of patients over a period following a meal. The vast majority of patients would show very few contractions since they would presumably be satisfied; they are represented by the highest part of the graph on the left. However a few people would show rather more activity and they are represented by the flattened tail of the graph to the right.

*Bimodal distribution (Fig. 5.13)*

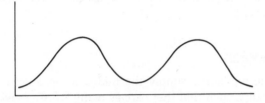

**Figure 5.13** Bimodal distribution.

This distribution is characterised by two distinct peaks and might have been obtained by plotting the vital capacities of a mixed group of smokers and non-smokers. The smokers would presumably be more likely to have smaller vital capacities and so would be represented by the left-hand peak, while the non-smokers, with larger vital capacities would be represented by the right-hand peak.

**Activity 5.1**  (Answers on pages 228–229)

In order to look at the consistency of measurements taken on a goniometer, you ask 15 physiotherapists to measure the knee joint mobility of a post-fracture patient. You obtain the results in Table 5.10.

**Table 5.10**  Number of physiotherapists recording a given degree of movement

| Degree of movement | No. of physiotherapists who recorded this score |
|---|---|
| 11–20 | 0 |
| 21–30 | 1 |
| 31–40 | 3 |
| 41–50 | 5 |
| 51–60 | 4 |
| 61–70 | 1 |
| 71–80 | 1 |
| 81–90 | 0 |

1 Draw (a) a histogram and (b) a frequency polygon to show these results.
2 In order to identify trends in the results, reduce the units along the horizontal axis and re-draw the frequency polygon.

## MEASURES OF CENTRAL TENDENCY

As has already been stated, any results from a piece of research must be presented in a way that can be clearly understood by the reader. Besides making tables of the results and drawing graphs, the data can be presented in terms of **measures of central tendency.**

Measures of central tendency involve describing a set of data in terms of the most typical scores within it. This approach may be valuable to the physiotherapist in three ways:

1. A comparison of some capacity of a group of patients with an established norm or standard for that capacity. For instance you may wish to compare the mobility of a group of hip replacement patients with the normal or average mobility of people of a comparable age group without hip trouble.

2. Establishing a standard or norm not previously known. For example, if a new piece of equipment was introduced to stimulate muscle contraction, which you thought might be useful for patients with muscular dystrophy, you would need to establish the level of stimulation provoked in normal muscles by the apparatus as well as in patients' muscles, in order to establish what could normally be expected from this piece of equipment.

3. Comparing different treatment techniques or different groups of patients, e.g. is clapping more effective than breathing exercises in increasing the vital capacity of cystic fibrosis patients?

In order to answer the questions three measures of central tendency can be used: the **arithmetic mean**, the **median** and the **mode**.

### Arithmetic mean

This is the average of a set of scores and is derived from adding all the scores together and dividing the total by the number of scores. It is usually denoted by the symbol $\bar{x}$. It is an extremely valuable concept in statistics, and enables the researcher to appraise a set of results at a glance.

For example, in the illustrations given above, the mean mobility for the hip patient group can be compared with the mean mobility for the non-patient group to see if there are any overall differences. Similarly, the mean vital capacity of the cystic fibrosis patients undergoing breathing exercises can be compared with the mean of those undergoing clapping, to give an estimate of which is more effective.

While the arithmetic mean is undoubtedly one of the most useful concepts in statistics, it can be misleading. Supposing you had the choice of giving a frozen shoulder patient one of two treatments. In order to help you make your choice, you turn to some statistics and find that treatment A produces an average 40% range of movement within 4 weeks, while treatment B produces 51% range of movement in the same period. From this information alone you would almost certainly favour treatment B. But let us suppose you were to look at the original data as shown in Table 5.11.

**Table 5.11** The results of two different treatment procedures for frozen shoulder patients

| Treatment A | | Treatment B | |
|---|---|---|---|
| Patient no. | Percentage range of movement | Patient no. | Percentage range of movement |
| 1 | 38 | 1 | 30 |
| 2 | 42 | 2 | 28 |
| 3 | 45 | 3 | 100 |
| 4 | 36 | 4 | 100 |
| 5 | 40 | 5 | 31 |
| 6 | 39 | 6 | 33 |
| 7 | 44 | 7 | 30 |
| 8 | 46 | 8 | 28 |
| 9 | 34 | 9 | 30 |
| 10 | 36 | 10 | 100 |
| $\bar{x}$ = | 40 | $\bar{x}$ = | 51 |

Although treatment A certainly produces, on average, less range of movement, the results are much more consistent than those from treatment B. Furthermore, with the exception of the three 100% scores, the remaining results from treatment B are lower than all the scores in treatment

A. In other words, the presence of three extreme scores in treatment B has distorted the mean and could have been misleading had you not looked at the original data. Having examined the raw data, you would probably now choose treatment A.

However, if you were conducting a large-scale survey, you might have thousands of data points and consequently it would be impossible to inspect the raw data thoroughly. Therefore, the arithmetic mean, while an essential component of statistics, is insufficient in itself to provide the necessary information about a set of results, and other forms of descriptive statistics are required as well.

## Median

The median is simply the mid-score in a set of results, such that there are as many scores above it as below it. To compute the median, arrange the scores in order of magnitude; then if there is an odd number of scores, the middle score becomes the median. So, for example, if you had five scores

14   9   28   5   11

you would arrange them in order of magnitude:

28   14   11   9   5

and the median is the third score from the end, i.e. 11. On the other hand, if there is an even number of scores, the median is the average of the two middle scores. So, if you had

14   9   28   5   11   18

you would arrange these in order of magnitude:

28   18   14   11   9   5

and the median is the average of the two middle scores, i.e.

$$\frac{14 + 11}{2} = 12.5$$

While the median obviously tells you the middle score out of a set of results, it tells you nothing about the range of the scores. For example, in the following sets of scores, the median in both cases is 10:

| 13 | 12 | 11 | 10 | 9 | 8 | 7 |
|----|----|----|----|---|---|---|
| 99 | 98 | 97 | 10 | 3 | 2 | 1 |

but the nature of the sets of scores is quite different, and the pattern of a set of scores may have important implications for their interpretation. For instance, if the first set of figures above referred to the ages of patients brought in with a particular disease, you may well think that the disease is one of childhood and early adolescence. You would not be inclined to think this if presented with the second set of figures. Thus, the nature of the scores is important in research if they are to be accurately interpreted.

So, the median alone gives insufficient information about the nature of a set of data. If it is used in conjunction with the mean, then more information can be derived about the total set of scores. For example, the more similar the mean and median, the smaller the range of scores. This can be illustrated with the above sets of figures. The first set has a mean and a median of 10 and the scores are all within a small range (13 – 7); however the second set of figures also has a median of 10 but a mean of 44.3 and a range of scores from 99 to 1.

While the median is not as valuable as the mean, if both techniques are used together they can be more useful in describing a set of data, especially where there are extreme scores.

## Mode

The mode is the most commonly occurring score in a set of data. So, in the following two sets of scores, 15 is the mode:

| 15 | 15 | 14 | 10 | 15 | 18 | 15 |
|----|----|----|----|----|----|----|
| 15 | 15 | 3 | 2 | 1 | 4 | 5 |

However, within any set of scores, you may have more than one mode. Its value lies primarily in its ability to answer the question 'which one event occurs most often?'. So, for example, you might want to ask: 'What is the commonest age of onset of motor neurone disease?'

To answer this question you would simply look at the ages at which the patients first presented with the symptoms of the condition and identify which was the most frequently occurring age.

## A comparison of the mean, mode and median

Comparing the value of the arithmetic mean, the median and the mode, the mean is the most commonly used statistic and provides more information about a set of scores than the median and the mode. This is due to the fact that the computation of the mean depends on the exact value of every score in a set of data and alteration of even one score will alter the mean. This is not necessarily the case for the median and the mode as illustrated by the following set of data:

| 3 | 14 | 10 | 19 | 8 | 5 | 15 | 20 | 3 |
|---|----|----|----|---|---|----|----|---|

The mean of this data is 10.8, the median is 10, and the mode is 3. If we alter the 20 to 40, the mean becomes 13, but the median and the mode stay the same.

In addition, the median and the mode may be totally unaffected by altering a large number of scores in a set of data. If the above set of figures is changed to:

| 3 | 34 | 10 | 39 | 2 | 1 | 45 | 17 | 3 |
|---|----|----|----|---|---|----|----|---|

although 6 out of 9 figures have been radically altered, the median remains 10 and the mode 3.

Conversely, the median and the mode may be drastically altered just by changing one figure. To take the above set of figures, if the first 3 is changed to 34, the median becomes 17 and the mode 34.

In other words, the median and the mode are less reliable than the mean when providing information about a set of scores because they may not be altered by radical changes to a lot of scores, or they may be changed by altering just one score. The mean on the other hand will alter if any score is changed, however minimally.

However, as already pointed out, the mean may be less useful than the median or mode if there are extreme scores in a set of data, because it is easily distorted by the presence of very large or small scores. However, although all three concepts can be used in descriptive statistics to provide information about a set of data, it is advisable always to calculate the mean, and then to decide whether the median and the mode will provide you with relevant information about your particular set of data.

Measures of **central tendency** are a form of descriptive statistics and allow the researcher to highlight features of a set of results in terms of the 'most typical values'. The three most commonly used measures of central tendency are:

- the **arithmetic mean:** the average of a set of scores
- the **median:** the mid-score in a set of results, such that there are as many scores above it as below
- the **mode:** the most commonly occurring score in a set of data.

**Activity 5.2**  (Answers on page 229)

1 Calculate the mean, median and the mode for the following sets of figures:
    (i) 91   87   90   76   51   48   72   76   80   44   89
    (ii) 25   39   17   41   24   17   37   31   27
    (iii) 44   43   51   54   60   71   39   41   55   43
2 Just by comparing the means and the medians, find out which of these sets of data have (a) the largest range and (b) the smallest range of scores.

## MEASURES OF DISPERSION

If you look back at the measures of central tendency, you will see that it is possible to obtain the same or very similar means for sets of scores which are quite different. For instance, the mean for each of the following two sets of figures is 10:

9   11   12   8   10   11   12   12   8   7
1   2   3   3   2   1   40   3   15   30

However, the scores in the first set are all quite similar to each other in that they only range from 7 to 12; the scores in the second set, however, range from 1 to 40. Just knowing the mean of a set of scores, then, can be quite misleading; we need to know how variable the scores are as well, in other words, what the spread of the data is. The statistics which describe the variability of scores are called **measures of dispersion** and are valuable to the physiotherapist for the same reasons as the measures of central tendency.

If you look back to page 39, you will see that the first reason given is that the researcher can compare a group of patients with an established standard to discover how far their capacity, mobility, skills or whatever resemble the norm. This can be carried out just using means, medians, and modes, but we have already seen that

similar means can be obtained from two totally different sets of scores. So, if we use the example on page 39, you might find that four out of five of your hip replacement patients had extremely limited mobility, while one had much greater mobility than the non-patient group. If you simply combine the mobility scores of these five patients and take the mean, you may well find that due to the one very mobile patient, the mean is very similar to that of the non-patient group and yet four of the patients were barely mobile. In other words you need to know what the spread of scores is.

Similarly if you wish to establish norms for a new piece of apparatus, it is insufficient just to use measures of central tendency, because they can be misleading unless you know how consistent the scores are. Obviously a piece of equipment which produces uniform results will be much more use than one which produces erratic results from poor to excellent even though the mean performances may be similar.

In addition, measures of dispersion can identify patients who respond particularly well or particularly poorly. This information may be useful when selecting treatments. And similarly, when comparing two or more treatment types, the treatment which produces homogeneous results, i.e. where the range of scores is small, will be regarded quite differently from the treatment which produces erratic results which cover an enormous range. So, in descriptive statistics, not only do you need to use measures of central tendency, you also need to describe the results in terms of how variable they are and to do this you use techniques called measures of dispersion. There are three measures of dispersion which are valuable to the physiotherapist: the **range**, **deviation and variance** and the **standard deviation**.

## Range

The range is quite simply the difference between the lowest and highest scores in a set of data. To compute it, simply find the smallest score in the set of data and subtract it from the highest score, thus in the following set of data

14   22   5   11   12   19   31   27

the range is

$$31 - 5 = 26$$

Obviously, when used in conjunction with measures of central tendency, it can provide useful additional information, in the way already outlined. However, the information produced by the range gives a limited picture since a range of 45 – 3 may describe a set of scores such as:

| 45 | 44 | 43 | 42 | 7 | 6 | 5 | 4 | 3 |

or

| 45 | 40 | 35 | 30 | 15 | 10 | 5 | 3 |

In other words, the range provides no insight into how the scores are distributed. One way of getting round this problem is to use deviation and variance measures.

## Deviation and variance

A description of the spread of scores, as we've seen, is important in understanding the implications of a set of data. A picture of the distribution of the scores can be presented by expressing the scores in terms of how far each one deviates from the mean.

In order to calculate the **deviation** of a set of scores, the mean is subtracted from each score. Thus, for the following set of scores:

| 10 | 15 | 21 | 8 | 11 | 12 | 14 | 5 |

the mean is 12, and the deviation of each score is:

$$10 - 12 = -2$$
$$15 - 12 = +3$$
$$21 - 12 = +9$$
$$8 - 12 = -4$$
$$11 - 12 = -1$$
$$12 - 12 = 0$$
$$14 - 12 = +2$$
$$5 - 12 = -7$$

In subtracting the mean from each score, you can find the position of each score relative to the mean. So, for example, the score of 15 is +3 deviation points above the mean.

However, as you can probably see, expressing each score as a deviation from the mean is just as long-winded as setting out all your scores and the mean. What is needed is some shorthand method

of expressing how varied and dispersed the scores are.

While many students assume that the obvious way would be to add together all the deviation scores, the answer is always 0 (try it for yourself and see), so this clearly tells us nothing. One way of getting round this problem is to *square* each deviation score (this obviously gets rid of all the plus and minus signs) and then to add these squared deviation scores up. The result is then divided by the *number* of scores you added, to give the mean. The result is called the **variance**.

If we compute the variance for the set of scores above, we get:

$$\frac{(-2^2) + (3^2) + (9^2) + (-4^2) + (-1^2) + (0^2) + (2^2) + (-7^2)}{8}$$

$$= \frac{4 + 9 + 81 + 16 + 1 + 0 + 4 + 49}{8}$$

$$= \frac{164}{8} = 20.5$$

The variance of a set of scores tells us by definition how dispersed or varied the scores are. Obviously, the smaller the variance, the more similar the scores, while the greater the variance, the more disparate the scores. If you look back to the example on page 40 about the frozen shoulder treatments, you can see that knowledge of the spread of scores would be a very useful piece of information here, since the smaller the variance the more reliable and consistent the treatment procedure.

## Standard deviation

Although the variance score gives you the total degree of variability in a set of scores, it has been obtained, obviously, by adding together such varied squared deviations as 81 and 0 (see the previous set of figures). Sometimes you may want to find out what the average or standard degree of deviation is for a set of scores, rather than the total degree of variation. To do this you need a very useful statistic called, not unreasonably, the **standard deviation** (or SD).

To calculate it, you simply take the variance figure (i.e. the total of the squared deviation scores; in the above case, 164), divide this by the total number of scores (to give the average squared deviation) and then take the square root of this, to give you the standard deviation of the scores from the mean. The formula then is:

$$SD = \sqrt{\frac{\Sigma(x - \bar{x})^2}{N}}$$

where

$\sqrt{\phantom{x}}$ = square root of all the calculations under this symbol

$x$ = the individual score

$\bar{x}$ = the mean score

$\Sigma$ = total, or sum, of every calculation to the right

$N$ = the total number of scores.

You may have realised that $\Sigma(x - \bar{x})^2$ is the variance score. So, for the figures above, the standard deviation is

$$\sqrt{\frac{164}{8}}$$

$$= 4.528$$

Sometimes you will find the SD formula given as

$$\sqrt{\frac{\Sigma(x - \bar{x})^2}{N - 1}}$$

The $N - 1$ is used if you want to infer the standard deviation of the *population* from which your sample is drawn, whereas using just $N$ gives the standard deviation of the *sample only*. However, in practice, this variation makes very little difference, so don't worry unduly about it.

This means that the standard degree of deviation of this set of scores from the mean is 4.528. Such information gives you a picture, in a single figure, of how dispersed or variable a set of scores is. As we've already pointed out, this is particularly useful in determining the consistency of a set of figures.

All of this may seem rather confusing to you when deciding how to describe a set of data. As a rule of thumb, I would recommend that you always calculate the mean, range and standard deviation of a set of scores and then decide which of the other measures provides you with information which is relevant to the aims of that particular piece of research.

**KEY CONCEPTS**

Measures of dispersion are a branch of descriptive statistics which allow the researcher to describe a set of data in terms of how variable the scores are.

The measures of dispersion which are of particular importance to the physiotherapist are:
- the **range**: the difference between the lowest and highest scores in a set of data
- the **deviation**: provides information about the extent to which each score deviates from the mean, and is calculated by subtracting the mean from each score.
- the **variance**: is the mean of the squared deviations. It is calculated by squaring each deviation score, adding the results up and dividing the total by the number of scores you added together.
- the **standard deviation** (SD) is the average amount of deviation and is computed by dividing the variance by the total number of scores and taking the square root of this results.

**Activity 5.3**   (Answers on pages 229)

1 Find the range, deviation, variance and standard deviation of the following sets of scores:

(i)  14   9  21  23  18  17  33  28  12
(ii)  71  50  48  64  80  81  79

2 You are concerned about one of the goniometers in use in your department, since you are not sure how reliable it is. How might you assess its reliability using descriptive statistics?

## Normal distribution

It was pointed out earlier that there are a number of frequency distribution shapes which occur commonly in statistics. The most common of all these is the so-called **normal distribution curve** (sometimes known as the Gaussian distribution, after Gauss, the astronomer and mathematician who investigated it). The normal distribution curve is a symmetrical bell-shaped distribution (Fig. 5.14).

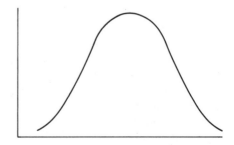

**Figure 5.14**   Normal distribution curve.

It possesses a number of important mathematical properties:

1. It is symmetrical.
2. The mean, median and mode all have the same value.
3. The curve descends rapidly at first from its central point, but the descent slows down as the tails of the curve are reached.
4. No matter how far you continue the tails of the curve, they never reach the horizontal axis.
5. The normal distribution curve occurs in data drawn from a wide range of subjects: mathematics, physics, engineering, psychology, etc. For example, height, IQ, and the life of electric light bulbs all have normal distributions. In other words, if we collected, for example, height data from a large number of people randomly drawn from the population and drew a frequency distribution of it, we would end up with something that resembled a normal curve.
6. If the mean and standard deviation of a normally distributed set of data are known, then we can draw the normal distribution curve. The reason we can do this is a result of the relationship between the standard deviation and the normal distribution curve.

### The standard deviation and the normal distribution curve

When a set of data is normally distributed, a fixed percentage of the scores always falls in a given area under the curve. If we take the central point of the curve shown in Figure 5.15 and then move one standard deviation above and below the mean, then 68% of the scores will *always* fall within this range. This is a constant fact of the normal distribution, i.e. that 34% of scores fall within 1 standard deviation above the mean, and 34% of scores fall within 1 standard deviation below.

If we move on, we find that a further 13.5% of the scores fall between standard deviations 1 and 2 above the mean, and 13.5% fall between standard deviations 1 and 2 below the mean. Thus, the two standard deviations on either side of the mean account for a total of 95% of the scores (13.5 + 34 + 34 + 13.5).

Going on to standard deviations 2–3 above and below the mean, we find that 2.36% of scores fall

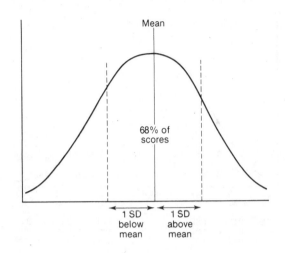

**Figure 5.15** The standard deviation and the normal distribution curve.

within each category, thereby allowing a total of 99.73% of the scores to be accounted for by 3 standard deviations above and below the mean (2.36 + 13.5 + 34 + 34 + 13.5 + 2.36 = 99.72, represented normally as 99.73 as a result of calculating further decimal places).

So, to take an example, if we know that the mean IQ of the population is 100 and the standard deviation is 20; then 68% of the population have IQs between 80 and 120; 95% have IQs between 60 and 140, and 99.73% have IQs between 40 and 160. We can see this more clearly in the normal curve in Figure 5.16.

### The value of the normal distribution

The value of the normal distribution is twofold. Firstly, it allows the researcher to describe a set of data and to predict (from knowledge of the properties of the normal curve) what proportions of people possess certain characteristics.

For example, if we know that the average heart rate is 72, with a standard deviation of 5, and that heart rate is normally distributed, we can draw the curve shown in Figure 5.17.

Now, because we know that 68% of people are accounted for by scores within 1 standard deviation either side of the mean, we know that 68% of the population must have heart rates between 67 and 77 beats per minute. Furthermore, we know that another 13.5% of people fall within

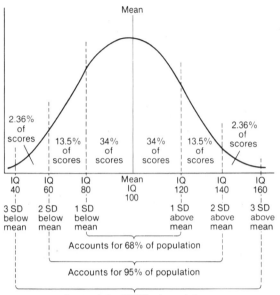

**Figure 5.16** Hypothetical normal distribution curve for IQ.

standard deviations 1 and 2 above the mean and another 13.5% fall within standard deviations 1 and 2 below the mean. This means 13.5% of the population have heart rates of 77–82 beats per minute and 13.5% have heart rates of 62–67 beats per minute. Finally, we know that 2.36% of the population fall within standard deviations

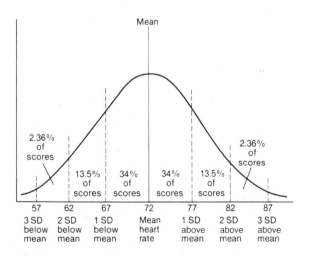

**Figure 5.17** Hypothetical normal distribution curve for heart rate.

2–3 above the mean and a further 2.36% within standard deviations 2–3 below the mean. This means 2.36% of people have heart rates of 82–87 beats per minute and 2.36% have heart rates of 57–62 beats per minute.

This information also allows us to 'work backwards'; if a patient presents with a heart rate of 86, then you can ascertain just how statistically unusual this is, since you know that only 2.36% of the population come within this range.

The second function of the normal distribution curve relates to its role in inferential statistics. Many of the tests used in inferential statistics require that the results being analysed are normally distributed (see section on 'parametric' statistics); if they are not, then these tests are inappropriate and other sorts of test (i.e. 'nonparametric') must be used. This will be explained in more detail in Chapter 9.

The normal distribution curve also underlies some of the theoretical assumptions of inferential statistics, although these need not concern us unduly here. However, the normal distribution will be referred to again in the Chapter on Estimation, as it is fundamental to understanding this concept.

---

**KEY CONCEPTS**

The **normal distribution curve** is a commonly occurring frequency distribution which possesses certain mathematical properties:

- If the mean and the standard deviation of set of scores are known, then the researcher is able to predict what proportion of the population have scores within a certain range. This is possible because a fixed proportion of the population will fall within a certain score range, as long as those scores are normally distributed.
- The normal curve is of fundamental importance in the theory behind inferential statistics.

---

**Activity 5.4** (Answers on page 229)

If we know that heart rate during weeks 10–20 of pregnancy is normally distributed, with a mean of 82 and a standard deviation of 8, then:

1 What percentage of patients will have heart rates between 66 and 98?
2 What percentage of patients will show heart rates of 99–106?
3 If a patient presents with a heart rate of 57, how common is this in terms of percentages?

# 6

# Testing hypotheses

We have briefly covered the topic of descriptive statistics, which provide the researcher with one method of presenting data. However, this approach is typically used to make sense of data derived from some form of survey, and is not always appropriate for analysing results from an experiment where an hypothesis has been tested. What is needed here, is a second branch of statistics known as **inferential statistics.**

There will be many occasions when you do not want simply to collect a mound of general information about a broad topic area, but wish, instead, to test out an idea; for instance, comparing the effectiveness of two treatment techniques, or monitoring the progress of a specific group of patients. In such cases, you would carry out an experiment and analyse the results from this using a statistical test. This sort of analysis is called inferential statistics, because it allows you to *infer* that the results you obtained from your experiment, using a small sample of people, may also apply to the larger population from which the sample was drawn. Look back to pages 13–15 to refresh your memory on this.

However, before you can reasonably start inferring anything from the results of an experiment, it is essential that the experiment is properly set up and designed, otherwise false inferences may be made. This chapter and the next are concerned with outlining the principles of good experimental techniques.

When carrying out any research which involves testing an idea or hypothesis, the following steps have to be taken:

- An hypothesis must be devised and stated clearly.

- A research project must be designed which will test the hypothesis.
- Results from the research have to be analysed using an appropriate statistical test.
- A report must be prepared on the research for future reference.

We shall deal with each of these stages in turn. The present chapter will be concerned with the principles involved in devising hypotheses and some basic concepts about research design.

## THE EXPERIMENTAL HYPOTHESIS

The starting point of any research is an idea known as the **experimental** or **research hypothesis**, sometimes referred to as $H_1$. This is usually based on some theory or observations that the researcher has made. You may, for instance, have noticed in the course of your work, that certain patients seem to respond better to particular types of treatment. An observation of this type would form the basis of an experimental hypothesis. Examples of experimental hypotheses include such ideas as the following:

1. Male physiotherapy students perform better in clinical assessment than female physiotherapy students.
2. Leg fracture patients make quicker recoveries with traction than with cast-bracing.
3. Job satisfaction is greater among community physiotherapists than hospital-based physiotherapists.

You probably have a number of such ideas that you are interested in looking at, and it would be useful to write them down at this stage.

If we look at the above hypotheses, we can see that what the experimental hypothesis does is to predict a relationship between two or more things, which are known as **variables.** Therefore, the first hypothesis predicts a relationship between gender of the physiotherapy student (male or female), and performance in clinical assessments. The two variables here, then, are gender of student and performance. The second hypothesis predicts a relationship between type of treatment (traction or cast-bracing), and speed of recovery. The two variables here are type of

treatment and recovery rate. The third hypothesis predicts a relationship between degree of job satisfaction and type of physiotherapist (community or hospital). The two variables, then, are job satisfaction and type of physiotherapist.

The relationship predicted in the experimental hypothesis is assumed to be a consistent and reliable one. So, if we take the second of the hypotheses above, the underlying assumption is that leg-fracture patients on traction will typically make more progress than those leg-fracture patients with cast-bracing, What we do *not* anticipate is a rather unpredictable outcome, such that sometimes traction patients do better, but sometimes they don't.

---

**KEY CONCEPTS**

The **experimental hypothesis** is the starting point of any research and predicts a relationship between two or more variables.

---

**Activity 6.1** (Answers on page 229)

Look at the following hypotheses and write down what the two variables are in each case.
1 Children with leg fractures progress faster on traction than adolescents with leg fractures.
2 Men and women with arthritis differ in their responsiveness to heat treatment.
3 Men are more likely to suffer chest infections following cardiothoracic surgery than are women.
4 Outpatients' clinics achieve better recovery rates for leg fractures than specific sports injuries clinics.
5 There is a difference in professional competence between physiotherapists who trained in hospital-based training schools and those who trained in university-based training schools.

Now think about the research project you would like to carry out. State the experimental hypothesis, making sure it predicts a relationship between the two variables. Write down what the variables are.

When formulating your experimental hypothesis, there are some points which would be useful to bear in mind. Firstly, your hypothesis should be *testable*. As an extreme example, you might have predicted that comatose patients experience less pain than non-comatose patients when undergoing the same physiotherapeutic treatment. How would you assess the pain levels of the comatose group? It would be an impossible task and consequently the hypothesis would not be testable.

Secondly, your hypothesis should be *realistic* in its aims. This means you should not be over-ambitious and, for example, try to compare the entire population of insulin-dependent diabetics with non-insulin-dependent diabetics for signs of neuropathy. A project of that size would be not only unnecessary but beyond the scope of any individual researcher or even of a robust cohort of researchers. Consequently, the aims of your experiment should be confined to something more do-able.

Thirdly, you must *define what your variables mean*. In the above example, 'comatose' patients is a very loose concept. Why are they comatose? What is their medical condition? How old are they? Who are they? You must be able to clarify exactly what your terms mean.

Finally, few researchers push back the frontiers of science with their projects. Most people for whatever reason, have to undertake small-scale studies, but this does not necessarily imply that their value is limited. Many such projects can have far-reaching implications for health care policy and practice and contribute a great deal to our knowledge base.

The next step is to find out whether the relationship predicted in your hypothesis does, in fact, exist, which means you must design and carry out a suitable project to test your hypothesis. Any results you get from the research are then analysed using the appropriate statistical test. But, before we move on to talk about how you proceed, one very important point must be made.

## THE NULL HYPOTHESIS

It must be logically possible for the relationship predicted in your experimental hypothesis to be wrong, otherwise there is no point in wasting your time carrying out any research. For example, anyone who hypothesised that all physiotherapists who were born in 1940 are older than those born in 1945 and then spent three days amongst the record books trying to support their hypothesis would be indulging in a pointless exercise, since there would be absolutely no possibility that their prediction would be wrong. Therefore,

to make any research project worthwhile, there has to be a chance that the predicted relationship does not exist.

To show that there is a possibility that the experimental hypothesis is incorrect, we have to state an alternative hypothesis called the **null hypothesis.** This is sometimes referred to as $H_0$. So, while the experimental hypothesis predicts that there is a relationship between two variables, the null hypothesis says there is no relationship and that any results you get from your research project are due to chance and not to any real and reliable relationship between the variables.

Let's take an example. Supposing in the course of your work you have noticed that patients are more likely to follow oral rather than written instructions for exercises following leg fractures. You decide to carry out some research to see if your hunch is right. The first step is to state the experimental hypothesis clearly, i.e. 'Patients are more likely to comply with oral exercise instructions than written exercise instructions following leg fractures'. So, you are predicting a relationship between the type of instructions given and degree of compliance. But because it is possible that your observations are wrong, you must also state the null hypothesis that there is no relationship between the type of instructions and degree of compliance. The null hypothesis also implies that should any differences in degree of compliance be found, then these are simply due to chance fluctuations and not to any real and consistent relationship. The usual way of stating the null hypothesis is simply to predict no relationship between the two variables. Therefore, here, your null hypothesis would be: 'There is no relationship between type of instructions and degree of compliance'.

If you ever get stuck when formulating the null hypothesis, the easy way to get round the problem is by:

1. Firstly identifying the relationship in the experimental hypothesis, by stating: 'There is a relationship between a and b'; (a and b being the two variables).
2. Changing the first part to 'There is no relationship between a and b'. This gives you your null hypothesis.

It is very important to note that the null hypothesis predicts *no relationship*; it does not predict the opposite of the experimental hypothesis. Many students get confused over this, and in the example just given would assume that the null hypothesis says the reverse of the experimental hypothesis, i.e. that written instructions are more likely to be followed than are oral ones. (Just refresh your memory and check that this is the opposite of our original hypothesis.) This assumption is incorrect, because if we look at it, a relationship is still being predicted between type of instructions and compliance. So, the null hypothesis says there is no relationship between the two variables; in this case, between type of instruction and degree of compliance.

**Activity 6.2** (Answers on page 229)

To see whether you are happy with this concept, look at the experimental hypotheses on page 48 and write down what the null hypothesis is for each one. State the null hypothesis for the research project you would like to carry out.

Why do we need to state the null hypothesis at all? Could we not just assume that there is a chance that our experimental hypothesis may be wrong without having to spell it out? The answer to this lies in a convention, which has its roots in the philosophy of scientific method. (For further details on this the reader is referred to Chalmers (1983).)

Essentially this convention states that when we carry out any research we do not set out to find direct support for our experimental hypothesis (or at least we shouldn't!) but, rather perversely, to falsify the null hypothesis. In other words we still hope to find the relationship we predicted in the experimental hypothesis, but we do this by stating the null hypothesis and setting out to reject it. It should be noted here that the words 'prove' and 'disprove' in relation to the hypotheses are not being used. This is because we cannot really ever prove or disprove anything in physiotherapy, psychology or whatever – all we can do is find evidence that supports or fails to support our prediction.

The intending researcher need not worry unduly about all this, since it is sufficient simply to state the experimental and null hypotheses at the outset of any experiment. The relevance of the null hypothesis will be discussed further in different parts of the book.

---

**KEY CONCEPTS**

The **null hypothesis** states that the relationship predicted in the experimental hypothesis does *not* exist, and implies that any results found from the research are simply due to chance factors and not to any real and consistent relationship between the two variables. In any research project, the experimenter sets out to support his/her prediction by rejecting the null hypothesis.

---

## BASIC TYPES OF DESIGN

Once you have sorted out the experimental and null hypotheses for your research project, you then have to decide on the best way to find out whether your predicted relationship actually exists.

In other words you have to design a suitable research project. It should be noted that there are often a number of designs that can be used to test an hypothesis, and it is up to the researcher to select the most appropriate one. As there is usually no single correct way of testing an hypothesis, the researcher must take into account a number of design considerations, and it is with these that this chapter and the following one are concerned.

There are two basic sorts of research designs: *experimental designs* and *correlational designs*. Both designs start off with an experimental hypothesis which predicts a relationship between two variables, but the aims and methods of each approach are different. These differences can be best illustrated by an example. Let's take the hypothesis that the professional rank of physiotherapist affects the degree of job satisfaction that is experienced. The relationship that is being suggested is between professional status of the physiotherapist and degree of job satisfaction. Let's see how experimental and correlational designs would each approach the problem of trying to find out whether this relationship does, in fact, exist.

## Experimental design: an example

The experimental design would take a group of senior physiotherapists (say 10 district physiotherapists) and a group of junior physiotherapists (say, 10 physiotherapists), measure the reported job satisfaction expressed by each group and compare the two groups to see if there was any *difference* between them.

We would have the following design.

Group 1
10 district
physiotherapists        } Compared on expressed job satisfaction for differences between the groups
Group 2
10 physiotherapists

## Correlational design: an example

The correlational design, on the other hand, would select a number of physiotherapists who represented the whole range of professional status, from physiotherapists through to district level, and measure their reported job satisfaction to see if there is any *similarity or association* between professional level and degree of job satisfaction, such that, for instance, the higher the status, the higher the corresponding job satisfaction.

The correlational design would be as shown in Table 6.1.

**Table 6.1** A correlational design investigating job satisfaction and professional rank

| Subject | Level of physiotherapist | Job satisfaction scores (on a 10-point scale) |
|---------|--------------------------|------------------------------------------------|
| 1 | District | 9 |
| 2 | Superintendent I | 8 |
| 3 | Superintendent IV | 5 |
| 4 | Senior | 4 |
| 5 | Physiotherapist | 4 |

The data on both status and job satisfaction would be examined to see if there is any pattern or association between them.

Experimental and correlational designs will be discussed more fully in the next two sections. It should be stressed, however, that for the hypothesis we are looking at, either design would be appropriate. This illustrates the idea that was mentioned earlier: for any hypothesis there may be a number of suitable designs to test it, and it is up to the researcher to think carefully about the aims, objectives and the relevant design considerations of the research, and to devise the most appropriate method of testing the hypothesis.

---

**KEY CONCEPTS**

- **Experimental** designs look for **differences** between sets of results.
- **Correlational** designs look for **patterns** between sets of results.

Therefore, each approach has a different objective and will consequently use a different method to test the hypothesis.

---

We will deal with the basic principles involved in each design separately, starting with experimental designs.

## EXPERIMENTAL DESIGNS

We have already noted that the experimental hypothesis predicts a relationship between two variables. The simplest way to find out whether this relationship actually exists is to alter one of these variables to see what difference it makes to the other. This is the basis of experimental design. This alteration is known as **manipulation of variables** and is actually something we do in everyday life, often without being aware of it.

This can be illustrated by a mundane example. Suppose you were babysitting for a friend and had decided to watch their televison. You turn it on and discover that the sound is too low. Because you aren't familiar with the controls on this set you aren't sure how to adjust the volume, but you think it might be the knob on the front right of the set. Unwittingly, you have formulated an hypothesis: that there is a relationship between the knob and the volume. In order to test this hypothesis, you have to manipulate one of the variables; in other words, you alter the knob to see what effect it has on the sound. You have just performed a very simple experiment, which involved hypothesising a relationship between two variables and manipulating one to see what difference it made to the other. This is the basis of experimental design.

These variables have names. The variable which is manipulated is called the **independent variable** or IV. The variable which is observed for any changes in it resulting from that manipulation, is called the **dependent variable** or DV. People sometimes get confused about which variable is which. The easiest way to identify the IV and the DV is to ask the question: 'Which variable depends on which'? In the above example with the television the question is: 'Does the knob depend on the volume or does the volume depend on the knob?' Clearly in this case the volume depends on the knob, and thus the volume is the dependent variable. The knob is therefore the independent variable.

Some important points emerge out of this. If, after turning the knob, the volume did increase, you might have concluded, (though perhaps not consciously) that twiddling the knob caused the volume to increase, and therefore the increase in volume could be seen as the effect of twiddling the knob. In this way, the IV can be thought of as the *cause* and the DV as the *effect*. In addition, any changes that you note in the dependent variable which result from manipulating the independent variable, constitute your data in an experiment.

Just to clarify this idea, let's take the hypothesis that leg fractures improve more quickly with traction than with cast-bracing. The two variables are (i) type of treatment and (ii) speed of recovery. Which variable is which? Does the type of treatment depend on speed of recovery? Or does speed of recovery depend on type of treatment? Clearly, the second suggestion is correct. Type of treatment is the independent variable and speed of recovery is the dependent variable because how quickly a patient recovers *depends* on the treatment received. What is meant here, then, when we talk about manipulating the independent variable is simply assigning some patients to traction and some to cast-bracing. Their progress is then compared.

However, the problem is not always quite as simple as this. Supposing we hypothesised that there is a difference between the responses of male and female patients to ultrasound. Here the dependent variable is the difference in response to ultrasound, so the independent variable must be the gender of the patient. But how does the experimenter manipulate the gender of the patient? Obviously in the previous example, it was easy (at least theoretically) for the experimenter to decide which treatment a fracture patient should receive, but in the latter case we cannot possibly take a group of patients and decide what gender they should be! In this case the experimenter would simply select two groups of patients, one male and one female, and compare their responses to ultrasound. The independent variable is still being manipulated but in a slightly different way. Obviously, this sort of manipulation is essential when the independent variable is of a 'fixed' nature, such as race, age, type of patient, etc. This point will be referred to again later.

One final point before moving on to discuss some basic principles of design. There may be many changes in your dependent variable that you wish to measure. For example, if we look at the hypothesis above, we predicted that there was a relationship between type of treatment for leg fractures (IV) and the speed of improvement (DV). Speed of improvement can be measured in several ways; how long it takes before the patient achieves a specified range of movement, how long before the patient walks a particular distance, levels of pain, etc. It would be legitimate to use any or all these measures as your dependent variable. In other words, you may have a number of outcome measures you wish to take – you don't have to confine yourself to just one.

---

**Activity 6.3**   (Answers on pages 229–230)

Look at the following hypotheses and decide which is the independent variable, and which is the dependent variable. When you have done that, decide how you would manipulate the independent variable. If you find that you are having difficulty deciding which variable is which, just ask yourself which variable depends on which.

1 Men and women differ in their tendency to complain about pain.
2 Walking frames are more effective than walking sticks in aiding the mobility of arthritis patients.
3 Absenteeism is greater amongst physiotherapists working in psychiatric hospitals than amongst physiotherapists working in general hospitals.
4 Physiotherapists are able to establish greater rapport with male patients than with female patients.
5 Physiotherapy schools which require 'A'-level physics have higher pass rates on the final exam than schools which do not require 'A'-level physics.

Experimental designs involve manipulating the **independent variable** and measuring the effect of this on the **dependent variable.** The independent variable can be thought of as cause and the dependent variable as effect.

## More than one independent variable

So far we have assumed that all experimental hypotheses have just one independent variable. However, as we mentioned earlier, this is not always the case and some more complex hypotheses may predict a relationship between more than one independent variables and the dependent variable.

An example of this sort of hypothesis would be a predicted relationship between the age of a patient and his/her response to one or more treatment types, e.g. that there is a difference in improvement rate of children and adolescents with cystic fibrosis to clapping or exercise techniques. Here the dependent variable is improvement rate, and the independent variables are the age of the patient and the type of treatment they receive. This hypothesis requires a rather more complicated design, which is outside the scope of this book, but the reader is referred to Greene & D'Oliveira (1982) or Ferguson (1976) for more details on experimental designs with more than one independent variable.

In this book we shall deal only with experiments which test hypotheses with just one independent variable.

## Some basic principles of experimental design with one independent variable

To recap, experimental designs require the experimenter to manipulate or alter the independent variable and to measure the effect of this on the dependent variable. In other words, you alter one variable and measure the difference it makes to the other. Hence experimental designs are said to look for differences. It is important to note that this applies only to experimental designs and not to correlational designs which we shall look at in the next section.

So, having formulated your experimental hypothesis and null hypothesis, the next task is to design a suitable experiment to find out whether the relationship predicted in your hypothesis exists. The basic concepts involved in this are best explained by an example.

Suppose you wanted to test the hypothesis that physiotherapists who did a psychology course run by the local college became more tolerant in their attitudes to patients. The independent variable is attendance on a course and the dependent variable is attitude change. To test this hypothesis you decide to give those physiotherapists who have completed a psychology course an attitude questionnaire. Therefore you would have the following design:

*Independent variable*     *Dependent variable*
Attendance on course    Measurement of attitudes

What could you conclude from the replies to the questionnaire? Could you assume that the physiotherapists' attitudes had changed or not? You have probably quite correctly decided that we cannot conclude anything from this study since we don't know what the physiotherapists' attitudes were in the first place. So an essential feature of an experiment is a pre-test measure, where possible, of the dependent variable. Let's revise our design to include this:

Pre-test          Attendance on       Post-test
measure of     course (IV)            measure of
attitudes (DV)                           attitudes (DV)

What could you conclude from this experiment now? You could certainly decide on the basis of some statistical analysis of the pre-test and post-test scores whether there had been a significant attitude change but you couldn't ascribe it necessarily to course attendance, since it is quite possible that there are other explanations for change. In other words, course attendance is not necessarily the cause of any observed change in attitudes.

**Activity 6.4**  (Answers on page 230)

Can you think of any possible alternative reasons for these results?

Certainly, it is conceivable that these physiotherapists might have become more tolerant anyway, simply because they were just a bit older, and a bit more experienced. They might also have changed jobs, got promotion or had any one of a number of experiences which might account for their attitude change. How, then, can we ever be sure that the results in our experiment are due to the independent variable? The only way to do this is to select another group of physiotherapists who do not experience the independent variable, that is, do not attend the course. We then have to make sure that the only difference between the groups is whether or not they experience the independent variable. So, going back to our example, we would select two groups of physiotherapists, of which just one group had attended a psychology course and we would compare their post-test attitudes. Our revised design looks like this:

*Group 1*  Physiotherapists who attend a psychology course

| Pre-test measure of attitudes (DV) | Attendance on course (IV) | Post-test measure of attitudes (DV) |
|---|---|---|

*Group 2*  Physiotherapists who have not attended a psychology course

| Pre-test measure of attitudes (DV) | No attendance on course (no IV) | Post-test measure of attitudes (DV) |
|---|---|---|

These two groups are given names: the group who receives the independent variable (in this case, attends a psychology course) is called the **experimental** group or condition. The group who does not receive the independent variable (in this case, does not attend a psychology course) is called the **control** group or condition. The control group is therefore a 'no-treatment' group. The pre-test and post-test scores from the two conditions are then compared using a statistical test to find out if there are any **significant differences** between them. Therefore, if the only difference between the two groups is the fact that one group experienced the IV and the other did not, then any differences in the attitudes of the groups at the end of the study must have been caused by the IV.

## Placebos

Sometimes a control group is used slightly differently. While the proper definition of a control group is a 'no-treatment' group, there may be occasions when it is more appropriate to give this group some 'pretend' treatment.

Let's take an example. Imagine a situation where community physiotherapy services for the elderly are being audited. A question arises as to whether there is any evidence to suggest that physiotherapy has any benefit for patients who have had a hip replacement, or whether this particular service could be carried out by a care assistant or community nurse in order to reduce costs. One way of testing this (as long as the ethics were acceptable), would be to have an experimental group receiving physiotherapy and a control group having no treatment. However, it occurs to you that one of the factors which may contribute to any benefits that might derive from the physiotherapy is the patient's *expectation* that they will improve if they are given some treatment. In other words, any improvement the patient demonstrates may be the result not of the physiotherapy itself, but rather of the power of expectation and auto-suggestion.

In order to establish whether or not this is the case, you decide to give the control group some dummy treatment which involves the same amount of one-to-one attention coupled with some exercises which have no value. If at the end of the study you found that the experimental group has made more progress than the controls, then you could conclude that physiotherapy was beneficial to these patients and the audit commission's question would have been answered.

The dummy treatment is called a **placebo**. This technique is used a lot in drug trials, where some patients are given the real drug and other patients are given a useless salt or sugar tablet. However, so great is the power of the mind and the patient's expectations that the group on the placebo usually shows a marked improvement, which is known as the **placebo effect.**

---

**KEY CONCEPTS**

The subjects in the **experimental condition** are subjected to the independent variable. The experimental condition can therefore be thought of as the 'treatment condition'. The **control condition** subjects are not subjected to the independent variable. The control condition can therefore be thought of as the 'no-treatment' group.
Sometimes the control group is given a dummy treatment called a **placebo**.

There are still many flaws in our design but we will talk about ways of eliminating them and refining the experiment in the next chapter. Nonetheless, the key concepts that have been outlined should give you an idea about some of the fundamental issues involved in experimental designs.

## Ethical issues

By now you might be wanting to raise some moral issues. The type of design described above is fine when we want to look at something like the effects of a psychology course on attitudes. In this instance, there is no real moral dilemma about not giving physiotherapists a psychology course. But supposing your hypothesis was that cystic fibrosis patients would improve significantly on a new exercise regime. The IV here is the treatment and the DV is the improvement. You select your two groups of patients, and you give the experimental group your new treatment, but according to the above principles of experimental design, the other group of cystic fibrosis patients should receive no treatment. Is this ethical? Surely we cannot possibly leave a group of patients with no treatment while we are busily testing out our ideas?

In cases such as this, you would compare *two* experimental groups rather than one experimental group and one control group. So, instead of comparing your new treatment with no treatment, you would compare it with the conventional treatment or another form of treatment.

Our design would look like this:

*Experimental condition 1*

| Pre-test measure of DV | New exercise regime (IV) | Post-test measure of DV |
|---|---|---|

*Experimental condition 2*

| Pre-test measure of DV | Conventional treatment | Post-test measure of DV |
|---|---|---|

In this case, both groups are subjected to the Independent Variable (treatment) and their progress compared, to find out whether there are any differences between the groups.

**Activity 6.5** (Answers on pages 230)

Look at the following hypotheses and set out the experimental design you would use in each case, using the sort of format and headings shown above:

1 Patients who are given information about the value of physiotherapy exercises are more likely to do those exercises than are patients who receive no information.
2 Physiotherapists who have been a hospital patient are more sympathetic than those who have not.
3 Physiotherapists who have qualified in the last 5 years are more motivated to do research than those who have been qualified for more than 10 years.

## More complex designs

The sort of design we have been looking at is the most simple experimental design of all: a pre-test measure of the dependent variable, manipulation of the independent variable and a post-test measure of the dependent variable. Two groups are used, of which one may be a control condition or alternatively, both groups may be experimental conditions.

However, you may become a bit more ambitious and decide that you would like to look at something a little more complex than this. If we look back to the hypothesis that cystic fibrosis patients make significant improvements on a new exercise regime, we used a design which involved the comparison of two experimental groups. But you could, if you wished, add further conditions to this design. If you managed to resolve any ethical problem in your mind, you might decide to add a control condition as well, and so your design would look like this:

*Experimental condition 1*

| Pre-test measure of DV | New exercise regime (IV) | Post-test measure of DV |
|---|---|---|

*Experimental condition 2*

| Pre-test measure of DV | Conventional treatment (IV) | Post-test measure of DV |
|---|---|---|

*Control condition*

| Pre-test measure of DV | No treatment (no IV) | Post-test measure of DV |
|---|---|---|

So you still have two experimental conditions, or *levels* of the independent variable, but you now have a control condition as well.

Alternatively, you might feel that it would be useful to compare three types of therapy instead of two, perhaps adding heat treatment to the exercise regime and conventional therapy.

Therefore, your hypothesis would be something like 'exercise, heat treatment and conventional therapy are differentially effective in helping cystic fibrosis patients'. The dependent variable is degree of improvement and the independent variable is still type of treatment, but this time we have got three types of treatment. Therefore, the independent variable has three experimental conditions or levels: exercise, heat treatment and conventional therapy. Our design would look something like this:

*Experimental condition 1*

| Pre-test measure of physical condition | New exercise regime (IV) | Post-test measure of physical condition (DV) |

*Experimental condition 2*

| Pre-test measure of physical condition | Heat treatment (IV) | Post-test measure of physical condition (DV) |

*Experimental condition 3*

| Pre-test measure of physical condition | Conventional therapy (IV) | Post-test measure of physical condition (DV) |

You could extend this further and add a control condition thus:

*Experimental condition 1*
*Experimental condition 2*
*Experimental condition 3*
*Control condition*
} Compared on the dependent variable to assess whether there are any differences between the conditions

Or you could go on adding experimental conditions involving different forms of treatment.

In all these cases we still have only one independent variable, i.e. type of treatment, but we have varying numbers of experimental conditions or levels of it.

So, it should be clear by now that hypotheses which predict a relationship between one independent variable and a dependent variable may be tested by comparing:

1. one experimental condition and one control condition
2. two experimental conditions
3. two experimental conditions and one control condition
4. three experimental conditions
5. three experimental conditions and one control condition
6. more than three experimental conditions etc.

Each of these designs requires a different statistical test to analyse the results, since unfortunately, there is no multi-purpose test for all experiments. Matching the design with the appropriate statistical test is something that we shall look at in Chapter 9 .

## CORRELATIONAL DESIGNS

Not all research has to take the form of manipulating an independent variable to see what effect it has on the dependent variable. Sometimes a researcher is not interested in looking for differences between groups or conditions in this way, but instead is concerned to find out whether two variables are associated or related. (Look back to page 51 to refresh your memory on the distinctions between experimental and correlational designs.)

Let's suppose we are interested in finding out whether there is a relationship between students' grades on clinical assessments and performance in theory exams, since we have noticed that students who get high grades on one tend to get high grades on the other. Our hypothesis might be that: 'There is a relationship between performance on clinical assessments and performance in theory exams, high marks on one being associated with high marks on the other'. The two variables are clinical assessment and theory exam performance.

A major difference in the research design needed to test this hypothesis is that the experimenter does *not* manipulate one of the variables, but simply takes a whole range of measures on one of the variables and assesses whether they show a pattern or relationship of some sort with the measurements on the other variable.

The correlational designs and analyses which will be covered in this book are only concerned with ordinal and interval/ratio data, since these levels of measurements provide a range or dimension for our data. It is possible to do a correlation with just nominal data, but such analyses are not always very informative and so they have been omitted from this text.

In our example, then, we might take a group of physiotherapy students and collect their clinical assessments and their theory exam marks to see if the two sets of scores are linked, e.g. high marks on one variable being associated with high marks on the other. Because the experimenter does not manipulate one variable, the concepts of independent and dependent variable are not appropriate in correlational designs.

Furthermore, because there is no manipulation of one variable and hence no measurement of the effect this has on the other variable, we cannot say, in a correlational design, which variable is cause and which effect. So returning to our example, we don't know whether clinical performance affects theory exam performance or vice versa. For instance, it may be that students who are good at clinical practice use their experience to answer their theory paper. Or it is possible that students who do well in theory use their knowledge in the clinical context. Alternatively, clinical performance and theory exam performance may both be related to a third variable. For example, good marks on both may be due to an 'easy' marker. Therefore, from any results we got from this study we do not actually know if:

> practice affects theory
>
> or
>
> theory affects practice
>
> or

another variable affects both theory and practice.

You can see from this that because we cannot ascertain which variable is having an effect on the other, there cannot be an independent or dependent variable or an identifiable cause and effect. Even in correlational studies where we feel we could make an educated guess as to which

variable is cause and which effect, we still cannot draw causal conclusions. For instance, a parent might observe that their child's eczema got worse when the child's behaviour got worse. However, while there might indeed be a pattern in the data such that the severity of the child's eczema and naughtiness seemed to go together, it could not be ascertained from this study whether:

> the eczema caused the bad behaviour
>
> or
>
> the bad behaviour caused the eczema
>
> or

both were caused by a third, unknown factor, such as problems at school.

Because of this inability to state categorically which variable is cause and which is effect in a correlational design, many researchers prefer the certainty of experimental designs. However, because the experimenter is not involved in manipulating anything (such as types of treatment), the correlational design is often thought to be more acceptable ethically.

As causal conclusions are often wrongly drawn from correlational studies this point will be explored again at the end of the next section.

---

**KEY CONCEPTS**

- Experimental designs covered in this book have two variables in the hypothesis, one independent and one dependent. The independent variable is manipulated by the experimenter, and the difference or effect this has on the dependent variable is measured. Thus in experimental designs we can ascertain cause and effect.
- Correlational designs also have two variables in the hypothesis but neither is manipulated. Therefore, there is no independent and no dependent variable. As a result it cannot be ascertained which variable is having an effect on the other. All that can be established is whether or not the scores on the two variables are linked in some way.

---

*Correlations between more than two sets of data; reliability measures*

Note that correlational designs are not confined to seeing how far just two sets of data are related; they can also be used to look at the degree of similarity between three or more sets of data.

Let's imagine you want to observe a child with

cerebral palsy on a number of activities, such as mobility, coordination, control, etc. If you observe the child just once, how will you know whether what you see is typical of what the child can do? Would it not be better to observe the child on a number of occasions in order to see whether there is a significant similarity in observed ability? This would mean that you need to assess the child on all the aspects of behaviour in which you're interested on several occasions. If you then analysed your data according to the principles of a correlational design, you would find out whether the observations were similar or not and from this you could get some reliable assessments of the child's capacities. This sort of 'self-checking' is useful in physiotherapy and is called an **intra-observer reliability measure.**

Let us take this idea a step further. Suppose you have been working with this child for several months and have grown very fond of her. This affection could bias your observations of her capabilities. Would it be useful, therefore, to have a number of independent physiotherapists (say five) observing the child, according to your checklist of activities, to see if they were in agreement? If you then analysed their scores using a test for correlational designs, and found that the ratings given by the independent physiotherapists were significantly similar, you would have a better and more reliable basis for making your statements about the child's capabilities. This form of 'other-checking' is called **inter-observer reliability,** and again is a valuable tool for physiotherapists.

## The correlation coefficient

It should be noted here that the degree to which each variable is associated in a correlational design is determined using an appropriate statistical test. We will deal with these tests in more detail in Chapter 9 but it is important to look at the underlying concepts here. To do this, let's return to our hypothesis and imagine that we have collected the students' clinical and theory exam marks; the next step is to find out whether there is a significant relationship between them, so we use the correct statistical test (see Ch. 9). When we have finished the calculations involved

in this test, we will end up with a number somewhere on a range from −1.0 through 0 to +1.0.

This figure is known as a **correlation coefficient.** The size of the correlation coefficient indicates the closeness of the relationship between the two variables. The closer the figure is to −1 or +1, the stronger the relationship, while the closer it is to 0 the weaker the relationship. This concept is illustrated by the continuum in Figure 6.1.

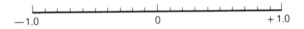

**Figure 6.1** The value of the correlation coefficient lies somewhere on a range from −1 to +1.

## The scattergram

Let's explore this idea a bit further, using the hypothesis about the link between clinical assessments and theory exam marks. Supposing you had collected the clinical assessments and theory exam marks from 30 students (so you would have two scores for each student) you could plot their scores on a graph, known as a **scattergram** (Fig. 6.2) to see if there is any association between the marks.

In order to do this, you need to take a student's pair of scores (say, for the dot ringed in Figure 6.2, 58% on the theory exam and 66% on the

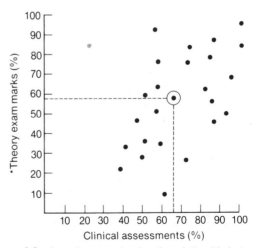

**Figure 6.2** A scattergram showing the relationship between theory exam marks and clinical assessments.

clinical assessment) and to move along each relevant axis until you had located their score. You make a mark at the intersection point. This is repeated for each pair of scores.*

**Activity 6.6** (Answers on page 230)

As practice, plot the scores in Table 6.2. as a scattergram. The hypothesis is that there is a relationship between the number of cigarettes smoked daily and the rate of recovery following cardiothoracic surgery.

**Table 6.2** Number of cigarettes smoked daily and number of postoperative days to discharge

| Subject | No. of cigarettes | No. of postoperative days to discharge |
| --- | --- | --- |
| 1 | 20 | 15 |
| 2 | 15 | 12 |
| 3 | 17 | 12 |
| 4 | 0 | 7 |
| 5 | 5 | 7 |
| 6 | 0 | 8 |
| 7 | 10 | 9 |
| 8 | 7 | 8 |
| 9 | 40 | 17 |
| 10 | 0 | 7 |

*In plotting a correlational graph, it does not matter which variable is plotted against the vertical axis and which against the horizontal one. However, should you ever wish to plot the data from an experimental design it is a convention that the independent variable scores are plotted along the horizontal axis and those from the dependent variable along the vertical axis.

## Positive correlation

When you have plotted a scattergram you can see whether there appears to be a relationship between the two variables by the nature of the pattern of dots. If the dots show a general upward or downward slope, it is likely that there is a relationship between the two variables. So in the example about theory and practice marks, it seems that there is a relationship, because the pattern of dots in Figure 6.2 shows a general upward slope. This is known as **positive correlation.**

A positive correlation means that high scores on one variable are associated with high scores on the other and hence low scores on one variable are linked with low scores on the other. For example, there is a positive correlation between weight and hypertension, such that the

higher the weight the higher the hypertension. So a scattergram pattern which shows a general upward slope like the one in Figure 6.3 indicates a positive correlation.

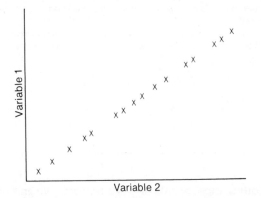

**Figure 6.3** The upward slope in this scattergram indicates a positive correlation between variable 1 and variable 2.

It should be noted that the perfectly smooth upward slope in the graph in Figure 6.3 shows a perfect positive correlation (i.e. there is a one-to-one relationship between high scores on one variable and high scores on the other). However, perfect correlations are extremely rare, if they exist at all. But, the smoother and straighter the upward slope, the stronger the positive correlation between the two variables. A positive correlation would be represented on our continuum somewhere around the +1.0 end, as in Figure 6.4.

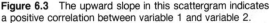

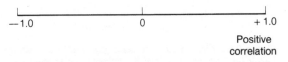

**Figure 6.4** The correlation coefficient has a value towards the +1 end for a positive correlation.

## Negative correlation

The correlation coefficient just mentioned would have been derived from a statistical analysis and the nearer to +1, the stronger the relationship. This, however, is not the only sort of correlation that can occur. Sometimes it is possible that *high* scores on one variable are associated with *low* scores on the other. For example we might hypothesise a relationship between body weight of an arthritic patient and distance that can be walked, such that the greater the body weight the shorter the distance. Our data may look like Table 6.3.

**Table 6.3** Body weight and distance walked in arthritic patients

| Patient | Weight (kg) | Distance (metres) |
|---------|-------------|-------------------|
| 1 | 74 | 12 |
| 2 | 59 | 20 |
| 3 | 64 | 15 |
| 4 | 67 | 15 |
| 5 | 72 | 10 |
| 6 | 80 | 5 |

Plotting these results on a scattergram, we end up with the pattern in Figure 6.5. There is a general downward slope in the pattern of dots.

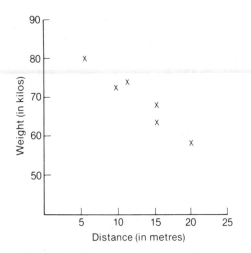

**Figure 6.5** This scattergram has a downward slope, as the higher the body weight in arthritic patients, the shorter the distance that can be walked.

When this sort of pattern emerges, it suggests that high scores on one variable are associated with low scores on the other. This is known as a **negative correlation** and would be represented on our correlation coefficient continuum near the − 1 end; the closer to − 1, the stronger the negative correlation (Fig. 6.6). On a scattergram, a negative correlation is indicated by the pattern shown in Figure 6.7. (Again this shows a perfect

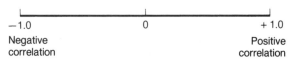

**Figure 6.6** A correlation coefficient value near to −1 indicates a strong negative correlation.

negative correlation, which is very unlikely ever to occur.)

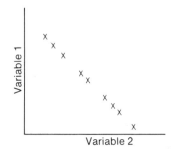

**Figure 6.7** A scattergram pattern indicating a negative correlation.

It is very important to note that a negative correlation does *not* mean *no* correlation. This is a point that confuses some students. A negative correlation indicates a relationship between high scores on one variable and low scores on the other, while no correlation means that there is no relationship at all between the two variables. The following example demonstrates this:

*Hypothesis*   There is a relationship between the age of driver and the number of road traffic accidents.

The data obtained are shown in Table 6.4.

**Table 6.4** Age of driver and number of road traffic accidents

| Subject | Age | No. of road traffic accidents |
|---------|-----|-------------------------------|
| 1 | 19 | 1 |
| 2 | 30 | 2 |
| 3 | 57 | 0 |
| 4 | 41 | 5 |
| 5 | 25 | 4 |
| 6 | 32 | 1 |

Plotting these on a scattergram we get the picture shown in Figure 6.8. This shows a fairly random scattering of dots, suggesting there is no

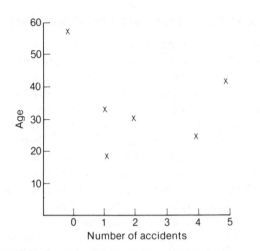

**Figure 6.8** This scattergram pattern suggests there is no link between the two variables.

link between the variables of age and the number of road traffic accidents.

In this case the correlation coefficient score from our statistical analysis would be around 0 (Fig. 6.9).

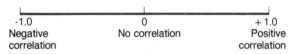

**Figure 6.9** A correlation coefficient value around 0 indicates little or no relationship between the two variables.

---

**KEY CONCEPTS**

- **Positive correlations** indicate that high scores on one variable are associated with high scores on the other.
  - They are represented by an upward slope on a scattergram.
  - They have a correlation coefficient near +1; the closer the coefficient to +1, the stronger the positive correlation.
- **Negative correlations** indicate that high scores on one variable are associated with low scores on the other.
  - They are represented by a downward slope on a scattergram.
  - They have a correlation coefficient of around -1; the nearer the coefficient to -1, the stronger the negative correlation.
- **No correlation** indicates that there is no relationship between the scores on the two variables.
  - They are represented by random clusterings on a scattergram with no obvious direction to the pattern.
  - They have a correlation coefficient of around 0, with the closer the coefficient to 0, the weaker the relationship between the two variables.

---

**Activity 6.7** (Answers on page 230)

1 Look at the following hypotheses and state whether they suggest positive or negative correlations between the variables. Also state how they would be represented on a scattergram, and where on a scale of -1 to +1 the correlation coefficient would be.
  (i) The older the patient, the longer the recovery time following lower leg amputation.
  (ii) The further from an outpatients' physiotherapy department a patient lives, the less the likelihood of keeping an appointment.
  (iii) The lower the 'A'-level results of physiotherapy students, the lower the exam mark in the final year.
  (iv) The higher the intake of dietary fibre, the lower the incidence of diverticulitis.
2 Look at the following correlation coefficients and rank them from the strongest relationship to the weakest:
  -0.73  -0.42  +0.61  +0.21  -0.17  +0.09

## A word of warning

It should be reiterated that even if you do find a strong positive or negative correlation, you still cannot conclude that the variables are causally related. However, many people do make this error. For example, when the AIDS problem started to reach public awareness a few years ago, one politician asked whether the condition was caused by Greek yoghurt, since he had noted that the amount of yoghurt appearing in supermarkets had risen alongside the number of reported AIDS cases. Almost certainly, had the data been analysed using the appropriate test, a positive correlation would have been found, but there is clearly no way in which Greek yoghurt was causing the epidemic.

Similarly, over the past year, a Sunday newspaper has been making a deliberate play out of statistical correlations. For example, it reported that over the previous few years the number of divorces had risen. Furthermore, it was noted that there had been an increase in the lofts that were being insulated. The paper concluded, tongue-in-cheek, that insulating lofts causes divorce. I'm sure you can see from this that just because data is correlated, does not mean that it is also causally related.

## Making predictions

However, if you do find that two variables are correlated together, you can make predictions about one variable from information about the other. Therefore, if you found that two variables were negatively correlated, you could predict high scores on one variable from knowledge of low scores on the other and vice versa. Equally, if you found that two variables were positively correlated, you could predict high scores on one variable from a knowledge of high scores on the other or low scores could be predicted for one variable from a knowledge of low scores on the other.

For example, you might have established that there is a negative correlation between the amount of pelvic floor exercise a woman does and the frequency of urinary incontinence. If a woman then presents with a specified incidence of leakage, then you would be able to predict from this knowledge how much pelvic floor exercise she was doing. This technique is known as **linear regression** and will be dealt with in more detail in Chapter 17.

## How close must the correlation be?

We have already said that the nature of the scattergram and the correlation coefficient indicate the strength of the relationship between the two variables and that there is unlikely to be a perfect correlation. Therefore how smooth must the scattergram slope be and how close must the correlation coefficient be to +1 or −1, before we decide that there is a relationship? Will + 0.63 do? or − 0.54? Because we cannot make an arbitrary decision like this, after we have calculated the correlation coefficient using a statistical test, we use a set of statistical tables to see whether the correlation coefficient is sufficiently big to indicate that the relationship between the two variables is significant. This will also depend on how many subjects you have used in your project. We will deal with these concepts in more detail in Chapter 17.

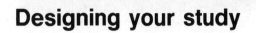

# 7

# Designing your study

## SOME BASIC CONCEPTS

### Definition of subjects

When you carry out any research you will almost certainly recruit people (perhaps patients or colleagues) to take part in it. The people who take part in research are called **subjects**, sometimes referred to as **Ss**. You will always have to decide what sort of subjects you need in your research, for instance, trainee physiotherapists, talipes patients or elderly amputees, and these participants must be defined carefully and clearly. It is insufficient, for example, just to state 'hemiplegic patients' since the term covers a range of causes of problem and types of person. So you must be clear as to the precise nature of your subjects.

### Generalisability

Whoever you decide to use, there is a very important point to note: you don't want your results to apply only to the small group or sample of people you used in your experiment, as you need to be able to generalise your results. This is a crucial feature of research and central to the topic of inferential statistics. For example, supposing you had compared the lung capacity of 20 cystic fibrosis patients treated by clapping with 20 patients treated by breathing exercises, and had found better results with the exercises group. It is important that these results do not just apply to the 20 subjects you used in your experiment, but that they are very likely to apply to other cystic fibrosis patients.

The point here is that if your results can be generalised in this way, then predictions can be made – and this is another essential feature of research. So , when you have to treat a new cystic fibrosis patient you can predict that breathing exercises are more likely to be effective than clapping on the basis of the generalisability of the results from your research, and consequently this knowledge confirms your choice of treatment.

But, short of carrying out your experiment on huge numbers of cystic fibrosis patients, how can you ascertain that your results are generalisable? We have already touched on this issue when the topic of inferential statistics was introduced; if you recall, inferential statistics allow the researcher to use a small sample of people in an experiment, and from the results of these experiments to infer that the same findings would apply to the larger population from which the sample comes. Now in order to be able to make this assumption, you must ensure that the sample you selected for study is sufficiently large and representative.

### Size of sample

The sample must be sufficiently large to ensure that it reflects the larger group or population from which it is derived. Let's consider the situation whereby the district physiotherapist is thinking about altering the number of hours in the day shift. If she asks one physiotherapist out of the 30 under her, then it is less likely that she will receive a view which reflects the opinion of the whole group (or **population**) than if she asks 15 of the 30. In other words the number of subjects you select for study must be sufficiently big for you to be able to generalise the results from your experiment.

What does this mean in practice? Although opinions on this vary, it is usually considered that 12 to 15 subjects per group or condition is the absolute minimum number required. Of course, if you're dealing, say, with von Recklinghausen's syndrome, it will be unlikely that you will get as many as 12, and you may want to consider a single-case study instead. There are also situations where more subjects are required. Where this is the case, it will be pointed out in the relevant chapter. Similarly, in some of the illus- trations quoted in later chapters, fewer than 12 subjects are used. This has been done simply for ease of calculation.

### A representative sample

The sample must be representative of the population from which they come and so, fairly typical.

The easiest way to ensure reasonable typicality is to select your subjects randomly, for instance, putting the names of all the cystic fibrosis patients you might have access to in a hat and randomly selecting 20. This point was covered in more detail in Chapter 3 and will be referred to again later in this chapter.

Before moving on though, it is important to recognise that you cannot always select your subjects randomly because there are insufficient numbers of particular patient types and you may just have to use everyone you find. If this is the case, then you must be aware of the limitations on generalising the results from such a study.

## TREATMENT OF YOUR SUBJECTS

A very important point should be noted concerning how you treat your subjects. You should *never* do anything to your subjects which would harm or upset them in any way. It is important that you treat your subjects well, that you do not deceive them or use your position to pressurise them to take part.

It is important that your subjects know what they are letting themselves in for before they agree to participate: in other words they give their informed consent. In all events, your research project should be referred to the ethical committee for consideration before you begin.

Failure to observe these guidelines would undoubtedly tarnish a researcher's reputation and could damage the participants physically or psychologically.

## TYPES OF EXPERIMENTAL DESIGN

Whatever sort of subjects are involved in your study, you will need to decide how to use them in the research design and this decision is a crucial one.

For example, if you look back to the hypothesis given on page 53, where it was predicted that physiotherapists who attended a psychology course would develop more tolerant attitudes than those who did not attend, you will see that to test this hypothesis it was suggested that two groups of physiotherapists were selected, one of which attended the course, and the other of which did not. In other words, two different groups of physiotherapists were used, one in the control condition and one in the experimental condition. However, not all hypotheses are best tested by comparing different groups of subjects in this way; sometimes it is more appropriate to use just one group of subjects and to measure them on two or more occasions.

When two or more different groups of subjects are used and compared in a project, it is called an **unrelated-, between-** or **different-subject design**. When just one group of subjects is used in all conditions it is called a **related, within-** or **same-subject design**. We will look at each of these more closely.

## DIFFERENT- (UNRELATED- OR BETWEEN-) SUBJECT DESIGNS

It was said earlier that hypotheses could often be tested in different ways, using different types of experimental designs, and that it was the job of the experimenter to decide on the most suitable design for a particular hypothesis. However, for some hypotheses there is really only one obvious way to test them. If you look again at the hypothesis about physiotherapists' attendance on a psychology course, two different groups of physiotherapists were used, one as a control condition and one as an experimental condition. The design looked like Figure 7.1.

Group of physiotherapists — Condition 1 (Experimental Condition) Attendance on course
Group of physiotherapists — Condition 2 (Control Condition) No attendance on course
} Groups compared for differences in attitude

**Figure 7.1**  A different-subject design.

At the end of the experiment the attitude change of the two groups would be compared to see if, in fact, the group who had attended the course became more tolerant.

This is a typical example of the sort of hypothesis which requires a different-subject design since it would have been totally inappropriate to use just one group for both conditions. If we think about this idea a bit more closely, it becomes clear that if we had selected just one group of physiotherapists, to be both the control (no course) condition and the experimental (attendance on course) condition, all sorts of problems would have emerged.

Let's explore this a bit further. There are two possible ways of carrying out this experiment, using just one group of subjects. You could either send your group of physiotherapists

a. on a course for 3 months (experimental condition)
   followed by
   'no course' for 3 months (control condition)

or

b. on 'no course' for 3 months (control condition)
   followed by a course for 3 months (experimental condition).

You can see from this that although there are control and experimental conditions in each design, the results from the second condition would always be contaminated by the results from the first because the group had done both conditions.

For example, in the first design, if we did find that there was a significant attitude change after going on a course for 3 months and that there was no further change after the 'no course' condition what could we really conclude about the control condition? It may be that the control condition had no effect because the group's attitudes had changed as far as they could by the end of the course, or because the control condition was a time for consolidating the attitude change already experienced. Alternatively, if we found that there was a change during the control condition this may be due to the continued effect of the course, or the effects of 3 months' more time and experience; but we wouldn't know which.

In the second design, any change in attitude found after doing the course might simply be due to the combined effects of the control and experimental conditions, or the passage of time on the experience, opinions and attitudes of these subjects and not to the course.

In other words, whatever the order these designs adopt, any results obtained would have more than one explanation because we have contaminated the outcome by subjecting the subjects to both conditions. This is known as an **order effect** and will be discussed in more detail in the next chapter.

Therefore, an hypothesis like this one requires a different-subject design in order to eliminate the confounding effects of participating in both conditions. It is important to note here that in this context, 'different' simply means 'separate'. In other words, in the previous example, while all the subjects were physiotherapists and were therefore similar to each other, they were split into two separate or different groups.

There are many other hypotheses in physiotherapy research which necessitate using two or more different groups of subjects. For example, any comparisons of different races, ages, sexes, type of patient, etc. all mean that different subjects have to be used. For example, if you wanted to compare muscle tone of Asian and African Caribbean children, you would have to use one group of Asians and another group of African Caribbeans. One subject group is quite obviously inappropriate here, since it is impossible for someone to be of both discrete racial origins.

In other words, if the manipulation of the independent variable simply involves the comparison of two or more inherently different groups of subjects (old vs. young, male vs. female, cardiothoracic vs. carcinoma patients, etc.) you must use a different-subject design.

Remember that you don't need to confine yourself to the comparison of just two different or separate groups. It is perfectly acceptable to compare three or more groups, although the type of analysis will be different.

While it is sometimes essential to use different groups of subjects in your experiment, there is a major disadvantage in the design: that of individual differences among the subjects. If we look at the example regarding differences in muscle tone between Asian and African Caribbean children, it is quite possible that some children would not really understand what they have to do in the experiment; others may just have had 'flu' and so be feeling weaker anyway; others may be really motivated to please the experimenter, yet others may be frightened. All these factors may influence how a subject performs in an experiment and so will affect the results. For example, the child who is frightened of the experimenter and the situation may have increased muscle tone due to fear. Therefore, his performance score may be high for reasons other than inherent muscle tone. While these individual differences may be evenly distributed among all the groups, thereby cancelling the effects out, it is also possible that more of the individual differences that affect the results may occur in only one of the groups and thus will artificially distort the results.

The problem of individual differences can be partly overcome by ensuring that the subjects are randomly selected and used. Randomisation can mean one of two things in different subject designs. Firstly, it can mean selecting a group of subjects (e.g. hip replacement patients) and randomly allocating half of them to one treatment and half to the other, in order to compare the effects.

Obviously, this cannot be done in our example about muscle tone, since it would not be possible to select a group of children and randomly allocate them to being Asian or African Caribbean. Here randomness means something different: that the subjects in each group should be a random, and therefore typical, selection of the group they represent. In other words, the children in the Asian group should be reasonably typical of Asian children as a whole, and not all particularly weak, strong, fit, athletic, motivated, awkward or anything else. The same should be true of the children in the African Caribbean group. The ways in which random selection can be achieved are outlined in Chapter 3.

## SAME- (RELATED- OR WITHIN-) SUBJECT DESIGNS

Some hypotheses, however, are not suited to using designs with different subjects in each condition. Some hypotheses are more suited to being tested by designs which use only one group of subjects, but this group is measured under all the conditions and its performance in each condition is compared.

For example, you might be interested in looking at the level of confidence a group of elderly patients had in uniformed vs. non-uniformed community physiotherapists. Here you would randomly select a group of patients and ask them to indicate how confident they felt (a) when being treated by a uniformed physiotherapist, and (b) when being treated by a non-uniformed physiotherapist. The design would look like Figure 7.2.

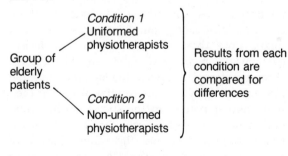

**Figure 7.2** A same-subject design.

Thus, one group of subjects is tested under both conditions and the two sets of ratings are compared to see if there is any difference between them.

It would be inappropriate here to use two groups of patients, one to rate the uniformed physiotherapists and the other to rate the non-uniformed, because the groups may differ inherently in a number of ways which would affect the outcome of the results. For example, one group may be generally more confident anyway, may love all uniforms, or may try harder to please the experimenter by inflating their ratings, etc., and we wouldn't know this because we have nothing against which to measure their ratings. Hence, there may be basic individual differences between the two groups which might affect the results and which would prevent us from establishing any baseline for comparison.

However, if we use just one group of patients then whatever their idiosyncrasies and personal characteristics, they will at least be constant over both ratings. Therefore, one important advantage of a same-subject design is the fact that it overcomes the problem of individual differences inherent in different-subject designs. Because of this, it is especially useful in 'before and after' type experiments, where the researcher wants to look at the effects of a treatment procedure on a group of subjects. A common example of this are the television advertisements for washing powder, showing viewers the dirty washing before being washed in the product and the same linen after being washed. The same clothes are used when the before and after assessments are made, and thus constitutes a same-subject design.

However, this design too has its snags. If we look at the example concerning physiotherapists' dress, supposing we gave all the subjects the uniformed rating-task first, and the non–uniformed rating-task second. It is quite conceivable that on the first task they didn't quite understand what was required of them and so filled in the questionnaire using the wrong criteria, while by the second task they had realised what they had to do. This may well distort the results. Alternatively, it could be argued that by the time the second task had to be completed, the subjects were bored or tired and so filled in lower confidence ratings. In other words, the results may have been affected by the order in which the tasks were carried out. Therefore to overcome this, half the subjects should do task A first, followed by task B, while for the remaining subjects, the order would be reversed. This is called **counterbalancing** and is discussed more fully in Chapter 8.

It should also be noted that one group of subjects can be tested on more than two occasions. For example, you might wish to look at the pain levels experienced by a group of women in the first stage of labour using TENS (transcutaneous electrical nerve stimulation). To do this, you decide to select one group of say, 20 women and you assess their pain levels before using TENS; 1 hour after using TENS; 2 hours after using TENS, and 3 hours after using TENS. Your design would look like Figure 7.3.

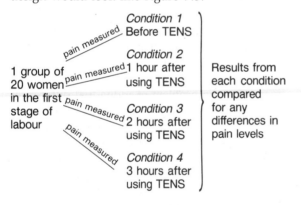

**Figure 7.3** A same-subject design, with the subjects being measured under four conditions.

You have here a same-subject design, with the subjects being measured under four conditions, to establish whether the use of TENS makes any difference to their pain levels.

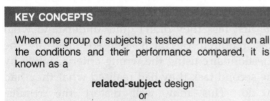

**KEY CONCEPTS**

When one group of subjects is tested or measured on all the conditions and their performance compared, it is known as a

**related-subject** design
or
**same-subject** design
or
**within-subject** design.

The advantage of this design is that it eliminates the distorting effects of individual subject differences.

However, it has two disadvantages: firstly, it cannot be used when 'fixed' differences such as sex, race, type of ailment are being compared, and secondly, any effects deriving from the order of the conditions may have to be counterbalanced.

## MATCHED-SUBJECT DESIGNS

One way of overcoming all the disadvantages of both different- and same-subject designs is to use two or more groups of subjects who are matched on a number of characteristics. Let's take an example. Suppose you wanted to compare the recovery times of leg fractures resulting from road traffic accidents (RTAs) and leg fractures resulting from sports injuries. Obviously you cannot use a same-subject design, since a patient's fracture cannot simultaneously be due to an RTA and sports injury, and if you use a different-subject design, you might find a number of individual differences in the subjects which predisposed one group to recover more quickly than the other. For example, the sports injuries patients may be younger, male, fitter and stronger, whereas the RTA patients may be less fit, older, diabetic and include females. In addition, the amount and type of treatment may be different for each group. All these factors may influence recovery rates. In such cases, then, it is necessary to try to identify the characteristics which may bias the results of the experiment and to ensure that the groups are matched on these factors.

The way in which the matching is carried out involves firstly, identifying all the possible characteristics which may influence the results, and then selecting a subject (for example, an RTA patient) and assessing how s/he rates on these characteristics. For example, in this case, you might note their age, sex, degree of fitness (perhaps by heart rate, pulse rate, blood pressure), previous fractures to the leg (and anything else you feel may bias the results). You must then find another patient in the sports injuries category who is the same age, sex, has the same fitness ratings, has had the same number of previous fractures to the leg and has other characteristics similar to the RTA patient. You then need to find the next set of 'twins' and so on. These patients do not need to be identical to the first pair selected, but they must be the same as each other. Therefore, in terms of the personal characteristics which are likely to influence the results from the experiment, each pair of subjects is like identical twins, with the only difference between them being the way in which the fracture occurred. Thus, for every subject in one group, there is an 'identical twin' in the other. However, the matching shouldn't stop there. You would also need to ensure that the quality, type and extent of treatment were also the same for each patient, together with any other factors which were likely to influence the study's outcomes.

When you are involved in comparing 'non-fixed' groups, e.g. the effects of the different treatments, you can match up a pair of subjects first and then randomly allocate one subject to one treatment and the 'twin' to the other treatment. Because of the similarity of the subjects, matched designs are treated like same-subject designs for the purposes of statistical analysis. Similarly, as with same-subject designs, the matched design overcomes the problem of individual differences, because of the 'twinning' of the subjects. Yet the matched-design has all the advantages of a different-subject design, since 'fixed' groups can be compared and there need be no order effects.

So why don't we always use matched designs if they're so good? I'm sure you will have realised already that it is often extremely difficult to match pairs of subjects in this way, usually because there are limited numbers of suitable subjects to choose from. Even if we allow ourselves a little leeway, say by matching an RTA patient aged 30 with a sports injury patient aged 28, there may still be many important differences between the subject pair that we either cannot identify or cannot match for, e.g. biochemical composition

of bones and blood that affect healing rates. Thus, while these designs are theoretically very desirable, in practical terms they are extremely difficult to implement properly.

It must be stressed that it is not adequate simply to select 20 RTAs and 20 sports injury patients, all of whom are male and under 40 and say that you've matched them. For every subject in one group, there must be a 'twinned' subject in the other, matched on all the relevant variables which may influence the outcome of the experiment. Therefore, because of the difficulties involved in matching people, caused largely through our lack of knowledge of which factors are relevant, it is usually desirable to use a same-subject design in preference to a matched-subject design. As one statistician says:

> A matching design is only as good as the Experimenter's ability to determine how to match the pairs, and this ability is frequently very limited.
>
> Sidney Siegel (1956)

While matched-subject designs can be used with more than two groups of subjects, because of the problems outlined above, it is very unlikely that you will ever be able to match subjects up in 'triplets' or 'quadruplets' , and so this may be better avoided.

---

**KEY CONCEPTS**

**Matched designs** involve selecting pairs of subjects, matched on every variable which may influence the outcome of the experiment, and allocating one of the pair to one condition and one to the other.

This design has all the advantages of same- and different-subject designs.

It has the major disadvantage that it is very difficult to match subjects in this way, because firstly it is not always possible to find subjects who are sufficiently similar, and secondly, you can never be sure that you have matched pairs of subjects on all the factors that may influence the results.

# 8

# Sources of error in research

There are a number of potential sources of bias or error which can creep into the design of an experiment. These may distort your results and therefore must be controlled for. We will look at each of these separately.

## ORDER EFFECTS

When a piece of research is carried out which follows an experimental design, the experimenter manipulates the independent variable and measures the effect of this on the dependent variable, in the hope that altering the IV will have a significant effect on the DV. Changes in the DV are called the experimental effect and constitute the data in your study.

Let's take an example. Suppose you had hypothesised that students perform worse on a neurological placement than on an orthopaedic placement during their second year of training; in other words you are predicting a relationship between type of placement (IV) and performance (DV). To test this, you set up the experiment shown in Figure 8.1.

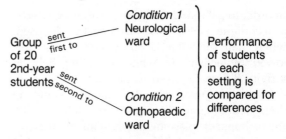

**Figure 8.1**  A same-subject design, with one group of subjects being measured on two occasions.

This is a same-subject design, with one group of students being measured on two occasions and their performances in both placements compared (using the appropriate statistical test) to see if they differ.

Let us assume that you did in fact find that students seem to do better on orthopaedic placements; can we conclude that the results are the effect of some inherent difficulty associated with neurological physiotherapy? Or might there be some other explanations?

One obvious alternative explanation that we've already touched on and you've probably thought of, relates to the sequence of the placements. If the students' first placement is on a neurological ward and their subsequent placement is on an orthopaedic ward, it is conceivable that their improved performance in the latter case may be due simply to the fact that it was second. In other words, the students may do better on any second placement (regardless of its nature) because they are more confident, more skilled, more familiar with hospital routines, etc.; they are more *practised*. Hence, this is known as a **practice effect**. It is, of course, equally likely that students do worse on their second placement because they are more jaundiced, more tired, less motivated etc. This is known as a **fatigue effect**.

Regardless of which way performance is affected, the general issue is the same: that order effects, rather than the nature of the placement itself, could be influencing students' performance. Order effects are a common problem in experiments where one group of subjects is compared on two or more conditions, i.e. same-subject designs.

### Counterbalancing

In order to get round the problem of order effects, a technique called **counterbalancing** is used, where half the subjects do activity A first, followed by activity B, while the other half do activity B first, followed by activity A.

In our example, then, 10 students would do their neurological placement first, followed by the orthopaedic placement, while for the remaining 10 the order would be reversed. At the end of the study, all the neurological ratings would be compared with all the orthopaedic ratings. You can select which students do which placement first by a number of methods: the first 10 students alphabetically, the first 10 names pulled out of a hat, alternate names alphabetically. While it doesn't really matter which method you use, do try to ensure that the students are randomly allocated. Don't put all your worst students into neurology first just to prove your point! The section on random selection (page 23) may clarify this point further.

So, by counterbalancing in this way, any bias in the results due to order effects is balanced out. One point is important here: we cannot eliminate order effects totally, because one activity must precede the other in designs like this. All we can do is to balance out the order effects as far as possible.

---

**KEY CONCEPTS**

If one group of subjects has to be measured in all the conditions then the order in which they do these conditions may influence the results. For example, they may perform better on the last activity because of **practice effects**, or they may perform worse on the last activity because of **fatigue effects.**

In order to eliminate these sources of bias, the order in which the subjects carry out the activities should be counterbalanced, such that half the subjects do activity A first, followed by B, while for the remainder, the order is reversed.

---

So, one explanation for the results from the experiment described above is the possible influence of order effects. However, even if you had counterbalanced these, there are still other variables which could account for your results.

## EXPERIMENTER BIAS EFFECTS

Suppose, like all experimenters, you are very committed to your research and are very keen that your hypothesis will be supported, in this case, that students will do worse on neurological wards. It is conceivable that in your anxiety and enthusiasm to obtain the predicted outcome, you will unwittingly influence the results.

I don't mean by this that you will cook the books, but that unawares, you may use a slightly different set of criteria when assessing the students on each placement, perhaps ignoring some negative things on the orthopaedic placement, or putting more emphasis on other factors while carrying out the evaluation. In other words, you may have a set of expectations about the outcome of the experiment which will influence what you perceive, how you behave, etc.

Alternatively, you may unconsciously influence your subjects' responses by using a set of non-verbal cues. Imagine in the present example, you had decided, as an additional outcome measure, to elicit the students' subjective evaluations of their placements. You interview the first student on the neurological placement and s/he starts to say how awful it was, how incompetent and deskilled they felt, etc. This is exactly what you want to hear because it supports your hypothesis! And when we hear something we like we automatically respond with a set of non-verbal cues which the other person quickly picks up; for instance, we might smile, nod our head, lean forward into the conversation and this encourages the other person to go on saying similar things. When we hear something we don't like, we might frown or lean out of the discussion and this has the effect of discouraging further comments of that type.

In addition, the subjects may take a dislike to the experimenter and so deliberately say things they know will not support the hypothesis; or they may like the experimenter and distort their responses to help him/her.

In all cases, there is the potential for bias, particularly where the data involves subjective report. Such influences are very common and are known as **experimenter bias effects**. Other sources of experimenter bias include the personal characteristics of the experimenter, such as status, sex, class, race, age and so on, all of which may have some effect on the subjects and their performance.

It should be emphasised that normally such experimenter influences are quite unintentional and unconscious, but there is a great deal of documented evidence to show that they exist. How can we get round this problem?

### 'Blind' procedures

The usual solution is to operate a **'blind' procedure**, whereby you ask someone who does not know what your hypothesis is to collect your data; in this case, to assess the students. Because they are not aware of what you have predicted, they will also not know how the students are meant to behave in each placement and so their evaluation of the students' performance should be much more objective.

Blind procedures may be of two sorts: **single-blind** procedures where either the subject *or* the person collecting the data is unaware of the hypothesis being tested, or alternatively, **double-blind** procedures where *neither* party knows what the aims of the study are. This sort of double-blind procedure is very common in medical research, particularly when carrying out drug trials. In these cases, one group of patients is given the drug, while another group is given a placebo. Neither the doctors assessing the outcome nor the patients themselves know who has been given which. In this way, the results cannot be biased by expectations, or deliberate or unintentional manipulation.

---

**KEY CONCEPTS**

Sometimes experimenters unwittingly influence the outcome of their experiment by the way in which they behave, appear or interact with the subjects. This is known as **experimenter bias**. Subjects sometimes distort their responses too.

To overcome this sort of problem in your research, you should use a **blind** procedure, whereby you ask someone who is absolutely unaware of what your hypothesis is to collect your data from subjects who may also be unaware of your hypothesis. In this way, any bias due to expectations and predictions will be eliminated.

---

However, there are still other variables which may influence our results, besides the manipulation of the IV even if we control for order and experimenter bias effects. These are called **constant errors** and **random errors**. Let's look at constant errors first.

## CONSTANT ERRORS

Constant errors are all the possible sources of bias and influence that will affect the results in a constant and predictable way.

If we go back to our example of comparing students' performance in two placements, we can identify a number of potential sources of constant error. Suppose the neurological ward had 50 patients, two qualified physiotherapists and 10 students, while the orthopaedic ward had 25 patients, five qualified staff and 10 students. Under such conditions, it is quite possible that students do less well on the neurological ward because (a) of greater patient-to-staff ratios, which would increase workload, pressure, tension, etc., and (b) they have fewer qualified physiotherapists available to teach and support them. Therefore, their poor performance may be the direct result of these variables and not to do with problems inherent to neurological work. Also, the superintendent physiotherapist at the neurological hospital may dislike the disruption caused by students and so may provide less constructive tuition and guidance. The neurological placement may also involve a more arduous journey (students arrive feeling fatigued), or longer shifts or any one of a number of other problems.

Note that each of these factors can be called a constant error because of the predictable way in which they would distort the results. For example, poor patient/staff ratios are more likely to depress students' performance than improve it and so the effect of this variable is constant; less tuition will also depress, not improve, performance, as will fatigue. Thus, each of these factors will have a similar effect on all the students and so will distort the results in a constant, predictable way.

It is your job as a researcher to try to identify all the possible sources of constant error in your experiment and either eliminate or control them. If you leave any constant error uncontrolled then your results may be explained by that, rather than by the manipulation of the IV. Taking the constant errors quoted as examples here, we can eliminate or control them as shown in Table 8.1. In other words, you must standardise all aspects of the experimental situation in each placement.

Thus, when designing an experiment you must try to highlight all the factors which will bias your results in a constant and predictable way, and then attempt to eliminate or control these factors by standardising the situation and procedures in each condition.

**Table 8.1** Control or elimination of constant errors

| Constant error | Solution |
| --- | --- |
| Different patient/ staff ratios | Ensure both placements have comparable ratios |
| Different numbers of qualified staff to act as tutors | Ensure ratios of students/qualified staff are the same in each placement |
| Different amounts of supervision times | Ensure students in each placement receive same amounts of clinical instruction |
| Different journey lengths | Either select placements which are equidistant or arrange transport to neuro hospital such that travelling times and problems are similar |
| Different shift times/lengths | Ensure students in each placement work the same number of hours at similar times of day |

## RANDOM ERRORS

Random errors are not as easy to deal with. As their name suggests, they are random: randomly occurring, randomly distributed and with a random and unpredictable impact on the results. If we look back to our example, we identified some factors that would influence our results in a very predictable way, but there are other factors, the random errors, which will obscure our results in a totally variable or chance way.

In the above example, the moods of the patients, staff and students will all have an effect on performance. If all the neurological patients were always in a bad mood and all the orthopaedic patients always in a good mood then moods would influence the results in a predictable way and so would be classified as constant errors. But moods aren't like that: they fluctuate up and down and interact with other people's behaviour, mood and attitudes. As a result they cannot be eliminated or controlled. Transitory changes in health among the patients, staff and students, their personalities, attitudes, beliefs, motivations, etc. are all examples of random error factors which will obscure the results in an unpredictable, chance way and about which we can do very little.

The only real precaution that we can take against random errors is to ensure as far as possible that the people involved in our research are drawn randomly from the population they represent. Therefore, our students should be fairly typical of physiotherapy students as a whole and not particularly deviant, disturbed, problematic, good, able or anything else. The neurological patients should be fairly typical of neurology patients as a whole and not particularly unusual, ill, well, independent, dependent, irascible, helpful, etc., and similarly with the orthopaedic patients and staff. In this way the random errors should be fairly evenly distributed across both the placements, and therefore should (at least theoretically) affect the students' performance in each setting in a similar, if random, way.

One other point is important here: if your subjects can be randomly allocated to conditions (e.g. to different treatments, or in this case, allocating students to a particular order of placements) so much the better, because the random errors should then be evenly distributed at least theoretically.

---

**KEY CONCEPTS**

- **Constant errors** are those factors that distort the results in a constant or predictable way. They can be eliminated or controlled by ensuring the procedures, conditions and other essential factors are similar.
- **Random errors** are those factors which obscure the results in a random or unpredictable way. They cannot be eliminated, although random selection and allocation of subjects will distribute them evenly across conditions (at least theoretically).

---

**Activity 8.1**  (Answers on page 231)

Look at the following hypotheses and identify the sources of constant and random error and their solutions:

$H_1$: Men are more likely to suffer respiratory complications following cardiothoracic surgery than are women.

$H_1$: Outpatients' clinics achieve better recovery rates for leg fractures than specific sports injuries clinics.

## PROBABILITIES

If we cannot get rid of random errors, how can

we be sure that the results from our experiment are due to some real and significant relationship between the variables, as predicted in the hypothesis, and not to the obscuring effect of random errors? The answer to this lies in the use of statistical tests. At a general level, when we use a statistical test to analyse a set of results, we end up with a numerical value. This value is looked up in a set of probability tables, to give us a probability or *p* **value**, which is expressed either as a decimal (e.g. 0.01) or as a percentage (e.g. 1%). **The *p* value tells us how probable it is that the results from our experiment are due to random errors.** It is very important to understand and remember this, as it is the basis of all statistical analyses.

Because this *p* value tells us how likely it is that the results from the experiment are due to random error (and not to the real and consistent relationship predicted in your hypothesis) then the smaller the *p* value, the smaller the possibility that random error or chance factors can account for your results. Therefore, by implication, the smaller the possibility that your results are due to random error, then the greater the possibility that they are due to the relationship you predicted in your hypothesis. Thus, the smaller the *p* value, the greater the implied support for your experimental hypothesis.

Do bear in mind that it is highly unlikely that you will ever get 100% support for your hypothesis, and so *p* will always have a value greater than 0. If your *p* value is very low, then you can reject the null (no relationship) hypothesis, and conclude the experimental hypothesis has been supported. (Remember! When we carry out an experiment we do not set out to support our experimental hypothesis directly, but instead, we try to reject the null (no relationship) hypothesis.)

Probability values, as we noted earlier, can be expressed either as a percentage or as a decimal. Therefore, if our *p* value was 5% (or 0.05) then we could say that there is a 5% chance that the results are due to random error. A *p* value of 3% means that there is a 3/100 chance that your results are due to the effects of chance or random error factors. Put crudely, then, the smaller the *p* value you obtain for your results the less the probability that random error can explain your findings, and consequently, the better it is for your hypothesis.

---

**Activity 8.2** (Answers on page 231)

Look at the following p values and order them in terms of greatest implied support for your experimental hypothesis. (Greatest support on the left, to least support on the right.)

$p = 5\%$  $p = 19\%$  $p = 7\%$  $p = 0.01\%$  $p = 15\%$  $p = 3\%$

When you have done this, convert each p value to a decimal.

---

**KEY CONCEPTS**

When you carry out a statistical analysis, you end up with a numerical value which you look up in a set of probability tables to give you a **p value**. The p value tells you how likely it is that the results from your experiment are due to random error or chance. The smaller the p value, the stronger the support for your hypothesis. The p values are expressed as percentages or decimals.

---

**Activity 8.3** (Answers on page 231)

Suppose you saw the following p values in physiotherapy articles, what do they mean, in percentage terms, about the possibility of chance or random factors being responsible for the results?

The probability that the results are due to chance:

$$p = 0.01$$
$$p = 0.07$$
$$p = 0.03$$
$$p = 0.05$$
$$p = 0.50$$

---

## SIGNIFICANCE LEVELS

It was said earlier that if your p value was very small you could reject the null (no relationship) hypothesis and conclude that your experimental hypothesis had been supported by the results. When the null hypothesis is rejected in this way, the results are said to be **significant**. But how small must your p value be before you can conclude that your results are significant? There is no simple answer to this as it depends upon the nature of the experiment you've carried out.

For example, suppose you had hypothesised that a new form of treatment was much more effective for bronchitis patients' vital capacity than the standard breathing exercises. In order to carry out this research you randomly allocate 20 patients to the new treatment and 20 to the old treatment, and after a month you compare their vital capacities, using the appropriate statistical test. Let's assume your resulting p value is 5%, which means that there is a 5% probability that your results are due to random or chance factors. You would probably be quite happy to recommend the better treatment in future if the 5% random error didn't cause any serious problems for your patients. On the other hand, if your recommended treatment produced nasty side-effects, you would be very reluctant to use it if 1 in 20 patients derived no benefit at all. Under these circumstances, you would need to consider reducing the significance level to 1 in 100 (1%) or even 1 in 1000 (0.1%) before the treatment was used more widely. In other words, the effect of the random errors determines how small your p value must be before you can conclude your results are significant.

We could compare this to placing a bet on Grand National Day. Supposing you've looked at the horses, and you've decided to place a bet on a particular horse; you've unwittingly formulated an hypothesis that there is a relationship between this horse and final placing. If you're only going to put 10p on this horse, you won't mind a fairly large significance level (or p value) because losing 10p is not too disastrous. However, if you've placed all your life-savings and assets on this horse, then you want to be very sure that it's going to win. In other words, you will want to ensure a small chance that random error will influence the outcome before you bet, since if you are wrong, the effects will be devastating.

The p value you decide upon in an experiment is called the **level of significance**. It is so-called because when you look up the results of your statistical analysis in a set of probability tables, you will find the p value for your results. If this p value is equal to or smaller than the significance level you have selected as being appropriate for your research, then your results are said to be **significant**. This means that you can reject the null (no relationship) hypothesis and accept that your experimental hypothesis has been supported. If the p value is larger than the significance level you have selected, your results are classed as not significant, which means you cannot reject the null hypothesis.

Therefore, it is up to you, the experimenter, to state what significance level you think is appropriate for a particular piece of research and the significance level you finally select will reflect the nature of your experiment. All this seems to leave the field wide open for you. However, a good rule-of-thumb if you're not doing anything that may have a disastrous outcome if you're wrong, is to use a cut-off point or significance level of 5%. So if you obtain a $p$ value of 5% or less, then you can conclude that your results are significant and that your experimental hypothesis has been supported.

This point will be referred to again later.

## MAKING ERRORS IN YOUR CONCLUSIONS REGARDING SIGNIFICANCE

When you have analysed your results and looked these up in the probability tables, you will obtain a probability or $p$ value which is a statement of how likely it is that your results are due to random error. Usually, if this $p$ value is 5% or less, the results are said to be significant and therefore support your experimental hypothesis. On the basis of such a conclusion, you would be in a position to make predictions and recommendations based on your findings.

However, it is possible to draw the wrong conclusions from your study and these errors are known as **Type I** and **Type II** errors.

## Type I errors

These refer to those situations when we conclude our experimental hypothesis has been supported when, in fact, it hasn't. Such errors can be avoided by two safeguards:

1. Ensuring that the selected significance level is appropriate; in other words, do not use a significance level of more than 5% for most research, and reduce this to 1% in cases where any errors in your conclusions could be disastrous (see previous section).

2. Replication of the study and its findings by independent researchers adds credibility to the original conclusions.

## Type II errors

These refer to situations when the experimental hypothesis is rejected in favour of the null (no relationship) hypothesis, when the data do, in reality, support the experimental hypothesis.

The chance of making this mistake can be reduced by:
1. Increasing the size of the sample.
2. Using a less stringent significance level.

It is essential when selecting a significance level that all the implications of any errors deriving from decisions about the results are considered. If they are not, then patient wellbeing could be at risk.

## STATISTICAL AND CLINICAL SIGNIFICANCE OF RESEARCH FINDINGS

It should also be pointed out that results are sometimes statistically significant but yet have very little clinical meaning.

For example, you might conduct a study of the relative strength of the pelvic floor muscles post-partum, dependent on the type of exercise regime the women undertook. One group of women might exercise for 30 minutes per day and the other group for 60 minutes. Let us imagine at the end of the study that this latter group was found to have pelvic floor muscles which were significantly stronger statistically, but yet they still suffered a high level of stress incontinence. It could be said that these results were statistically significant but were clinically meaningless.

Therefore, while significance levels are essential guides to deciding whether or not your data support your hypothesis, it is important to remember that these results should be considered in conjunction with their physiotherapeutic implications.

## KEY CONCEPTS

The **p value** states the probability of your results being due to chance or random error. If the $p$ value is very small you can conclude that your results are significant. This means you can reject the null (no difference) hypothesis and conclude that your experimental hypothesis has been supported. The experimenter decides upon how small the error margin must be before the results are said to be significant.

The size of the error margin is called the **significance level**. The decision about the size of the significance level is based on the effects of the error. If the error is likely to be disastrous, then the significance level is reduced. If the effects are not likely to be terrible, then the significance level can be increased. A good rule-of-thumb is to use a 5% significance level as long as you are not doing anything dangerous.

# 9

# Matching the research design to the statistical test

## DECIDING WHICH STATISTICAL TEST TO USE

The previous chapters have all been concerned with how to design a piece of research to test an hypothesis. Once you have designed and carried out your research, you need to analyse your data to find out whether the results do, in fact, support your hypothesis. The analysis involves using statistical tests. Essentially, what this means is that you apply a particular formula to your data and then work through the formula to get the answer. This answer is then looked up in the probability tables to see whether it supports your hypothesis.

However, there is no single all-purpose test which you can use to analyse your results, since each experimental design has an appropriate statistical test. Therefore, one of your tasks as a researcher is to match up the appropriate statistical test with your research design. If you select the wrong test to analyse your data, then your conclusions will be vitiated – it's as critical as that. Unfortunately, many people become very worried about this matching task, but as long as you ask yourself some basic questions about your design, you shouldn't have too much trouble.

A word of warning first, though: when you are planning your research project, do ensure that you know which statistical test you will be using. All too often people carry out their experiment without doing this first and then find that they don't know how to analyse the results, or that they need a complicated computer programme which they can't get access to. So, make sure at the planning stage that you know which statistical test you will need for your design.

To decide on which statistical test to use with an experimental design, the following questions must be asked:

1. Is the design experimental or correlational?
2. How many conditions are there?
3. If the design is experimental, is it same–, matched– or different-subject? We will now look at these questions in more detail.

## Is the design experimental or correlational?

To answer this, it is usually easier to look back at your hypothesis and decide whether you were predicting differences in your results (for example, between patient groups, types of treatment, males and females) or whether you were predicting similarities or patterns between sets of data. If you were predicting differences, you will have used an experimental design, while if you were predicting similarities, you will have used a correlational design.

Since this is often a focus of confusion for some people, it may be useful to go over the concepts again.

If you look back to Chapter 2, you will see that in an experimental design, we manipulate one variable (the independent variable) and measure the effect of this on the other variable (the dependent variable). So, if you were hypothesising that clapping is more effective than breathing exercises for cystic fibrosis patients, your IV would be type of treatment and the DV would be effectiveness. Typically, you would design an experiment whereby you gave one group of patients breathing exercises and another group clapping (manipulation of the IV), and after a fixed period you would compare the progress of the two groups. (You measure the effect on the DV of manipulating the IV.) Here then, you would be looking for differences between the two groups in terms of the effectiveness of the two treatments.

On the other hand, in some hypotheses you may predict patterns or similarities between the two variables (look back to pages 56–62): these require a correlational design. In these hypotheses you are predicting either:

a. that as scores on one variable go up, so the scores on the other variable will also go up (positive correlation)

or

b. that as scores on one variable go up, so the scores on the other variable will go down (negative correlation).

For example, if you hypothesised that physiotherapy students who do well on theory exams also do well on their practical assessments, you would take a group of students and look at their performance in both situations, on the assumption that the higher the theory mark, the higher the corresponding practical mark. This is called a positive correlation.

Alternatively, you may predict a link between the amount of dietary fibre eaten daily and the incidence of diverticular disease, such that the higher the amount of fibre, the lower the corresponding incidence of diverticulitis. This is called a negative correlation.

In these correlational designs you do not manipulate one variable to see what effect it has on the other; instead you take a whole range of scores on one variable and see whether they are related to a whole range of scores on the other variable. If you are still unclear about the differences between experimental and correlational designs, re-read Chapter 6.

## How many conditions are there?

### Number of conditions and correlational designs

If you have a correlational design, you need to ask whether you are comparing two sets of results, or more than two sets. Once you have answered this, you need only ask yourself about the levels of measurement you have on each variable. This point is dealt with in Chapter 17, which covers analysis of data deriving from correlational designs.

*Number of conditions and experimental designs*

If you have an experimental design, however, you need to decide how many conditions you have (see pages 54–56) since designs with only two conditions in total require a different type of statistical test from those with more than two conditions. For example, if you compared two groups of patients, one of whom had received some treatment (experimental condition) and the other whom had received no treatment (control condition), then you would have two conditions. If you had compared two types of treatment (i.e. two experimental conditions) you would again have two conditions. On the other hand, if you had compared the effectiveness of three treatment procedures, you would have three conditions.

Look back to pages 54–56 to refresh your memory on this.

## If the design is experimental, is it same-, matched- or different-subject?

What type of experimental design was used? For example, did you use just one group of subjects for all conditions (e.g. comparing the attitudes of one group of physiotherapists to paraplegic vs. hemiplegic patients). Or did you use two or more totally different groups of subjects and compare them in some way (e.g. a comparison of attendance levels, at an outpatients' department, of Asian vs. African Caribbean patients?). Or did you use two or more groups of subjects who were matched on certain key features (e.g. a comparison of the quality of newly qualified physiotherapists from three different training schools, which would necessitate matching the subjects on such variables as 'A'-level grades, attendance levels, etc.). (See Ch. 7.)

Remember, for the purposes of statistical analysis, matched and same subject designs are treated alike, so you only have to decide between:

same-/matched-subject design

or

different-subject design.

## Choosing the appropriate test

The above questions can be set out as a decision chart like those in Figures 9.1 and 9.2.

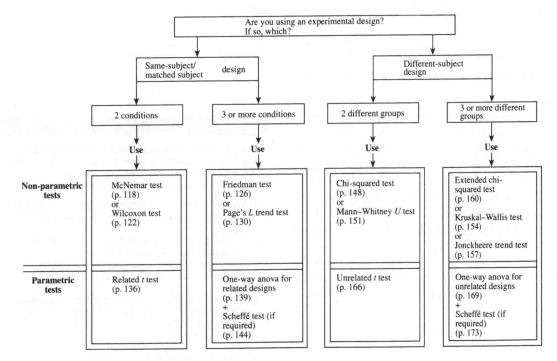

**Figure 9.1**   Choosing the correct test for an experimental design.

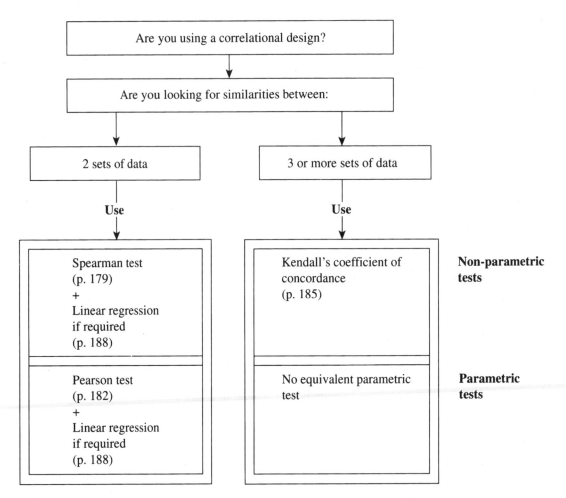

**Figure 9.2** Choosing the correct test for a correlational design.

Note that the names of the appropriate statistical tests are given in the boxes on the charts. You can see from these charts that sometimes the names of two or three tests are given. This does not mean that any one of them can be selected, but that instead each requires slightly different conditions for use, for example, a different level of measurement. These differences are outlined in the relevant chapter.

You will also notice that you are given the choice of 'non-parametric' or 'parametric' tests. The differences between these will be outlined in the next section.

**KEY CONCEPTS**

Every experimental design has its own statistical test(s) which must be used to analyse the data. In order to select the appropriate statistical test for your own design you must ask yourself a number of questions:

1. Were you looking for differences (i.e. an experimental design) or patterns/similarities (i.e. a correlational design)?
2. If you had a correlational design, you must also ask: 'How many sets of data did I have?'
3. If you had an experimental design, then you must ask: 'How many conditions were there?' (Two or more than two)
4. If you did, did you use the same or matched subjects in each condition? Or did you use different subjects in each condition?

## PARAMETRIC AND NON-PARAMETRIC TESTS

You will notice that the statistical tests in Figures 9.1 and 9.2 are classed as 'Parametric tests' and 'Non-parametric tests'. Essentially, for most of the designs you are likely to use, you have a choice of using a parametric test or a non-parametric test. What is the difference?

Basically, a parametric test is a much more sensitive tool of statistical analysis. If, for example, you are comparing responses to two different kinds of treatment, and there *are* differences in responsiveness, the parametric test is more likely to find them than is the non-parametric test. Perhaps the point can be clarified by an analogy. Supposing you were making a cake and you wanted to weigh out the ingredients. You have two weighing machines in the house; the bathroom scales and the kitchen scales. You could use your bathroom scales to weigh out your 8 oz of sugar, but they will give you a less accurate and less sensitive reading than your kitchen scales. The non–parametric test is like the bathroom scales as it will analyse your results but it will not be as fine or as sensitive as the analysis of the parametric test (the kitchen scales).

If parametric tests are so good, then why do we bother with non-parametric tests at all? Like most things that are good, there are prices to pay and conditions to fulfil, and so it is with parametric tests. Before you can use one to analyse your results, four conditions have to be satisfied.

The first of these is critical: your data must be of an interval/ratio level of measurement, since parametric tests cannot be used on nominal or ordinal data. This condition cannot ever be violated.

The other three conditions are not quite as important, and may be waived to some degree. The first of these is that your subjects should be randomly selected from the population they represent.

Second, your data should be normally distributed. As you will probably remember from Chapter 5 a normal distribution looks like an inverted-U shape and you can plot your data on a graph to find out whether it is (more or less) normally distributed.

Third, the variation in the results from each condition should be roughly the same. This means that the range of scores in each condition should be more or less similar. If, for instance, the scores in one condition ranged from 20–120, while for the other they ranged from 60–80, the degree of variation in each condition's scores would be too dissimilar for a parametric test to be used. On the other hand if they ranged from 50–100 in one condition and 60–90 in the other, this would be acceptable.

To each of the last three conditions we would add the caveat 'within reason', because parametric tests are said to be 'robust'. Essentially, what this means is that it does not matter too much if you cannot fulfil the last three conditions; as long as your data is of an interval/ratio level, and there are no glaring deviations with respect to the other three conditions, you can use a parametric test.

Table 9.1 may help to clarify this point.

**Table 9.1** Levels of measurement for parametric and non-parametric tests

| Level of measurement | Type of test which can be used |
| --- | --- |
| Nominal | Non-parametric |
| Ordinal | Non-parametric |
| Interval | Parametric and non-parametric |
| Ratio | Parametric and non-parametric |

If you're ever not sure as to whether you've satisfied the conditions adequately, then use a non-parametric test, since this is an error to caution. So, when in doubt, use the non-parametric test.

**KEY CONCEPTS**

The results from any research design may usually be analysed either by a parametric or a non-parametric test. A parametric test is much more sensitive and will identify significant results more readily than a non-parametric test. However, before you can use a parametric test, four conditions must be fulfilled:

- the data must be on an interval/ratio level
- the subjects should have been randomly selected
- the data should be normally distributed
- the variance in the results from each condition should be similar.

The first condition is essential.
The other three can be violated to some extent.
Non-parametric tests do not require these conditions to be fulfilled and can be used with any level of measurement.

## ANOTHER WAY OF DECIDING WHICH TEST TO USE

Alternatively, some students prefer to make this decision by using diagrammatic representations of the design. These are set out with examples in Tables 9.2–9.4. You should note that in Examples 2, 4 and 6 you can use more than three groups or conditions and still apply the same test.

## Experimental designs

**Table 9.2**  Same-subject designs

| | | Test | |
|---|---|---|---|
| | | Non-parametric | Parametric |
| *Example 1* | | | |
| One group of Ss *takes part in* Condition 1 *takes part in* Condition 2 | Compared for differences between conditions | McNemar test (if data is nominal) or Wilcoxon (if data is **other** than nominal) | Related *t* test (if data is interval/ratio) |

H₁  Elderly patients develop more rapport with uniformed physiotherapists than with non-uniformed physiotherapists.
Method  Select a group of elderly patients and measure rapport;
(1) with uniformed physiotherapists and
(2) with non-uniformed physiotherapists,
i.e. one group of patients measured under both conditions.

| | | | |
|---|---|---|---|
| *Example 2* | | | |
| One group of Ss *takes part in* Condition 1 *takes part in* Condition 2 *takes part in* Condition 3 | Compared for differences between conditions | Friedman or Page's *L* trend (if data is **other** than nominal) | One-way anova for related designs (if data is interval/ratio) + Scheffé test if required |

H₁  The attitudes of a group of physiotherapists to 3 (or more) types of patient differ significantly.
Method  Select a group of physiotherapists and measure their attitudes to 3 types of patient,
i.e. one group of physios measured under 3 different conditions.
(It can be seen that this design is an extension of Example 1.)

**Table 9.3**  Different-subject designs

| | | Test | |
|---|---|---|---|
| | | Non-parametric | Parametric |
| *Example 3* Subject group 1 ———takes part in——— *Condition 1* ⎫ Compared for differences between conditions Subject group 2 ———takes part in——— *Condition 2* ⎭ | | Chi-squared test (if data is nominal) or Mann–Whitney *U* test (if data is **other** than nominal) | Unrelated *t* test (if data is interval/ratio) |

    H₁   Men are more likely to experience respiratory complications following cardiothoracic surgery than are women.

Method   Select a group of male cardiothoracic patients and a group of female cardiothoracic patients and compare degree of respiratory complications, i.e. two different groups of Ss compared.

| | | Test | |
|---|---|---|---|
| *Example 4* Subject group 1 ———takes part in——— *Condition 1* ⎫ Compared for differences between conditions Subject group 2 ———takes part in——— *Condition 2* ⎬ Subject group 3 ———takes part in——— *Condition 3* ⎭ | | Extended Chi-squared test (if data is nominal) or Kruskal–Wallis or Jonckheere trend (if data is **other** than nominal) | One-way anova for unrelated designs (if data is interval/ratio) + Scheffé test if required |

    H₁   There is a difference in responsiveness to interferential treatment of middle-age stress incontinence in women with no children, 2 children or 4+ children.

Method   Select 3 groups of women: 1 with no children, 1 with 2 children and 1 with 4 or more children and compare their responsiveness to treatment, i.e. 3 different groups of Ss compared.

(This is an extension of Example 3.)

**Table 9.4**  Matched-subject designs

| | | Test | |
|---|---|---|---|
| | | Non-parametric | Parametric |
| *Example 5* Subjects **matched** on key variables<br>Subject group 1 ——takes part in—— *Condition 1*<br>Subject group 2 ——takes part in—— *Condition 2* | Compared for differences between conditions | McNemar (if data is nominal) or Wilcoxon (if data is **other** than nominal) | Related *t* test (if data is interval/ratio) |

$H_1$  Cast bracing is more effective than traction in the treatment of leg fractures.

Method  Take two groups of leg fracture patients, matched on key variables such as age, sex, prior fractures, and fitness and treat one group with traction and the other with cast-bracing. Compare their progress, i.e. two groups of Ss **matched** on certain critical factors, and compared for progress.

| | | Non-parametric | Parametric |
|---|---|---|---|
| *Example 6* Subjects **matched** on key variables<br>Subject group 1 ——takes part in—— *Condition 1*<br>Subject group 2 ——takes part in—— *Condition 2*<br>Subject group 3 ——takes part in—— *Condition 3* | Compared for differences between conditions | Friedman or Page's *L* trend (if data is **other** than nominal) | One-way anova for related designs (if data is interval/ratio) + Scheffé test if required |

$H_1$  To extend the hypothesis in Example 5, you add a further treatment group which uses plaster of Paris.

Method  You select a further group of leg fracture patients matched with groups 1 and 2 on age, sex, prior fractures and fitness and compare the progress of the 3 groups, i.e. 3 groups of Ss **matched** on certain critical factors, and compared for progress.

# Correlational designs

**Table 9.5** A correlational design where two sets of scores are involved

| | Test | |
| --- | --- | --- |
| | Non-parametric | Parametric |

*Example 7*

These may predict:

a. positive correlation, i.e. high scores on one variable are associated with high scores on the other (Fig. 9.3).

Spearman (if data is **other** than nominal) + Linear regression if required

Pearson (if data is interval/ratio) + Linear regression if required

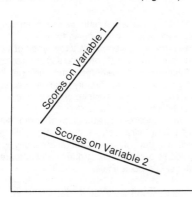

**Figure 9.3**

H₁   There is a correlation between age and recovery time following gall bladder removal, such that the older the patient, the longer the recovery time.

Method   Select a whole age range of cholecystectomy patients and note their recovery time from operation to discharge.

b. negative correlation, i.e. high scores on one variable are related to low scores on the other (Fig. 9.4).

Spearman (if data is **other** than nominal) + Linear regression if required

Pearson (if data is interval/ratio) + Linear regression if required

**Figure 9.4**

H₁   There is a correlation between vital capacity and number of cigarettes smoked, with high numbers of cigarettes being associated with low vital capacity.

Method   Select a whole range of smokers (e.g. non-smokers to 80+ per day and measure their vital capacity).

**Table 9.6**    A correlational design where more than two sets of scores are involved

| | Test | |
|---|---|---|
| | Non-parametric | Parametric |

*Example 8*

Where you are looking for the degree of similarity between 3 or more sets of scores (Fig. 9.5).

Kendall coefficient of concordance (if data is **other** than nominal)

There is no parametric test

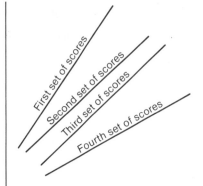

**Figure 9.5**

(Here you can only predict a positive correlation; see Ch. 17 for the reason why.)

H₁    There is a positive correlation among physiotherapists' judgements of the handicapping nature of various clinical conditions.

Method    Select 4 physiotherapists and ask them to rank order 6 clinical conditions (blindness, lower leg amputation, deafness, emphysema, osteoarthritis of the hip, carpal tunnel syndrome) for their assumed handicapping impact on the patient.

---

**Activity 9.1**    (Answers on page 231)

Using the decision guidelines presented earlier, look at the following brief descriptions of some research projects, and decide which statistical tests you should use. (Quote both the parametric and non-parametric alternatives where relevant, since at this stage you would not know whether your data would allow you to use a parametric test.)

1 In order to compare the speciality preferences of a group of newly qualified physiotherapists and a group of senior physiotherapists, you select two groups of 30 subjects to represent each group and ask them to state whether they prefer geriatric or paediatric work.

2 To find out whether leg fracture patients progress faster on hydrotherapy or suspension, you select two groups of 15 Ss, matched on certain key features such as age, sex, prior fractures, etc. and compare their progress after 4 weeks' treatment.

3 On the assumption that seniority in the physiotherapy profession is related to high absenteeism rates, (the higher the grade, the greater the absenteeism) you look at the number of days off taken by all grades of physiotherapist at a large general hospital.

4 To find out whether social class is related to compliance with exercise regimes following laminectomy operations, you select 30 patients from social classes 1 and 2 and

30 from social classes 4 and 5 and compare their reported compliance, on a 5-point scale.

5 To compare the effectiveness of three types of walking aid for hip replacement patients, you select three groups of Ss, matched on key variables, such as age, fitness etc. and give one group Zimmer frames, the second group walking sticks and the third group crutches. Their mobility after 3 weeks is compared.

6 In order to compare the attitudes of three different grades of physiotherapist to a new set of shift hours, you select a group of 15 superintendent physios, 15 senior grade IIs and 15 basic grades and compare their attitudes, using a point scale.

## LOOKING UP THE RESULTS OF YOUR ANALYSIS IN THE PROBABILITY TABLES

Let's suppose you have designed and carried out your experiments and have analysed the results using the correct statistical test. As you will remember, it was stated earlier that a statistical test will give you a result which you look up in a set of probability tables in order to find out whether your results are significant and support your hypothesis. This process will be described more fully in the chapters which deal with the particular statistical tests, but an outline of the general principles will be given here.

When you have worked through the appropriate statistical test or formula, you will end up with a number which you look up in a set of probability tables for that particular test. It is important to note that each statistical test has its own set of probability tables, which you will find at the back of this book. Thus, the Mann–Whitney $U$ test will provide you with a numerical value which is looked up in the probability tables for the Mann–Whitney test (see Tables A2.7 (a–d)). The Wilcoxon test provides you with a numerical value which is looked up in the probability tables for the Wilcoxon test, and so on.

More details on this will be given with the description for each statistical test.

## Degrees of freedom

Before you can look up the numerical value mentioned above, some tests require an additional value: either the number of Ss you used or a number called the **degrees of freedom (df)**. This concept which is quite a complex one to understand refers to the degree of potential variability in the data. (The reader is referred to Ferguson (1976) for a discussion of this.) However, although the concept is hard to understand, the 'df' is very easy to calculate. The details of how to do this will be given in the description of the tests which require the df.

However, before you can conclude whether your numerical value represents a significant result from your experiment, you require one further piece of information: namely whether you have a one- or two-tailed hypothesis.

## One- and two-tailed hypotheses

The way in which you state your hypothesis has implications for how you look up your numerical value in the probability tables.

### One-tailed hypotheses

Some hypotheses are stated very specifically in that they predict precisely what the outcomes will be. For example, if the hypothesis was: 'elderly patients experience more rapport with uniformed rather than non-uniformed physiotherapists', we are predicting a very precise outcome in that we are saying that the patients will experience more rapport with uniformed physiotherapists. Again, if we hypothesised that: 'leg fractures improve faster with traction than with cast-bracing', we are making a precise prediction, because we are assuming faster progress with traction. These are known as **one-tailed hypotheses or tests** because the results are expected to go in one particular direction. The following are all examples of one-tailed hypotheses:

1. Women are more likely to experience complications following cholecystectomy operations than are men.
2. Ultrasound is more effective than megapulse for arthritic toe joints.
3. Social classes 4 and 5 are less likely to keep to exercise regimes than are social classes 1 and 2.
4. Children with lower leg amputations are less likely to suffer from negative body image than adolescents with lower leg amputations.
5. Male physiotherapy students are more likely to fail the clinical assessment than are females.

### Two-tailed hypotheses

However, hypotheses can be stated much more vaguely, without any precise predictions. For example, it might have been hypothesised that elderly patients experience different degrees of rapport with uniformed and non-uniformed physiotherapists. In contrast to the one-tailed hypothesis which predicted more rapport with uniformed physiotherapists, this hypothesis allows for the possibility that more rapport could be experienced either with uniformed or with non-uniformed physiotherapists, because it simply predicts differences in rapport, without specifying what these differences might be. Similarly, if we predict that leg fractures respond differently to traction and cast-bracing, we are not specifying how they respond, but simply that there is a difference in response, which could mean leg fractures improve more either with cast-bracing *or* with traction.

These hypotheses are known as **two-tailed hypotheses or tests** because the results could go in either of two directions. The following are examples of two-tailed hypotheses:

1. Senior and basic grade physiotherapists differ in their absenteeism rates as a result of stress.
2. Student physiotherapists with 'A'-level physics differ from students without 'A'-level physics, in terms of their theory exam marks.
3. Interferential and exercise techniques are differentially effective in treating stress incontinence.
4. Zimmer frames and walking sticks afford different degrees of mobility for patients with ankylosing spondylitis.
5. Patients who are given preoperative respiratory exercises differ in their incidence of postoperative complications from patients who are given no preoperative respiratory exercises.

---

**Activity 9.2**   (Answers on pages 231–232)

Look at the following hypotheses and identify which are one-tailed and which are two-tailed:

1 Praise is a more effective motivator for mobilising exercises, when used in group rather than one-to-one situations.
2 Paraffin wax and hot soaks are differentially effective as a preparation for mobilising exercises in post-fracture patients.
3 Patients who attend for rigorous exercise regimes in back schools make fewer complaints following treatment, than patients who attend for heat treatment.
4 There is a difference in the strength of muscle contraction of a selected muscle group when preceded by 2 minutes infrared radiation as opposed to 2 minutes specific warm-up.
5 The application of lumbar traction diminishes vital capacity.

Look back at the examples of one-tailed hypotheses and convert them to two-tailed hypotheses.

Then look at the example of two-tailed hypotheses and convert them to one-tailed hypotheses. (It does not matter in which direction you predict the results will go.)

---

## One-tailed or two-tailed: why does it matter?

Why is this important? Supposing you had stated a one-tailed hypothesis, (i.e. that your results will go in one specific direction) and having done your experiment and statistics, had ended up with a $p$ value of 1%. This means that there is a 1% chance that your results are due to random error. However, had your hypothesis been two-tailed instead, you would be predicting that your results could go in either of two directions. Therefore, because your results could go in either of two directions, there will be twice the possibility that random error could account for your results, and so for exactly the same data your $p$ value would be doubled to 2%, i.e. a 2% chance that your results are due to random error.

Let's illustrate this with an example. Suppose you had hypothesised that exercise is more effective than clapping for increasing lung capacity in cystic fibrosis patients (i.e. you have stated a one-tailed hypothesis), you would probably have selected two groups of patients, one of which received exercise and the other clapping. You would expect that the lung capacities of the exercise group following treatment would be generally larger. Suppose again, that your results suggest this is the case, and you end up with a $p$ value of 5%. This means that there is a $5/100$ chance that your results are due to error.

However, had you simply hypothesised that clapping and exercise are differentially effective in increasing lung capacity then you would expect either the exercise group or the clapping group to do better. This is now a two-tailed hypothesis, because you have allowed for the possibility that the results could go in either of two directions. You carry out exactly the same study and achieve exactly the same results, but your $p$ value would now be 10% (i.e. doubled) because if your results are expected to go in either of two directions, there must be twice the possibility that random error can account for the results. Let's see how this works in practice by turning to Table A2.2 (Wilcoxon).

At the top of the table you will see two headings: 'Level of significance for one-tailed tests' and 'Level of significance for two-tailed tests'. You can see that every level of significance for a two-tailed test is twice the corresponding level for a one-tailed test, i.e. 0.10 is twice 0.05; 0.05 is twice 0.025; 0.02 is twice 0.01; 0.01 is twice 0.005.

### Should a hypothesis be one-tailed or two-tailed?

Many students ask how they should decide on whether an hypothesis should be one- or two-tailed. The answer to this lies in the background theory associated with the research you are carrying out. For example, if you are concerned with the relationship between smoking and bronchitis, the background reading that you will have done, prior to embarking on this research, will probably have revealed that:

- smoking is related to lung cancer
- bronchitis is associated with particular atmospheric pollution

and therefore, it would be reasonable to predict that heavy smokers are more likely to get bronchitis (i.e. a specific one-tailed prediction). Thus, the existing research and literature will guide your prediction here.

If, however, you were interested in looking at the effects on patients' feelings of physiotherapists wearing uniform, you may well have found background literature which suggests that some patients are more comfortable with uniformed physiotherapists, while others prefer the informality of the physiotherapist in 'civvies'. Thus, because the background research is less clear cut here, you would probably not wish to make a specific prediction about patients' attitudes to uniformed vs. non-uniformed physiotherapists, and would therefore formulate a two-tailed hypothesis. In other words, existing research knowledge and theory should guide you when making predictions in the hypothesis.

## A CHECKLIST OF STAGES INVOLVED IN SETTING UP YOUR RESEARCH PROJECT

Let's recap on the essential guidelines that have been covered so far, and are involved in designing a piece of research. Please note that this checklist only applies to studies which are involved in hypothesis testing.

1. Have you formulated an experimental hypothesis which clearly predicts a relationship between two variables? Have you stated your null (no relationship) hypothesis?
2. Are you going to test this hypothesis using a correlational design (i.e. are you predicting that as scores on one variable go up, so scores on the other variable go up or down accordingly)? Or are you going to use an experimental design which will test for differences between conditions or subject groups?
3. If you are using a correlational design, what level of data do you have on each variable?
4. If you are going to use an experimental

design, have you sorted out what you are going to measure (i.e. what is the DV?). Have you decided when you will take the pre-test measures of the DV and the post-test measures? What level of measurement are you using?

5. Are you going to use a different, same- or matched-subject design? Are you sure that this is the most appropriate design for your hypothesis? Why?

   If you are going to use a matched-subject design, have you identified the critical variables on which the Ss have to be matched?

6. Will you be using a control group? Is this ethically acceptable?

   If you are not using a control group, how many experimental conditions have you decided upon?

7. Who are your subjects going to be? Can you select them randomly? How many will you need?

8. Is there any need to counterbalance the conditions to overcome order effects?

9. Have you controlled for experimenter bias?

10. What are the sources of constant error? Have you controlled or eliminated them? Have you taken account of the random errors as far as you are able?

11. Is your experimental hypothesis one- or two-tailed?

12. What test will you need to analyse your results?

# 10

# Putting the theory into practice

Everything that has been said so far is theory. To carry out a piece of research, you need to put this theory into practice. This Chapter is concerned with providing some practical guidelines to help you set up your research project.

## PREPARATION FOR RESEARCH

### 1. Stating your aims and objectives

It is essential that you clarify in your own mind what the object of your research is to be. All too often students say rather vaguely 'I'd like to do something on back pain/fractures/torticollis' etc. without having any idea what exactly they want to investigate. While a general topic area like this is a good starting point, since it defines your area of interest, you will need to develop a more precise idea of what you are trying to find out before you start your research. In some cases, this will involve collecting large amounts of data for a survey.

Alternatively, you may wish to test a specific hypothesis at the outset. If this is the case, ensure that the hypothesis conforms to the principles outlined on pages 48–50, in that it makes a clear prediction of a relationship between two variables, and that it is a testable hypothesis. Some topics in which you are interested may simply not be researchable because the necessary skills, techniques, procedures, etc. are not available or ethically acceptable, or because the project would involve major policy changes, which are out of the control of the researcher or would take too long or involve too many people. So do ask yourself whether the hypothesis is testable and feasible.

Furthermore, do define the terms in your hypothesis clearly and unambiguously. Using terms like 'safe practice', or 'effective' or 'improvement' are too vague as they stand, and you must have a clear idea of what they mean in real terms.

Even if you are interested in a particular area and simply want to explore it fully without formulating any hypothesis (i.e. some form of survey technique) you will still need to clarify your aims and terms so that you can define the area to be studied precisely.

## 2. Reviewing the background research

Once you have formulated your hypothesis or defined your survey area, you will have to review all the relevant literature relating to the area you want to investigate. The purposes of this activity are to:

- Acquaint yourself fully with the theoretical background to the topic, so that you have a full understanding of the issue.
- Familiarise yourself with all the existing research that has been carried out in the area, firstly to ensure that your own project has not been conducted before, and secondly to provide a context for your experiment. These points are particularly important if you want to write up your research project for publication in a journal.
- Consider the possible methods and techniques of conducting your research.

However, having just said that one of the purposes of reviewing the research literature is to ensure that your intended study has not been carried out before (i.e. it is an original piece of work), there will be occasions when you simply want to replicate someone else's experiment in order to see whether their results apply to your own professional setting. In such a case, the process is slightly different, in that your aim or hypothesis will be identical to that of the study you wish to replicate, and the entire experimental procedure will also be the same. You will still need to acquaint yourself with the background literature so that you are familiar with the theories and related studies, but its purpose is obviously not to ensure the originality of your project.

It should be pointed out that it is perfectly acceptable to replicate an existing study as long as this is your real intention and not just the result of your not being aware of what has already been done in the area!

Do not underestimate the importance of a really thorough search of the literature: there is nothing more infuriating than carrying out a superb(!) piece of research with earth-shattering results, only to be told by a colleague that Bloggs et al. performed an identical piece of research a year ago. A full search of the literature will prevent time wastage and disappointment. That having been said, there are a number of practical tips to remember when searching through the literature.

### The Index Medicus

Use the Index Medicus in your hospital/university library. The Index Medicus is, as it suggests, a medical index citing all the medical research which has been published in over 3000 journals. However, it should be pointed out that it does not cover physiotherapy journals. It is produced monthly, and a cumulative volume is issued annually.

There are two stages to using the Index Medicus. The first stage involves using a volume called MeSH (Medical Subject Headings) which contains all the official subject headings under which articles are classified in the Index Medicus itself. It is essential to consult MeSH before proceeding, for two reasons:

1. You could waste a considerable amount of time searching through the Index Medicus for a topic heading which is not officially used. For example, you might be interested in hemicrania. Thus you would look this up in MeSH. You would find the following:

Hemicrania *see* Migraine

This tells you that hemicrania is classified as migraine in the Index Medicus and that you should refer to this heading instead.

2. MeSH provides a list of related topics in which you might be interested, e.g.

Mental Health Services
*see related*    Halfway Houses
             Hospital Psychiatric Departments
             Hospitals, Psychiatric

Once you have identified all the subject areas which may be relevant to you, move on to the Index Medicus itself. The first half of the Index Medicus volume has an alphabetical list of research topics, which is followed by titles of articles published in the area, the author (s) and a reference to the journal where the article was originally published. The second half has an alphabetical list of researchers followed by what they have published and where the article can be located.

Thus, if you just want to find out what has been done on prolapsed intervertebral discs over the last decade, you simply find out the official listing of this topic in MeSH and then look this up in the last 10 issues of the Index Medicus and make a note of all the relevant articles, so you can go and read them in the original journal. Alternatively, if you know that Legge is famous for his work on amputations, you would look up Legge in the name section of the Index Medicus to find out what he's published recently. You would similarly make a note of where to find the relevant articles and go and read the original. If when reading the article, it does appear to be relevant, make a note of it (see next point) and its content. You might also want to look at the list of references at the end of the article to see if there are any important ones which you have missed.

You will find that the journal title is given in abbreviated form. If you're not sure about the abbreviations, you will find a list of all the journals referred to, together with their shortened form in the January issue of the Index Medicus.

In addition, many articles, although having English titles, are written in a foreign language. These articles can be identified by the square brackets which enclose the title. The language of the original paper is provided at the end of this, together with information on whether or not an English abstract is available.

If you are just starting a literature search on an area which is fairly new to you, articles which review subject areas are particularly useful, since they provide you with an excellent résumé of the topic as well as a list of useful references. Review papers are listed at the front of each monthly issue of the Index Medicus and in the first volume of the annual publication.

A particularly easy way of carrying out your literature search is an online computer facility, which many medical libraries run. Medline is the major computer database and is the CD-ROM version of the Index Medicus. It has details of articles from 3000 of the world's most important journals in the areas of nursing, medicine and dentistry. Many medical libraries offer courses in how to use Medline fully; alternatively you could seek help from library staff. Computer searches are especially valuable if you are interested in a particularly esoteric topic, such as 'exercise techniques for elderly prostatectomy patients following bladder infections'. However, you do have to pay for this facility and the cost will depend on the number of articles produced. Information about the availability of this service should be obtained from your library. (It should be noted that there is an International Nursing Index which works according to the same format, but has the drawback of referring to numerous journals which are not available in this country.)

Do remember – if you are not sure how to use the Index Medicus, ask the librarian.

### Physiotherapy CATS

There is also an abstract system for physiotherapy journals, running along similar lines, which is called Physiotherapy CATS (Current Awareness Topic Search). This is published monthly, and is divided into two parts. The first part comprises a subject index; under each subject heading is a list of authors who have produced work in the area, the title of their articles and the journal in which it was published. The second part is an author index, similar to that in the Index Medicus. All the journals covered are indexed at the back of the volume. There is also a Keyword Index at the back which, like MeSH, gives the official subject classifications which are used in CATS. Each subject classification has some numerical references which relate back to articles quoted in the first part of the volume.

So, a very easy way of carrying out a literature search is simply to identify the official classification in the Keyword Index, make a list of all the associated numbers, and then turn to the front of the volume to find out whether the articles referred to by these numbers are relevant to you.

However, because CATS has only been introduced relatively recently, it will not be a completely comprehensive reference point. Therefore, you may need to search earlier physiotherapy journals by hand. Other sources of information may throw up useful literature. There is also available an online database called AMED (Allied and Alternative Medicine) and a CD-ROM database called CINAHL (Cumulative Index to Nursing and Allied Health) both of which might provide useful information.

These systems, while an invaluable source of information on the available literature are by no means exhaustive, since there may be research projects on the fringe of conventional medical approaches which are not included or which are thought to be more appropriately classified elsewhere. It is a good idea, therefore, to browse through any professional journals which you think may contain relevant articles, as well as textbooks on the topic.

It is worth noting that the Chartered Society of Physiotherapy (14, Bedford Row, London WC1R 4ED; telephone 071–242–1941, fax: 071–831–4509) has an Information Resource Centre which holds a large number of journals; it can also provide literature searches and allied information and advice. Appointments should be made in advance if you want to visit the Centre.

### Reference information

Keep a card index of all the references you think are useful. For each relevant reference use one large index card and include, for journal articles:

- the full name of the author
- the date of the journal
- the precise title of the article
- the precise title of the journal where the article appears

- the volume (and part if relevant) of the journal
- the first and last page numbers of the article
- a résumé of the article with all the relevant details.

For chapter references in a book, where the book has an editor, include:

- the full name of the author of the chapter
- the date of publication of the book
- the title of the chapter
- the full name of the editor
- the full title of the book
- where the book was published
- the name of the publisher
- a résumé of the chapter, with all the relevant details.

For references to a book which has an author rather than an editor, include:

- the full name of the author
- the date of publication of the book
- the full title of the book
- where the book was published
- the name of the publisher
- a résumé of the relevant information.

You may think this is rather fussy, but I can assure you that a fully detailed card index file is worth its weight in gold. All too often researchers assume (and I have been amongst them) that if they need a particular reference again, they'll know where to find it and so then fail either to make a note of it at all or they make an insufficiently detailed note of it. I can guarantee that by the time you've completed your project and you're ready to write it up, your memory for references will have let you down, and you will consequently waste hours in libraries trying to track down a piece of information which you're sure you saw on the top right-hand page of a newish blue book!

Shortcutting references really isn't worth the time, frustration and energy so do keep a full card index of all relevant references as you go along. And, in addition, if you continue to research a topic, such a fund of references will be used time and again.

## 3. Deciding how you will carry out the project

Once you have completed a thorough literature review and made sure that your proposed project has not been carried out before, you must then decide on the best method of proceeding with your research. Are you going to conduct a survey, whereby you collect a large quantity of data and then use some form of descriptive statistics to highlight important features of it (Ch. 5)? Or are you going to use a correlational design whereby you measure two (or more) variables to see whether they co-vary in some predicted way (Ch. 6)? Or is an experiment more appropriate for the particular project, which will involve manipulating one variable to see what effect it has on the other (Ch. 6)?

There follows a brief re-cap on the salient issues involved in each approach.

Survey methods involve collecting a large quantity of data on a particular subject and using descriptive statistics to highlight the important aspects of the data. Surveys can be used for a number of purposes:

- To describe the topic area, e.g. how many patients suffer lower leg amputations as a result of circulatory defects, their ages, sex, social class, previous health, occupation , length of time in hospital etc.
- To pinpoint problem areas. If, in the above example, you found that 50–60-year-old men who worked in the brewery trade were more likely to have lower leg amputation, this might point the way to further research on any possible causal links. This might then give rise to an experimental study where you tested this hypothesis.
- To identify trends, both past and present. Is there, for instance, an increased tendency towards these lower leg amputations over the last decade? If so, it is conceivable that this trend may continue. If it does, then this might point the way towards developing physiotherapeutic expertise in the area of lower limb amputation and rehabilitation.

Remember, though, that survey techniques may be unsuitable for testing specific hypotheses.

For this, experimental and correlational designs are needed.

Experimental designs are used to test whether the relationship predicted between the two variables in the hypothesis actually exists. To do this one of the variables must be manipulated and the effects of this on the other variable are then measured. Such an approach has to be carefully designed and controlled, which may involve the researcher in a considerable amount of effort. The results of this approach have to be analysed using statistical tests (see Chs 13–17). If the experiment has been carried out properly, the results can provide very useful answers, by identifying causes and effects of certain events. The approach can also establish which of a number of treatment procedures is more effective, which types of patient respond best to particular therapies etc. and so may be especially useful in streamlining and systematising professional practice.

However, it does, of course, have its disadvantages. Experiments can be complicated and time-consuming to carry out and they may be entirely unsuitable if any ethical issues are involved. For example, it would be of dubious ethical value to look at the effects of psychoprophylactic relaxation techniques during childbirth on length of labour by comparing a group who had been trained in the technique with a group who had no preparation for childbirth at all. In such cases, alternative approaches must be considered. One such is the correlational design.

Correlational designs are used to test hypotheses where it would be unethical to manipulate deliberately the independent variable (in the latter case, relaxation techniques) to see what effect it had on the dependent variable (length of labour). In correlational designs, the researcher simply takes a range of measures on each variable to ascertain whether they vary together in an associated way. For example, are high scores on one variable associated with high scores on the other? Or alternatively, are high scores on one variable associated with low scores on the other? Because the technique does not involve any artificial manipulation of patients or treatments, it is easier to carry out than experimental procedures and can more easily be used in naturalistic settings. However, it is for the same reason that cause and effect cannot be established using a correlational design, and therefore cannot provide the same degree of conclusive evidence.

You must decide which of these approaches is most suited to the topic you wish to research.

## 4. Preparation for the research: writing a research proposal

Once you have decided on your research topic, carried out a literature review and established which general approach to the project would be most appropriate, it is a good idea to write out a fairly detailed research proposal, so that you can plan the structure and specifics of the project. Many people consider a research proposal to be a waste of time unless they are trying to obtain financial support from some organisation, when a proposal is absolutely essential. However, writing up a research proposal has three important functions:

• It helps the researcher to plan the project and to focus attention on all the essential issues, such as aims, methods, analysis and relevance.

• In medical and paramedical research, it is often necessary to check the suitability of a project with ethical and related committees before beginning. For this, a research proposal is vital, since it not only provides the necessary details of the project so that the ethical issues can be fully evaluated, but also demonstrates the researcher's competence, expertise and understanding of the topic area; an important consideration when a patient's health and wellbeing may be affected.

• On occasions, the research you wish to do will require more time, staff or equipment than is readily available and it may, therefore, be necessary to obtain financial support for your project (see next section). In order to apply for funding you will need to provide the potential sponsors with a fairly detailed research proposal, so that they can assess its value, viability and relevance.

Thus, for these reasons, it is good practice to prepare a research proposal prior to starting your project. No great detail about writing proposals will be given here, since a lot of the content will

be similar to that contained in the next chapter on writing up research for publication. Where this is the case, it will be indicated. Nonetheless, the following information should be included in a proposal in the order given:

1. The title of the research project (see next chapter) which should be clear and succinct.

2. Background theory and the research context for the project (similar to the 'Introduction' in the next chapter).

3. A clear statement of the aim or hypothesis under investigation.

4. The method of conducting the research should be clearly outlined. This is very similar in content to the 'Method' section of an article (see next chapter) and should include a statement of the design of the project, the subjects (type, number etc.) materials, apparatus and actual procedure. In addition, any relevant information about how the public relations aspect will be handled should be included here (i.e. feedback of results to patients, anonymity of the subjects, security of the data, cooperation with other members of the hospital staff, etc.).

5. The type of statistical analysis to be used for the results should be included.

6. The implications and relevance of the study must be highlighted, particularly if the proposal is to go to an ethical committee or a funding body. It is pointless merely to outline an experiment without indicating its direct application and worth to the patients/hospital/staff/funding body, etc.

7. The estimated length of time required to carry out each section of the research, as well as the overall time involved, should be included, since this will obviously influence the feasibility and finances of the study; 100 Dupuytren's contracture patients might be difficult to find in a fortnight! Obviously, you cannot be exact in your time predictions because all sorts of unforeseen circumstances will crop up which will delay completion. Hence, it is better to be pessimistic rather than optimistic on this one. If you can draw some sort of chart showing the sequence and timing of the main events, this would be invaluable, both in setting an overall idea of the project and in guiding its execution.

8. If the proposal is to be presented to ethical or funding, bodies, then it will be necessary to include details of any personnel (including yourself) who may be involved in the project, either existing personnel or staff recruited specifically for the purpose of the project. There are usually three types of personnel involved in research work:

—Research supervisor or director. This is the person who takes overall responsibility for the project's execution, directing and rescuing as necessary. If you are the person generating the ideas and submitting the proposal for consideration by ethical and financial committees, the odds are you will also be the research supervisor.

—Research workers. These people carry out the everyday running of the project, collecting data, administering the treatments etc. They usually have some grounding in research methods or at least receive some training prior to the start of the project. Obviously, careful thought needs to be given to the qualifications and skills required of the research staff.

—Support staff. These are quite often the lynchpin on which the whole project depends. They include secretarial and clerical staff, computer operators, technicians, etc.

In a research proposal, it is a good idea to name the participants involved, together with their qualifications, work and research experience and particular expertise for the job. If you need to recruit anyone specially for the project, you will need to specify the sort of person you want, how long you want them for and what the cost will be. Always remember when you specify the salary range that the appointee will probably only be on a short-term contract and so should be paid slightly more than usual. In addition to the cost of the salary, you will need to add the employer's national insurance (N.I.) contributions, superannuation, additional costs and overheads.

Even if you are not applying for any funding it is still a good idea to work out the cost of the project, even if only approximately. You may find that an outcome of limited impact may not justify

the expense of new equipment, staff time, computing, etc. However, if you are applying for outside money then you should itemise the following costs, overall or per annum, if the project is to last longer than 12 months:

1. Salaries, superannuation, N.I. of all staff to be employed on the project.
2. Any capital outlay on equipment, together with revenue expenditure on any apparatus etc.
3. Travel and subsistence costs; if anybody needs to travel to other hospital departments, patients' homes etc., these costs should be incorporated.
4. Stationery costs, postage, telephone, typing, computing, etc. must be estimated. If you are proposing to handle a large amount of data, your computing costs may be fairly high. It is worthwhile having a preliminary chat with the computing centre you intend to use about estimated costs and the types of statistical analysis available.

Two words of caution, though. Firstly, don't forget to build in some allowance for inflation. Too many promising projects have had to be abandoned before completion simply because the money ran out. And secondly, check out the sort of financial information your potential sponsors require and the format they wish to receive it in before you submit your proposal. A familiar layout and content can go a long way towards getting your proposal seriously considered.

Allied to this is the length of the proposal. Many ethical committees and funding agencies have specific criteria for proposal formats and length and it is always wise to find these out and stick to them. Skimpy, underworded proposals look superficial and ill-thought-out, while excessively verbose ones will lead to boredom and irritation in the readers. Consequently, you should pay close attention to any recommendations laid down by the appropriate body.

Before taking off on your research, do ensure that not only does it have the approval (if necessary) of the ethical committee, but that it has been discussed and given the go-ahead by all the necessary people. This may involve your superintendent, the relevant consultant, housemen, colleagues, etc. It does little for staff relations for a senior colleague to find suddenly that there is a major research programme starting tomorrow, which will involve a total reorganisation of the department. So, do discuss your proposals with all the relevant personnel from the outset. This is a critical stage in any research project and should never be overlooked.

## 5. Obtaining financial support

Some research projects can be extremely expensive in both time and money, and you may, therefore, need to apply for financial aid in order to carry out your research. Sources of financial support are many and various and all should be considered as possible sponsors at the outset. Undoubtedly, the easiest avenue through which to apply for money (though not necessarily to obtain it!) is your own organisation's research fund. Many hospitals, district or regional health authorities have money available for research, although its existence is not always widely known. However, a relevant research programme carried out on home ground, with direct value to the sponsoring institution or organisation is often a tempting cause and you may find the money forthcoming.

Beyond this immediate channel, there are outside sources, such as the Medical Research Council, pharmaceutical companies, manufacturers of apparatus and the like, all of whom may be suitable targets for your application for money.

In order to decide which of these is likely to be most profitable, it is worth doing some homework. Some agencies obviously favour certain types of research and these inclinations will be indicated by the sort of project they have supported in the past, as well as the nature of their own activities. Obviously, a manufacturer of traction beds is unlikely to sponsor research into the impact of wearing uniforms versus civvies by physiotherapists, unless the project has some direct impact on their product. Some funding bodies even lay down specific guidelines as to the sort of project they will consider sponsoring.

Once you have decided who to approach, have an informal discussion with them about your ideas, and if they are interested, get the relevant application forms from them, together with any general information they might provide to guide intending applicants. These must be read thoroughly and completed in accordance with any regulations laid down by the organisation.

Some words of advice. The funding bodies are only likely to concern themselves with novel, useful and relevant pieces of work. Projects which are run-of-the-mill or contentious are usually avoided for obvious reasons. Therefore, before applying for money, do think carefully about the nature and implications of your research and how likely it is to fit in with the overall flavour of the sponsor's interest. Also, check the final presentation of your research proposal, ensuring that it is typed, and without errors. Omissions, incorrect spelling and poor syntax will do little to create a favourable impression of your professional competence!

If your proposal is turned down in the end, try to find out why and whether the sponsors would reconsider it if amendments were made. If, on the other hand, it is accepted, then you must keep your sponsor happy. This will involve you in three activities. Firstly, do try to keep within your time and financial budget: funding agencies are rarely pleased with requests for more money or time extensions. Secondly, do send regular progress reports so that they can be satisfied that all is going according to plan (or if it isn't that they are informed about the problem and what you're doing about it). And thirdly, do provide a detailed final report on time, with clear conclusions, implications and recommendations. (You might even consider inviting someone from the sponsoring organisation to be on a steering committee for the project. In that way, the sponsors can be kept fully informed at all stages.)

All this may seem like a lot of time and effort which perhaps could be better spent on the actual research project itself. Undoubtedly, there are borderline cases where you're not sure whether it really is worth the trouble to make an application for money. This is something only you and the other researchers can decide. However, if you do decide to apply for funding, remember that the sponsors are being asked to invest a lot of money in you and they will obviously want to assure themselves that it will be money well spent.

## 6. Planning the details of the study

If you write a proper research proposal, many of the details of the study will have been considered and decided upon. Even if you decide against a research proposal, you must make a detailed outline of your plans and ideas for your own benefit, since when you come to write up the research report (probably a considerable time after the completion of the project) you will be surprised at how difficult it is to remember why you actually decided on one approach rather than another. So keep detailed notes for yourself as you go along as to the reasons for choosing each methodological or design approach of your research.

At this juncture, if you are using an experimental design, you should also address, in detail, the following points:

- Any instructions you will be giving to your subjects during the course of the experiment should be prepared verbatim, and typed up.
- Prepare sufficient score sheets on which to record the data; if your subjects are to be asked to make written replies during the experiment, ensure that you prepare enough response sheets for them.
- If you are going to randomise the order of presentation of the experimental conditions, or the order of subjects' participation, make sure this is done in advance.
- If you are keeping the subjects anonymous and just assigning them numbers, do keep a record of any relevant details of all the subjects (age, health, sex, experimental condition) on a separate sheet with the appropriate number attached. This is essential if you are to contact them with the results of the experiment.
- How you will select your subjects and who they will be.
- Prepare for yourself and any other researchers who will be working with you, a worksheet which outlines detailed instructions of what should happen when, and how it should be carried out.
- Make sure that you know how to analyse the data, and, if it requires a computer, where and how you can obtain appropriate computing facilities.

- If you are going to use someone else to run the experiment, because you suspect there will be some experimenter bias if *you* carry it out, then make absolutely sure that the substitute experimenter has only the relevant details (i.e. exactly how to carry out the project) and not what the predicted outcome will be, otherwise the possibility of experimenter bias will remain.
- If you have to write to people to ask them to participate as subjects, do enclose a stamped, addressed envelope for their reply, and do check just before the start of the project that they are still able and willing to come.
- Do run a pilot study, before carrying out the experiment proper, to iron out any problems in advance.

If you are conducting a survey, you must decide:

- How you will collect your data, e.g. by using a questionnaire, by post, in person, etc.
- How to design your measuring instrument, i.e. your attitude scale or questionnaire. This must be piloted before you run the full survey.
- What instructions for completion you will append to the questionnaire.
- How you are going to select your subjects.
- How you will ensure an adequate response rate if you are using a postal survey.
- How you are going to analyse your data.

## 7. Carrying out the study

A number of points are important here:

1. If you are using any apparatus do double-check before you start that it works properly. It is extremely irritating to collect your subject sample from far and wide only to discover when they arrive that the necessary equipment is out of order and they have to go away again. This is the way in which you lose subjects, time, patience and motivation. Also, do make sure you know how to use the equipment properly. While this may seem a ludicrously obvious point to make, it has been known for experimenters to spend a considerable time fiddling about with the apparatus, attempting to find the necessary switches. Trying to convince the subjects of your competence thereafter becomes a major task.

2. Always, always, always run some pilot trials before you begin the experiment proper. Pilot trials simply mean running through the experimental procedure with a few subjects to see whether there are any practical hitches. By doing this, you can establish:

(i) Whether your procedure is appropriate.
(ii) Whether the tasks you've set your subjects are of the right level; if they're too hard or too easy they can be adjusted.
(iii) Whether you've allocated a reasonable amount of time for the tasks.
(iv) Whether your instructions can be clearly understood by the subjects.
(v) Whether there are any practical problems in the project.

If you do find any hitches or difficulties at this stage, you can iron them out before beginning the real experiment.

3. Do familiarise yourself totally with the experimental procedure, and what should be done when. It does not inspire the confidence of subjects to see the experimenter scrabbling around for scraps of paper or trying to find out what to do next. So make the running of the experiment as smooth and automatic as possible. The pilot trials should help in this.

4. Treat your subjects well. They are the cornerstone of your study and must be looked after. This means keeping them informed (as far as is reasonable) of the purpose of the study and of the outcome. Should it ever be necessary to keep your subjects in the dark over the aim of a study, because their knowledge of this would bias the results, do debrief them when the project is over. Also tell them in advance, if possible, what is required of them and how long it will take. Do not do anything which will cause distress or embarrassment. People are understandably apprehensive about any form of research, so it is in their, and your, best interest, to try to achieve some rapport with them and an easy, pleasant atmosphere. Lastly, try to minimise the amount of inconvenience subjects experience during the course of the study. If they have to make lengthy and expensive journeys at unsociable hours of the day or night, they are unlikely to turn up. Quite simply, try to keep your subjects happy, particularly if they are patients when not only their psychological, but also their physical, well-being may be at stake.

## 8. Interpreting and disseminating the results of your research

There is no value in simply analysing your results and then forgetting all about them: they must be interpreted fully in terms of their relevance to the profession. What is the meaning of the outcome? How does it relate to current physiotherapy practice? What are the implications for policy changes/therapeutic procedures? And so on.

However, even this is not enough. If only you are aware of the nature and implications of your results then they are of limited value. The information must be disseminated to other members of the profession. And the easiest way to do this is by writing up the research either as an article for publication in a professional journal, or as a report produced within your department for circulation. While the former method will reach a greater audience, both require the same sort of format and approach.

With the increasing emphasis on research-based clinical practice within the health care professions, together with reductions in resources, it is essential that the results of sound research projects are published. Without this knowledge clinicians will not be able to make informed decisions, practice will not be accountable on objective grounds and patients' welfare will not be optimised through the best intervention procedures. Publication of results is an essential final stage of research, and is a moral obligation for any physiotherapists who have conducted good research with potentially useful findings. Guidelines for writing up research are given in the next chapter.

And finally, remember that there is no such thing as a perfect piece of applied research. In designing any study involving human subjects, compromises will have to be made in the design. However, these considerations must be informed and well judged. As long as the researcher can make reasoned, judicial adjustments to their design in order to accommodate the practical problems surrounding their study, the research will still be valid.

# 11

# Writing up the research for publication

Sometimes you will want to carry out a piece of research just for your own satisfaction or to resolve some issue that exists in your own work. However, there will be occasions when your experiment produces such an interesting and useful outcome that you will want to publish it so that the results can be disseminated to other related professionals. Hence you will need to prepare an article for publication in a suitable journal. I would urge you always to consider publishing your research however, for two main reasons. Firstly, if you have some interesting findings there is a moral obligation to share these with other physiotherapists so that they can integrate them in their practice. And secondly, if patient care is to be improved through the use of research results then it is essential that these are widely disseminated to other practitioners.

A word of caution, though. Good scientific journalese comes with practice. Even if you follow the guidelines provided here you will probably not be terribly satisfied with your first attempt at writing up a piece of research. I would recommend that you don't despair and throw it in the bin, but instead put the first draft away for a week or two and forget about it. When you re-read it afresh you will probably find a number of points that could be expressed more clearly or succinctly. If you're still not satisfied after doing this, repeat the process. You will soon find that you are able to produce a written style which is suitable for scientific journals at the first attempt.

## GENERAL GUIDELINES FOR WRITING UP RESEARCH

1. Always bear in mind that the aims of writing up research for publication are to inform readers of (a) the purpose of your study (i.e. the aims or hypothesis); (b) the results; (c) how you came by them (i.e. the procedure you adopted for your experiment), and (d) what the implications of your results are.

More details of the basic structure of a report are given in the next section.

2. Always write in the third person, not in the first or second person. In other words, use phrases such as 'The subjects were required to . . .' rather than 'I asked the subjects to . . .'.

While this is easy enough when describing the experimental procedure, many students find it more difficult when discussing the implications of their results, tending to write phrases such as: 'I think the results can be explained by . . . '.The 'I think' would be better replaced by phrases such as 'it is suggested/posited/hypothesised that the results etc. . . .' or 'One possible explanation for the results is . . . . or 'The results can be explained by . . .' etc. If you have difficulty in writing in the third person, it's often a good idea to take a passage from a book which is written in the first person and simply rewrite it in the third person, for practice.

If all this sounds unnecessarily pedantic, remember that any research should be objective and disinterested. If you start including 'I', 'me' 'my', 'personally', etc. the report begins to look highly subjective and consequently not very scientific. Use of the third person is a much better style for journal articles (and gives you a greater chance of publication!).

3. Keep your sentences clear and simple and try to convey just one idea per sentence. Remember that your report may well be read by someone unfamiliar with the field, so confronting them with complex grammar or sentences with several adjectival clauses will keep them unfamiliar with it! Clarity of style is easier to attain if you do not assume your reader had any prior knowledge of the specific area. (However, don't fall into the trap of writing as though the reader is a halfwit!) And finally, if you are going to use abbreviations, give their meaning in full at the first mention. For example:

> Twenty patients with leg fractures as a result of Road Traffic Accidents (RTAs) were selected for study etc.

4. Do not include any anecdotal evidence in the report, however relevant and interesting it may appear. Science is too formal, theoretical and empirical for personal experience to be introduced.

5. Try to make your article clear, logical, succinct and free of irrelevancies. Remember always that the purpose of any article is to provide information. Therefore, if someone unfamiliar with your area of research is to understand the article then it is essential that it is clear and logical. Similarly, in order to get the essential points across to the reader, it is important not to wrap them up in irrelevant information. The colour of the subject's pyjamas is rarely apposite, although I have seen it included in one student's report!

6. It is important to quote relevant research in your article for a number of reasons. Firstly, it shows the reader that you are familiar with the research area and that you have a number of important facts at your fingertips. Secondly, it adds weight to any argument you produce: if you simply say that 'the administration of lumbar traction restricts vital capacity' the reader may think 'who says?' On the other hand if you state that: 'Bloggs & Smith (1982) found that back pain patients commonly demonstrate restricted vital capacity during lumbar traction', your argument carries more credibility. (You will note that I have quoted the surnames of the researchers here, together with the date of their publication on back pain. Some journals specify different formats when quoting research; do check what is required by your intended publisher.) And thirdly, you need to refer to some plausible theory when explaining your results. As you might imagine, theories by identifiable authors carry more weight than anonymous theories which cannot be checked out.

7. There is no one correct way of writing up a report, since each journal tends to have its own format and requirements. It is therefore impor-

tant to look at the journal's specifications (usually inside the front or back cover) and to read a couple of articles produced in it before starting your own. That having been said, the following subheadings should provide you with a structure for presenting the essential information from your experiment; you can leave out the subheadings when a particular journal does not use them.

## DETAILED GUIDELINES FOR STRUCTURING AN ARTICLE

### The title

This should convey succinctly to the reader the essential point of your experiment. For an experimental report it is often easier to construct your title from the relationship predicted in your experimental hypothesis.

For example, if your experimental hypothesis had been: 'Vital capacity is diminished during administration of lumbar traction for back pain', then the predicted relationship would be between lumbar traction and vital capacity. Your title could then be:

An investigation into the relationship between lumbar traction and vital capacity in back pain patients.

To practise producing pithy and clear titles, you could turn back to the hypotheses on page 48 and construct titles from them.

### Abstract or summary

The abstract or summary is a short précis of the experiment or study. Usually around 10 lines or 100–150 words long, the abstract includes:
- the aim or hypothesis of the study
- a brief summary of the procedure
- the results, stating their level of significance if appropriate
- a brief, general statement of the implications of the results.

Therefore, the abstract for an experiment testing the previous hypothesis might be:

In order to investigate the relationship between lumbar traction and vital capacity in back pain patients [aim and hypothesis] 20 subjects between the ages of 40 and 55 were measured for vital capacity before receiving lumbar traction and again during the receipt of lumbar traction, over a number of treatments [brief experimental procedure]. Using the related $t$ test to analyse the data, the results were found to be significant ($t = 2.912$, $p < 0.01$) [brief results].
The implications of the findings are discussed with respect to the treatment of patients with reduced vital capacity [implications].

Obviously, though, you do not include the words in square brackets, and you would continue from one section to the next, without starting a new line. (You should also note that all the illustrations are fictitious and not derived from any actual research evidence!)

While not all journals require abstracts, they are very useful, not only to the reader who can find out whether the article will be worth reading in full by simply looking at the abstract, but also to the writer who is forced to summarise the critical points of the research in a few lines. This usually focuses the author's mind on the basic structure of the article.

## Introduction

The point of the Introduction is to put your study into a theoretical context. There are five main topics you should include:

1. It should start off with a general description about the background to the research area. In the above example some reference could be made to any relevant work which has been carried out on vital capacity and back exercises/general traction. You might start off by stating something like:

Over the last few years there has been increasing evidence of links between vital capacity and degree of shrinkage in the vertebral column.

In other words you have defined the topic area.

2. The next stage is to review the relevant literature which relates to this , by briefly quoting appropriate research work. So, you might continue with, for example:

Brown & Green (1989), in a study of osteoarthritis patients, found that vital capacity increased following back extension exercises. Similarly, Black

& White (1993) compared the vital capacity of cervical spondylosis patients and patients with prolapsed intervertebral discs during traction and found vital capacity was smaller in the latter group than in the former.

3. The third stage involves providing the reader with some theoretical explanation for these findings. Thus:

One possible explanation for these results comes from the work of Bloggs (1994) who suggested that the effects of the mechanical restriction by the traction harness reduce vital capacity.

4. The next part of the Introduction provides a rationale for your own research, so the previous two stages of the Introduction should be structured in such a way as to highlight the need for your study. Most reported research is original; that is to say, the study has usually investigated previously unexplored areas. Therefore, the initial part of your Introduction should present any relevant work which has been carried out, and should involve some statement as to where there was a gap in the research. For example, you may find that a particular treatment has not been tried out with a specific patient group, or that a variation on a treatment procedure has not been evaluated. This gap provides you with the rationale for your experiment. Therefore, you might conclude the previous section with:

However, while numerous studies have looked at the effects of exercise or cervical traction on vital capacity, to date no work has specifically looked at the effects of lumbar traction on vital capacity *during* treatment. This provided the focus for the present research.

5. Finally, you need to state clearly what your experimental hypothesis was, i.e.

The hypothesis under investigation, therefore, was that there is a relationship between vital capacity and lumbar traction in back pain patients.

If you now read just the parts in smaller type, you can get the overall idea of what the Introduction should look like.

Bear in mind that the literature you quote in the Introduction should be comprehensive, up-to-date and critically evaluated if appropriate. Include any seminal works in the area.

# Method

The aim of the method section is to tell the reader exactly how the study was carried out. It has to be so clear that anyone reading your method section would be able to replicate your research exactly, without having to ask for clarification on any point.

It is usually subdivided into the following sections (but once again, you should check the journal first).

## Design

The independent and dependent variables in your experiment are usually defined here (if appropriate), together with a statement of whether you used a same-, matched- or different-subject design (again if appropriate). Furthermore, if you have eliminated any sources of error by counterbalancing, randomising the allocation of subjects to conditions, using a double-blind procedure etc., you should say so in this section. If you have conducted a survey, you might include here any essential decisions concerning your questionnaire design, how the questionnaires were distributed and why you chose this method. You might state, then, for this section:

The independent variable was traction, while the dependent variable was vital capacity. A same-subject design was used, with subjects being measured on vital capacity before and during traction. Each subject's vital capacity was measured by three different physiotherapists on nine separate occasions, in order to eliminate any bias in procedure.

## Subjects

You should describe your subjects succinctly, giving all the relevant details, e.g. age, sex, medical condition, mean length of time ill, previous treatment, occupation and how they were selected. If you just asked the first 20 patients who required treatment for back pain, say so. However, it is important to specify whether they volunteered, were press-ganged, paid, etc., since it makes a difference to the way in which they react. Therefore, in the above example, the subject section might read:

Twenty subjects, 10 male and 10 female, were

randomly selected from a back pain clinic. All were aged between 40 and 55; they had been experiencing back pain for at least 6 months and all had been diagnosed as having non-specific back problems. There were no smokers among the subject sample. None of the subjects had received any previous treatment for their complaint and all took part in the experiment on a voluntary basis.

### Apparatus

Any apparatus used should be referred to in sufficient detail so that anyone wanting to replicate your experiment can obtain the same equipment. Thus, manufacturer's name, make and type of apparatus, plus a brief description of its capacities should be included. If the equipment has been made specially for you, it should be described in detail and should be accompanied by a diagram showing its main features.

In the above example, then, the apparatus section might be:

> Two pieces of apparatus were used in the experiment. The first was an Akron traction-bed and the second piece of equipment was an electrical spirometer used for measuring vital capacity (Vitalograph).

### Materials

Any non-mechanical equipment used should be included in this section, e.g. score sheets, record cards, etc. If a questionnaire or attitude scale was used, you should describe the measure in detail. In addition, it is often appropriate to include a copy of it in an appendix at the end of the article. Here, the section would read something like:

> The materials used in the current experiment included patient record cards to keep records of the treatment and graphs from which vital capacity could be calculated.

### Procedure

This subsection of the method is very important and should include a detailed description of what you did when you actually carried out the study. It should be clear and logical and should provide the reader with something akin to the method part of a recipe, i.e. a step-by-step account of what was done in the appropriate order. Remem-

ber that although this part, like the rest of the report, should be relevant and succinct, it should also be sufficiently detailed that anyone who reads the procedure could go away and replicate what you did, to the letter.

The word 'relevant' is important as well: you should only include those details which might have some influence on the outcome of the experiment. For example, the height of a chair a patient sat in to carry out the experiment would not be relevant unless you were carrying out research into an area which related to ergonomics or the ability to get in and out of chairs. It is not always easy at first to include just the right amount of detail, but it is a skill which develops over time.

Details which should be included here are things like order of presentation of tasks, and standardised instructions to the subject (which should be reproduced verbatim), how the dependent variable was measured and at what time intervals, number of treatment sessions, etc. Therefore, the procedure section here might be:

> Each subject's vital capacity was measured in the standard way prior to beginning treatment using the spirometer. The results were noted on the appropriate graph. Each patient then received 15 minutes traction three times a week for 3 weeks (9 treatment sessions in total). Constant traction was given for a period of 15 minutes and was identical for every subject. During the last 5 minutes of every treatment session, vital capacity was measured. Pounds weight on the traction bed were increased in relation to body weight in the usual way. The treatment sessions all took place during the morning and were carried out by one of three senior physiotherapists. The subjects were randomly assigned to therapists in a prearranged order, such that every patient was treated three times by each therapist. At the end of the 3 weeks, the 9 vital capacity scores for each patient were averaged.

## Results

The actual scores derived from your study do not need to be presented in this section, but may be included in an appendix, if this is appropriate. However, it is necessary to include the mean scores for each group or condition. If you present a graph, ensure that it conforms to the guidelines outlined in Chapter 5.

Perhaps the most important part of this section, though, are the results of the statistical analysis performed on the scores. While it is unnecessary to include the workings-out you do need to say:

1. what statistical analysis you used
2. what the result was
3. what the level of significance was (if inferential techniques were used)
4. (a point many people forget) a brief statement of what these results actually mean. It is insufficient to just say: 'The results are significant at the 0.01 level'. You must interpret this for the reader.

So, in the above example, the results section might be (the numbered points refer to the list above).

The mean pre-test score for the subjects was 4.21 litres, while the mean vital capacity score during treatment was 3.13 litres. The results were analysed using the related $t$ test [1] and were found to be significant ($t$ = 2.912, df = 19 [2], $p < 0.01$ (two-tailed [3]). These results suggest that there is a significant decrease in vital capacity during traction [4].

## Discussion

1. This section starts off with a re-statement of the outcome of your statistical analysis (usually a varient on the last sentence in the results section), and may add a comment as to whether or not they support the experimental hypothesis (if this is appropriate). For example:

The results of the present experiment indicate that the vital capacity of the patients diminished significantly during traction, thereby supporting the experimental hypothesis.

2. You should then go on to make some statement about how your results fit in with the findings from other related research. This can incorporate studies which produced contradictory as well as corroborative findings, as long as you provide some plausible explanation for the discrepancy. Here, then you might say:

These results accord with those of Brown & Green (ibid), Black & White (ibid) as well as those of Grey (1993). Grey found in a study of patients wearing lumbar surgical supports that vital

capacity was reduced by 20% due to limitations of diaphragmatic movement. However, work by Gold and Silver (1992) provided contradictory findings. Their results indicated that traction had a negligible effect on vital capacity. However, all the subjects in their sample were smokers and it is conceivable that the existing limitations in vital capacity as a result of smoking minimised the effect of the traction.

3. You must produce a cogent theoretical explanation for your results and also some comment about their practical implications. For instance:

The results of the present experiment can be explained by Bloggs' Mechanical Restriction Theory (ibid). However, the work of Barnes & Bridges (1989) is also relevant. They suggest that when the thoracic cavity is elongated, even marginally, then the lung capacity is restricted. Given that lumbar traction alters the length of the spinal column, it is conceivable that there is a consequent elongation of the thoracic cavity, thereby accounting for the present results.
Furthermore, Gold & Silver (1992) have convincingly demonstrated that any fear-inducing treatment procedure, such as that involving large mechanical apparatus, causes shallow respiration and a consequent reduction in vital capacity. Taken together these two theories could account for the present results. These findings, however, have important implications for the treatment of back pain patients who also suffer from chronic respiratory conditions in which the vital capacity is already low. In such cases, alternative therapeutic procedures should be considered.

4. Next you should include any additional analysis which you carried out and which produced some interesting results, together with some comment on these (ideally their theoretical and practical relevance). For example, you might compare male vs. female subjects; older vs. younger subjects; social class or occupational groups, etc. In the present example:

Further analysis of the results suggested that the vital capacity differences were greater for men than for women ($t$ = 2.103, df = 18, $p < 0.05$, two-tailed). This finding may be interpreted in terms of the generally larger physique of males, thus accounting for the relatively greater difference in vital capacity.

5. You should then acknowledge any limitations of your study, design flaws, unforeseen practical problems that you encountered (e.g.

patients not turning up, apparatus breaking down etc.), variables which you failed to control for etc. While this may look as though it is condemning your experiment to the waste bin, it isn't, as long as there are no major methodological flaws which would totally vitiate your results. Most research (especially applied research like physiotherapy) will have some minor faults since the perfect experiment is all but a fantasy. However, if you acknowledge the problems and recommend ways of overcoming them were the study to be repeated in future, then your work will not be dismissed as nonsense. The researcher who thinks his/her study is perfect is the one who is more likely to be rejected. For example:

> The experiment highlighted a procedural flaw, in that traction weights were not identical, but related to body weight instead. While this may have only limited impact on the results since a same-subject design was used, it might have been better to use patients with similar body weights and standardised traction weights.

6. Finally, if your study throws up any ideas for future research, say so. Here you might suggest:

> While the study has demonstrated that vital capacity diminishes during traction, it would be interesting to ascertain whether this is a continuous process or whether there is a point in the treatment when there is a sudden reduction. In addition, the permanency of the reduced capacity needs investigating. These areas could form the basis of a future research project.

## References

Every researcher you have quoted in your report must be included in the reference section in order that the reader can follow up ideas and theories in the area by going back to the original article or book. Usually, all the names are quoted in alphabetical order and you must give the full reference.

While many journals have their own formats (which you should check first), there are standard ways of presenting references for books and journal articles. For books, the author's surname is quoted first followed by initials, date of publication, title of the book (underlined), where it was published and by whom.

Therefore, the reference would look like:

> Bloggs A.B. (1984) <u>Mechanical Restriction Theory</u>. Oxford: Oxford University Press.

However, you must check the journal's requirements first, because if the above reference was listed in a book published by Churchill Livingstone, it would appear as follows:

> Bloggs A B 1984 Mechanical restriction theory. Oxford University Press, Oxford

For journal articles, the format is similar: surname, initials, date of article, title of article, title of journal (underlined), volume of journal and first and last page numbers of the article. Therefore, a journal article would be:

> Black, C. & White, R. (1993) A comparison of the vital capacities of cervical spondylosis and prolapsed intervertebral disc patients. <u>Therapeutic Medicine</u>, 14, 15–22.

In the example quoted throughout, all the cited research would have to be referenced in alphabetical order, using the correct format. You would therefore have:

> Barnes, M. & Bridges, P. (1989) etc.
> Black, C. & White, R. (1993) etc.
> Bloggs, A.B. (1994) etc.
> Brown, D. & Green, F.A. (1989) etc.
> Gold, E. & Silver, S. (1992) etc.

Do note though, that some journals require that authors are referenced not in alphabetical order, but in the order in which they appeared in the report. The cardinal rule is: check the journal's requirements on format of article and reference presentation.

If you go back and read just the sections in smaller type you should get an idea about the style and format of a journal article, although I would stress again that prior to writing up your research, you should select a journal which specialises in your research area and check the details of presentation it requires.

## SUBMITTING ARTICLES FOR PUBLICATION

Finally, just a few tips on submitting articles for publication:

• Do not submit the article to more than one journal at a time. If the journal of your choice turns it down, then send it off to another one, but never submit simultaneously. (And always keep a copy!)

• If you carried out the research with colleagues, then it may be appropriate to include their names as authors. Where there is multiple authorship of an article, the person quoted first is usually assumed either to be the most senior contributor (in terms of professional status) or alternatively to have carried out the bulk of the work. However, there is no fixed precedent for the order of names, and trouble frequently arises when the most senior author has done least work but still wants to take first place. So, sort out the issue in advance.

• Throughout the course of any research project many individuals will have helped, e.g. by sponsoring the research or helping with any computing. Those people who have made significant contributions should be acknowledged at the end of the article.

• You might consider asking the editor of the journal if your article can be refereed 'blind' since there is some evidence that this produces a fairer and more objective evaluation. Remember that getting research published may be something of a game (if you're interested to know just what sort of game, you might like to read Peters & Ceci 1982). However, if you observe the rules of the game as outlined above you should be successful in having your article accepted for publication.

### Some morale boosters

• Don't be disheartened if your article is rejected: even the most seasoned of researchers regularly experience rejection. Try to use the referees' comments to improve your article before sending it off to another journal. In other words, use the rejection as a learning exercise.

• Bear in mind that getting something published takes a long time. It may be months before the editor comes back to you with the referees' views, and if adjustments have to be made, the referees may need to see the article again, which will add to the time it takes for your report to be accepted formally. Added to this is the time lag before the article appears in print once it has been accepted, and this can run into months or sometimes years.

• Seeing your article in print is always gratifying, however many times you have experienced it before. It makes all the effort in its production worthwhile.

• Don't ever lose sight of the fact that a sound piece of research, however small, may have the power to influence patient care radically. You have a moral imperative to put up with the problems of publication, given the potential benefits to physiotherapy practice at all levels.

# 12

# Reading published research critically

If physiotherapy practice is to become increasingly research-based, then three essential requirements must be fulfilled. Firstly, physiotherapists must carry out sound research which has the capacity to influence service delivery; secondly, this research must be published, and thirdly, the published reports must be read and evaluated prior to any findings being implemented into clinical practice.

While it is neither appropriate nor realistic to expect that all physiotherapists will become research-active, it is imperative that they become research-minded. This means (a) that well-carried out research is universally acknowledged to be of value to the profession as a whole and to the patients it serves, and (b) as a consequence of this, that physiotherapists keep themselves updated on relevant research findings, with a view to modifying their practice if it is appropriate to do so in the light of those findings. This, of course, means that they should be in a position to assess the quality of the research they read and the validity of its conclusions before implementation into service delivery.

Many physiotherapists express concern at the prospect of evaluating published research, particularly if it has appeared in a reputable journal. Such diffidence may in part be a function of our society's traditional belief that anything which appears in print must be true, but it is often also the result of physiotherapists' lack of confidence about how to go about evaluating published research. Clearly, where patients' physical and psychological wellbeing may be adversely affected by unquestioningly implementing the results of a poorly conducted study, it is self-evident that physiotherapists should have a working knowledge of how to assess what they read. This will also mean that they will need to be familiar with some of the concepts outlined earlier in this section of the book, since without this information, their judgements may not be fully informed.

This chapter is concerned with providing general guidelines on how to make informed assessments of published research. It may be useful to read Chapter 11, on presenting research for publication prior to reading this one, since it gives a fairly detailed account of what should normally go in a research report.

## ASSESSING PUBLISHED RESEARCH

### The title

When you first look through a journal, you need an at-a-glance knowledge of what the contents are to see if they have any relevance for you. Consequently, the title of the article will be your first point of contact. Therefore, the title should be a clear statement of what the research project was about so the first question you need to ask is:

1. Is the title a clear and succinct statement of the research study?

### Abstract or summary

The abstract is a short statement of the aims, methods, findings and conclusions of a research project. While not all journals use abstracts as a means of providing a summarised overview of the research, where they do, you should ask

2. Does the abstract provide a clear statement of the aims, methods, results and conclusions/implications of the study?
3. After reading the abstract, are you clear in your mind about the nature of the study?

A negative answer to either question may constitute a flaw. Certainly if no clear aim is stated then it may be impossible to evaluate the rest of the abstract, since it would not be obvious whether the method adequately tests the aims, nor whether the results and conclusions support them.

## Introduction

The introduction to a piece of research should give a clear statement of the context and general background to the study, since this will give the reader an idea as to the importance and relevance of the project; it should provide a comprehensive and up-to-date critical review of the research literature, since this will demonstrate the researcher's knowledge of the topic area and enhance the credibility of the project as a whole; it should provide a rationale for why a further piece of research was necessary and it should plug a gap in existing physiotherapy knowledge; and it must give an unambiguous statement of the aims, or hypothesis to be tested. Without this, it will be impossible to assess whether the study is a proper test of the aims. Therefore, the questions concerning the introduction are as follows:

4. Is there an adequate description of the general context for the study?
5. Is the literature review thorough, relevant, recent and properly used to provide a structured argument leading to the reason for conducting the reported piece of research?
6. Is the hypothesis (if appropriate) clearly stated, and the predicted relationship between the variables apparent?
7. If the research does not test the hypothesis, are the aims of the study clear?
8. Are the aims or hypothesis useful to physiotherapy?
9. Is the project likely to be of value to physiotherapy?

If the answers to these questions are 'no' then doubt must be cast on the quality of the project.

## Method

The general format of the method section varies from journal to journal. However, the actual content is usually very similar. The method section should tell the reader exactly what was done; how it was done; the order in which it was done; why this approach was chosen, and with whom the project was conducted.

After reading this section, you should know all the relevant details and be in a position to replicate the study exactly if you so wished. If you have to ask any questions or you need clarification on anything at all, then this section is not adequate, and the report must be considered flawed.

So the questions concerning the method section are:

10. Has the design of the study been properly described?
11. Has the researcher made it clear why this design was chosen?
12. Is the design appropriate for the aims/hypothesis stated in the Introduction?
13. Are sources of error acknowledged and controlled?
14. Is the sample suitable? of an appropriate size? fully described? properly selected?
15. Were any sources of bias or error evident in the sample and/or in the process by which they were chosen?
16. Would this impact upon the study's outcome?
17. Was any mechanical apparatus used in the study and if so, was it properly described? Was it suitable for the project?
18. Were any other materials used, such as questionnaires, score sheets, attitude scales etc?
19. Were these described fully and/or included in the Appendix, if appropriate?
20. Were any questionnaires or scales which were used properly constructed and adequately tested before using them in the study? Were they suitable for their purpose?
21. Is the description of what was done absolutely clear?
22. Does it state the order in which things were done?
23. Does it provide a verbatim report of any instructions given to the subjects? Were the instructions clear?
24. Were the sources of error dealt with appropriately?
25. Was the method of data collection clearly described and appropriate?
26. Were the data a suitable measure of the dependent variable (if the study tested an hypothesis) or of the information required by the survey's aims?
27. Were the subjects treated well, their rights and confidentiality protected?
28. Was the study ethical?
29. Could you repeat this study to the letter, if it was considered necessary?

If the answer to the last question in particular was 'no' then the method section does not fulfil its purpose. Other negative answers in this section would suggest not only a report beset by omissions and obscurities, but might also reflect a poorly conducted piece of research.

## Results

The results section should summarise what was actually found in the project. While it does not typically include raw data or the workings-out of any statistical analysis, both these elements can be summarised. Raw data can be presented by tabulating means, standard deviations etc. and the results of any statistical analysis by the numerical value obtained as a result of performing the correct statistical test. This should be accompanied by a $p$ value and an interpretation of this.

Whatever the nature of the study, the meaning of the results should be made clear to the reader.

The questions relating to this section then are:

30. Are the graphs (if provided) clear, self-explanatory and useful?
31. Are the tables (if used) clearly labelled and constructed and with an obvious relevance to the study?
32. Are the statistical tests used the correct ones for the project's design?
33. Is the selected level of significance appropriate for the topic area?
34. Is the $p$ value clearly stated and correct for the hypothesis as stated (i.e. one- or two-tailed)?

If the analysis at any level is incorrect this will invalidate the study and conclusions. Therefore, positive answers to every question in this section are critical.

## Discussion

The discussion section of a research report should do just as it says: it should discuss the findings from the project in relation to other research work in the area, thus providing a broader context for the project's results.

In addition, some theoretical explanation for the results should be provided, as theory and practice should go together. Sometimes results do not tie in with findings of existing research and some convincing reason for this discrepancy must be put forward, otherwise doubts must inevitably be cast on the methodology and analysis used in the study.

The conclusions drawn in the discussion should reflect the results. They should not be extravagant and extend beyond what was actually found. Neither should the conclusions be incomplete and refer only to those parts of the data which confirm the researcher's original aims, while ignoring results which oppose those aims. Such selective discussion has the potential to be every bit as misleading as incorrect analysis and interpretation.

In addition, the discussion section offers the researcher an opportunity to acknowledge flaws in the study, together with suggestions for how these may be rectified in the future. Unconditional acceptance of the design of a research project may mean that the results are given more credence than they are due. Field research is never perfect and it is essential that the researcher recognises that, in order that the results can be interpreted with due caution.

Lastly, a good research project should spawn ideas for other studies. If it doesn't, then it is possible that the original project was too narrow and limited to be of much real value.

So the questions relating to this section are:

35. Are the results and conclusions clearly stated?
36. Are they related to other studies in the area, thereby putting them into a broader research framework?

37. Is a cogent theoretical explanation for the findings provided?
38. Are the results interpreted fully and correctly, or selectively and/or extravagantly?
39. Are any flaws in the study's design highlighted, together with recommendations for improvement?
40. Are the results interpreted with these limitations in mind?
41. Are any practical ramifications of the results discussed?
42. Do any ideas for future projects emerge?

The answer 'no' to any of the questions must produce reservations about the overall quality of the project.

## References

Every piece of work or research quoted in the report must be fully acknowledged and recorded in the reference section. These references should give the full name of the author, the date of the work, its title and where it was published (see section on references, page 109).

Omissions in the references are suggestive of sloppiness, and may then reflect adversely on the rest of the study.

Therefore:

43. Is every article, study, research report and book quoted in the reference section?
44. Do these references give all the required information?

## Overall considerations

Finally there are some general questions which need to be asked:

45. Was the project a worthwhile one, contributing to the knowledge base of physiotherapy?
46. Was it clearly written, so that the content was easily accessible to the reader?
47. Is the report scientific and objective both in the way in which it was conducted as well as the way in which it was analysed and written up?

48. Is the article devoid of jargon?
49. Has the research project advanced physiotherapy in any way?

These questions may seem pedantic and tedious, but a poorly reported project may suggest a poorly conducted project. Remember, that no research project is perfect. What is important though, is that the researcher recognises this, justifies why design and analysis decisions were taken, and interprets the results in the light of these. Asking the above questions of an article means that patient wellbeing will be safeguarded to some degree, since the reader will be in a position to make sound assessments of a research project before deciding whether to implement the findings into his/her practice.

# SECTION 2

# Statistical tests

It is essential that the data from any research project are properly analysed. Where research involves testing a hypothesis, through the use of either an experimental or correlational design, it is critical that the correct statistical test is used to find out whether the results support the prediction made in the hypothesis. Using the wrong test gives invalid results and conclusions, which is potentially very damaging in an area like physiotherapy where patient well-being is involved. Ways of choosing the correct test were outlined in Chapter 9. This section is concerned with how to carry out those tests.

# 13

# Non-parametric tests for same- and matched-subject designs

## INTRODUCTION

As was mentioned in Chapter 9, the results from most of the designs you are likely to use can be analysed using either a non-parametric or a parametric statistical test. Each test does essentially the same job, but the parametric test is rather more sensitive. However, in order to use a parametric test, certain conditions have to be fulfilled (see Ch. 9). If you cannot fulfil these or if you have any doubts then you should use the equivalent non-parametric test. All the tests in this chapter are **non-parametric for same- and matched-subject designs.** In the next chapter, the equivalent parametric tests for the same designs will be covered.

So, the statistical tests covered in this chapter are appropriate for any experimental design which involves either: one group of subjects which is used in two or more conditions (same-subject design); or alternatively two or more groups of subjects, each of which is used in one condition only, but who are matched on certain key variables (matched-subject design). (Have a look back to the examples given on pages 84 and 86 in Chapter 9.) Therefore, the sort of designs we are talking about are:

1. **Same-subject design:** One group of subjects used in two or more conditions.

   a. Two conditions (Fig. 13.1).

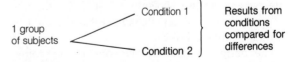

**Figure 13.1** Same-subject design: one group of subjects and two conditions.

or

b. Three or more conditions (Fig. 13.2).

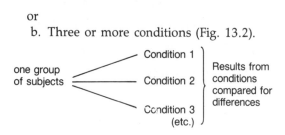

**Figure13.2** Same-subject design: one group of subjects and three or more conditions.

2. **Matched-subject designs:** two or more groups of matched-subjects, each of which is used in one condition only.

a. Two matched groups only (Fig. 13.3).

| Subject group 1 | takes part in | Condition 1 | } Results from conditions compared for differences |
| Subject group 2 | takes part in | Condition 2 | |

**Figure 13.3** Matched-subject design: two groups of matched subjects each taking part in one condition.

or

b. Three or more matched groups (Fig 13.4).

| Subject group 1 | takes part in | Condition 1 | |
| Subject group 2 | takes part in | Condition 2 | } Results from conditions compared for differences |
| Subject group 3 (and so on) | takes part in | Condition 3 | |

**Figure 13.4** Matched-subject design: three or more groups of matched subjects each taking part in one condition only.

The designs which involve one group doing two conditions (Design 1a), or two matched groups doing one condition each (Design 2a) are analysed using the **McNemar** test if the data is only nominal, or the **Wilcoxon** test if the data is ordinal or interval/ratio.

The designs which involve one group doing three or more conditions (Design 1b) or three (or more) matched groups doing one condition each (Design 2b), are analysed using either the **Fried-**

**man** test or the **Page's _L_ trend** test. Pages 128–135 will explain which of those two you should select, since each one requires slightly different conditions. This is summarised in Table 13.1.

**Table 13.1** Non-parametric tests for related- and matched-subject designs

| Design | Non-parametric test |
| --- | --- |
| 1a. One group of Ss taking part in two conditions. Results from conditions compared for differences | McNemar test if the data is nominal or Wilcoxon test if the data is ordinal or interval/ratio |
| 2a. Two groups of matched Ss each taking part in one condition only. Results from conditions compared for differences | McNemar test if the data is nominal or Wilcoxon test if the data is ordinal or interval/ratio |
| 1b. One group of Ss taking part in three or more conditions. Results from conditions compared for differences | Friedman test or Page's _L_ trend test (see pp. 128–135 for which one to use). Both these can be used with ordinal or interval/ratio data |
| 2b. Three or more groups of matched Ss, each taking part in one condition only. Results from conditions compared for differences | Friedman test or Page's _L_ trend test (see pp. 128–135 for which one to use). Both these can be used with ordinal or interval/ratio data |

# NON-PARAMETRIC TEST: SAME- AND MATCHED-SUBJECT DESIGNS, TWO CONDITIONS AND NOMINAL DATA

## McNemar test for the significance of changes

Just to remind you, this test is used when either you have one group of subjects who are measured or tested on two conditions (a same-subject design) and the two sets of results are then compared for any differences between them; or when you compare two groups of subjects who are matched on all the critical variables which might influence the results (i.e. a matched group design). Each group is tested in one condition and the results are compared for differences between them. In other words you would use this test if you had either experimental design 1a or 2a on pages 119–120.

The McNemar test is particularly suitable for 'before and after' type situations. However, there is one very important feature of this test: it is used with *nominal data*, that is, a level of measurement which simply allows you to allocate people or responses to named categories. Essentially what the McNemar test does is to record the changes from one category to the other, across the two conditions, to see if these changes are significant. When you calculate the McNemar test, you find a numerical value called 'Chi-squared', written as $\chi^2$, which you then look up in Table A2.1 (page 209) to see if this figure represents significant differences between the two conditions or the two matched.groups.

## Example

Let's imagine you've noticed over the years the degree of fear most women experience prior to having a hysterectomy. It occurs to you that a preoperative talk to explain what will happen, and to allow them to express any doubts or anxieties, may go a long way towards reducing their tension. You decide to try this and see whether your hunch is correct.

Your experimental hypothesis is:

$H_1$  A preoperative talk will reduce fear levels in hysterectomy patients

What would your null hypothesis be?
Is this a one-tailed or two-tailed hypothesis?

You select 20 pre-hysterectomy patients and note whether they are frightened about the operation. You classify them as either:

1. little or no anxiety or
2. high anxiety.

This is nominal data because you are simply allocating patients' responses to a named category. You then spend some time explaining to the patients what will happen, discussing any issues and problems they have etc. Following this session, the patients are asked whether their anxiety levels have reduced. According to their response, you again allocate them to one of the categories, as before.

You therefore have the design shown in Figure 13.5.

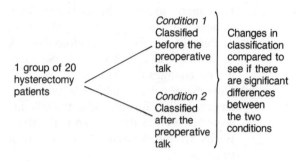

**Figure 13.5**  Design for experiment to assess effectiveness of preoperative talk for hysterectomy patients.

You have all the conditions required by the McNemar test, that is, a same-subject design and nominal data.

You obtain the results shown in Table 13.2.

**Table 13.2**  Patient anxiety about hysterectomy; $\phi$ = little or no anxiety, X = high anxiety

| Patient | Before talk | After talk |
| --- | --- | --- |
| 1 | $\phi$ | $\phi$ |
| 2 | X | $\phi$ |
| 3 | X | $\phi$ |
| 4 | $\phi$ | $\phi$ |
| 5 | X | X |
| 6 | X | $\phi$ |
| 7 | X | X |
| 8 | $\phi$ | $\phi$ |
| 9 | X | $\phi$ |
| 10 | X | $\phi$ |
| 11 | X | X |
| 12 | X | $\phi$ |
| 13 | $\phi$ | $\phi$ |
| 14 | $\phi$ | $\phi$ |
| 15 | $\phi$ | $\phi$ |
| 16 | X | X |
| 17 | X | $\phi$ |
| 18 | X | $\phi$ |
| 19 | X | $\phi$ |
| 20 | X | $\phi$ |

## Calculating the McNemar test

1. You must first of all record the changes that

occurred from one testing to the other. In other words you must count up:

(a) How many patients changed from 'little or no anxiety' to 'high anxiety' as a result of the talk, i.e. from '∅' before the talk to 'X' after. In the above example there are no changes of this kind.

(b) How many patients had very little or no anxiety both before and after the talk, i.e. were '∅' before the talk and '∅' afterwards. In this example, there are 6 such patients.

(c) How many patients had high anxiety both before and after the talk, i.e. were 'X' before and 'X' after. Here there were 4 such patients.

(d) How many patients changed from feeling high anxiety before the talk to feeling little or no anxiety after, i.e. changed from 'X' before the talk to '∅' afterwards. Here there are 10.

2. These figures now have to be put in a table like Figure 13.6.

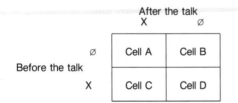

**Figure 13.6**   Table used in calculating the McNemar test.

Cell A represents those patients who changed from ∅ to X (little anxiety to high anxiety, i.e. 0). This is calculation (a) above.

Cell B represents those patients who had little or no anxiety before and after the talk (stayed at ∅, i.e. 6). This is calculation (b) above.

Cell C represents those patients who had high anxiety before and after the talk (stayed at X, i.e. 4). This is calculation (c) above.

Cell D represents those patients who changed from high anxiety to low anxiety (changed from X to ∅, i.e. 10). This is calculation (d) above. So, if we enter these figures into the cells, the table looks like Figure 13.7.

Remember! You must organise your cells in the way indicated above, otherwise your calculations

will be incorrect. In other words, whichever category is on the left-hand cell for the 'After'

|  | After the talk |  |
|---|---|---|
|  | X | ∅ |
| ∅ | 0 | 6 |
| X | 4 | 10 |

Before the talk

**Figure 13.7**   Table of Figure 13.6 with data entered.

condition, the other category should be at the top for the 'Before' condition. The numbers in the cells should add up to the same as the number of patients tested. In this case, the number is 20.

3. Find the value of $\chi^2$ from the formula:

$$\chi^2 = \frac{([A - D] - 1)^2}{A + D}$$

where A = the value in cell A (i.e. 0)
D = the value in cell D (i.e. 10)

If we substitute our figures we get:

$$\chi^2 = \frac{([0 - 10*] - 1)^2}{10}$$

$$= \frac{(9)^2}{10}$$

$$\frac{81}{10}$$

Therefore $\chi^2$ = 8.1

(*If you get a minus figure in the square brackets, ignore the minus and treat the figure as a plus; i.e. − 10 becomes 10)

4. Before looking up the results to see if they represent a significant change in fear, you need a further value: the df value. In the McNemar test, it is always 1.

### Looking up the value of $\chi^2$ for significance

To see whether this value of 8.1 represents a significant difference in fear levels, turn to Table A2.1, which is the probability table associated with the McNemar test (and the Chi-squared or $\chi^2$ test, see later). Down the left-hand column you will see df values from 1 to 30. To their right are five numbers, called **critical values of** $\chi^2$.

To find out whether our $\chi^2$ value is significant, look down the df column until you find our df value of 1. To the right you will see 5 critical values:

$$2.71 \quad 3.84 \quad 5.41 \quad 6.64 \quad 10.83$$

Each of these figures is associated with the probability value at the top of its column. For example, the critical value of 2.71 is associated with a probability value of 0.10, for a two-tailed test. You will notice that this table only refers to two-tailed hypotheses. Where you have a one-tailed hypothesis, look up the results in the way outlined, and simply halve the $p$ value (see pages 89–90).

For our $\chi^2$ value to be significant, it has to be *equal to* or *larger than* one of the critical values to the right of df = 1. Our $\chi^2$ value of 8.1 is larger than 2.71, 3.84, 5.41 and 6.64. We therefore take the value of 6.64 which is associated with a probability value of 0.01 for a two-tailed hypothesis, and therefore 0.005 for a one-tailed hypothesis (i.e. half 0.01). (If you look back to our hypothesis, you will see that we are predicting a specific direction to our results, i.e. preoperative counselling will reduce fear levels; therefore, our hypothesis is one-tailed.)

Now to be significant *exactly* at the 0.005 level, our $\chi^2$ value must *equal* 6.64. Our $\chi^2$ value is *larger* than 6.64, so that means that the probability of our results being due to random error is *even less* than 0.005. This is expressed as:

$$p < 0.005 \; (< \text{means 'less than'})$$

Had our $\chi^2$ value been exactly 6.64 we would have expressed this as:

$$p = 0.005$$

### Interpreting the results

Our results are associated with a probability of less than 0.005 or 0.5%. This means there is less than 0.5% chance of the results being due to random error. If you remember, a $p$ value of 5% or less was a standard cut-off point for claiming results to be significant. As 0.5% is less than 5% our results are significant.

However, before going on to explain what this

means, you must check that the changes in fear are in the direction you predicted, that is

| high fear before the talk | changed to | low fear after the talk |
|---|---|---|

It is possible to get significant results which are in the opposite direction to those predicted. In this case it would mean

| low fear before the talk | changed to | high fear after the talk |
|---|---|---|

These results, while significant, would not support your hypothesis.

If you look at the data in the table, you will see that the changes are in the predicted direction, and we can reject the null (no relationship) hypothesis and accept the experimental hypothesis.

We can state this in the following way:

Using a McNemar test on the data ($\chi^2$ = 8.1, df = 1), the results were found to be significant at $p < 0.005$ for a one-tailed test. This suggests that preoperative talks significantly reduce the fear of hysterectomy patients.

It is very important to note, though, that there should be significant numbers involved to compute the McNemar test. If (Cell A + Cell D) ÷ 2 comes to less than 5, you cannot use the McNemar. In such a case, it would be worth your while to collect sufficient data to satisfy the above requirement.

---

**Activity 13.1** (Answers on page 232)

1 To practise looking up $\chi^2$ values for the McNemar test, look up the following and say whether you would classify them as significant.
   (i)  $\chi^2$ = 3.98   df = 1   one-tailed $p$
   (ii)  $\chi^2$ = 6.71   df = 1   one-tailed $p$
   (iii) $\chi^2$ = 5.41   df = 1   two-tailed $p$
   (iv) $\chi^2$ = 2.59   df = 1   one-tailed $p$
   (v)  $\chi^2$ = 10.96  df = 1   two-tailed $p$
   (vi) $\chi^2$ = 4.82   df = 1   two-tailed $p$

2 Calculate a McNemar test on the following data:
As a district physiotherapist, you wish to alter the 'on-call' duty rotas, but have so far met with opposition from the physiotherapists in the district. In fact on the last poll, only 5 out of 30 were prepared to alter their duties. You decide to send round an explanatory fact sheet, in the hope that presenting the reasons for your change might alter their views. At the end of the fact sheet you simply ask the physiotherapists to indicate whether or not they would

accommodate the altered duties. Your hypothesis is:

H₁ Providing extra information about the reasons for changing on-call duty hours will modify the opinions of the physiotherapists involved.

Is this a 1- or 2-tailed hypothesis?

You obtain the results shown in Table 13.3.

**Table 13.3** Effect of extra information on opinions of physiotherapists; √, for the change; X against the change

| Physiotherapist | Opinions prior to receipt of factsheet | Opinions after the receipt of factsheet |
|---|---|---|
| 1 | X | √ |
| 2 | X | √ |
| 3 | X | X |
| 4 | X | √ |
| 5 | √ | √ |
| 6 | X | X |
| 7 | X | √ |
| 8 | X | X |
| 9 | X | √ |
| 10 | X | X |
| 11 | X | √ |
| 12 | X | √ |
| 13 | X | X |
| 14 | X | X |
| 15 | X | √ |
| 16 | √ | √ |
| 17 | X | √ |
| 18 | √ | √ |
| 19 | X | X |
| 20 | X | √ |
| 21 | X | X |
| 22 | X | √ |
| 23 | X | X |
| 24 | √ | √ |
| 25 | X | X |
| 26 | X | X |
| 27 | √ | X |
| 28 | X | √ |
| 29 | X | √ |
| 30 | X | √ |

State what your $\chi^2$ value is and what your $p$ value is. Write this out in a similar format to that given on page 121.

# NON-PARAMETRIC TEST: SAME- AND MATCHED-SUBJECT DESIGNS, TWO CONDITIONS AND ORDINAL OR INTERVAL/RATIO DATA

## Wilcoxon signed-ranks test

To recap, this test is used when you have two conditions (either one control condition and one experimental condition or two experimental conditions) and you have either one group of subjects doing both conditions, or two groups of matched subjects, one group doing one condition and the other group the other condition (see Designs 1a and 2a on pages 119–120). The data for this test must be ordinal or interval/ratio.

Essentially what the Wilcoxon test does is to compare the performance of each S (or pairs of matched Ss) in each condition to see if there is a significant difference between them. When you calculate this test, you end up with a numerical value called 'T', which you then look up in the probability tables for the Wilcoxon test, to see if this value represents a significant difference between the conditions.

### Example

Let's take an example. The issue regarding the wearing of uniform by physiotherapists seems unresolved. Some physiotherapists are of the opinion that uniforms increase the psychological distance between the patient and therapist and thus discourage the development of rapport. Others feel that the nature of the physiotherapist's job can be very stressful and intimate; the uniform sanctions such activities and makes the patient feel more comfortable. Obviously central to this issue is the patient–therapist relationship, a factor of major importance in long-stay patients. You decide you will assess the effects of physiotherapists wearing uniform on the degree of confidence experienced by a group of long-stay patients. Therefore you decide to test the following hypothesis:

H₁ Long-stay patients experience greater confidence when being treated by uniformed physiotherapists than when treated by non-uniformed physiotherapists.

What would your null hypothesis be?
Is this a one- or two-tailed hypothesis?

You devise a questionnaire which simply asks the subject to indicate on a 5-point scale (ordinal data) how confident they feel when being treated (a) by a uniformed physiotherapist, and (b) by a non-uniformed physiotherapist. On your scale, a score of 1 means 'not at all confident' while 5 means 'very confident'. You give this questionnaire to 15 paraplegic patients. Thus, you have the design shown in Figure 13.8.

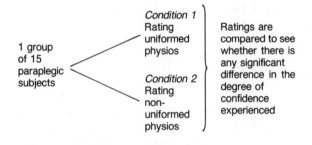

**Figure 13.8** Design to test effect of physiotherapists' wearing uniform on patient confidence.

You have all the conditions required by the Wilcoxon, i.e. a same-subject design and ordinal data.

You administer your questionnaire to the 15 Ss (having, of course, included all the essential prerequisites for such a design, See Chs 7 and 8) and you end up with the results shown in Table 13.4.

### Calculating the Wilcoxon test

In order to find out whether these ratings differ significantly for each condition, you must take the following steps:

**1.** Add up the total ($\Sigma$) for the uniformed condition A:

$$\Sigma A = 60$$

**2.** Add up the total ($\Sigma$) for the non-uniformed condition B:

$$\Sigma B = 38$$

**3.** Find the mean ($\bar{x}$) for each condition

$$\bar{x}A = 4 \quad \bar{x}B = 2.533$$

**4.** Calculate the difference (d) for each pair of scores by taking A – B, remembering to put in the + and – signs. Therefore for S1 you would have 5 – 3 = + 2 and so on. Put the results in column 3 (d = A – B).

5. You must then rank order these differences, in column 4, by giving a rank of 1 to the smallest difference, 2 to the next smallest and so on. When you do this, you must ignore the plus and minus signs. However, where the difference between a pair of scores is 0, you omit this pair altogether from any further analysis. Therefore, in this example, subjects 5, 6 and 11 are now excluded from any further analysis and we are reduced to 12 subjects.

You will also note that there are a number of d values which are identical, e.g. Ss 2 and 7 both have a d of +1, Ss 1, 8, 9, 10, 12 and 14 all have a d value of +2. Where this happens a special procedure is used – the 'tied rank' procedure.

### Tied rank procedure

To carry out the tied rank procedure, rank the scores as usual, giving a rank of 1 to the smallest, 2 to the next smallest (remember: we omit the 0s and ignore the + and – values).

Continue this procedure until you come to the tied scores. Here, Ss 2 and 7 both have d values of 1. These two scores are the lowest and should therefore occupy the two lowest ranks, i.e. ranks 1 and 2. So we add up these two ranks (1 + 2) and divide this by the number of d values that are the same score (i.e. 2 d values of 1):

$$\frac{1+2}{2} = 1.5$$

Therefore, the d values of 1 are both given the ranks of 1.5 (see column entitled 'Rank of d').

We now find there are 6 d values of 2. These values occupy the next lowest ranks, i.e. 3, 4, 5, 6, 7 and 8, because ranks 1 and 2 have already been used up.

Therefore we add these ranks together:

$$3 + 4 + 5 + 6 + 7 + 8 = 33$$

and divide this by the number of d values which have the value of 2 (i.e. 6 d values of 2):

$$33 \div 6 = 5.5$$

**Table 13.4**   Results of questionnaire and calculation of Wilcoxon test

| Subject | Results | | Calculations | | | |
|---|---|---|---|---|---|---|
| | 1<br>*Condition A*<br>Uniform | 2<br>*Condition B\**<br>Non-uniform | 3<br>d =<br>A – B | 4<br>Rank order of<br>d | 5<br>Rank of<br>+<br>differences | 6<br>Rank of<br>–<br>differences |
| 1 | 5 | 3 | + 2 | ( + ) 5.5 | + 5.5 | |
| 2 | 4 | 3 | + 1 | ( + ) 1.5 | + 1.5 | |
| 3 | 5 | 2 | + 3 | ( + ) 9.5 | + 9.5 | |
| 4 | 2 | 5 | – 3 | ( – ) 9.5 | | – 9.5 |
| 5 | 4 | 4 | 0 | exclude | | |
| 6 | 3 | 3 | 0 | exclude | | |
| 7 | 5 | 4 | + 1 | ( + ) 1.5 | + 1.5 | |
| 8 | 5 | 3 | + 2 | ( + ) 5.5 | + 5.5 | |
| 9 | 4 | 2 | + 2 | ( + ) 5.5 | + 5.5 | |
| 10 | 4 | 2 | + 2 | ( + ) 5.5 | + 5.5 | |
| 11 | 2 | 2 | 0 | exclude | | |
| 12 | 3 | 1 | + 2 | ( + ) 5.5 | + 5.5 | |
| 13 | 5 | 1 | + 4 | ( + )11.5 | + 11.5 | |
| 14 | 4 | 2 | + 2 | ( + ) 5.5 | + 5.5 | |
| 15 | 5 | 1 | + 4 | ( + )11.5 | + 11.5 | |
| Σ | 60 | 38 | | | + 68.5 | – 9.5 |
| $\bar{x}$ | 4 | 2.533 | | | | |

*It does not matter which condition is called A and which B.

Thus, all the d values of 2 are assigned the rank 5.5.

We now find there are 2 d values of 3 (Ss 3 and 4). These are the next two lowest scores and they would occupy the next two lowest-ranks, i.e. 9 and 10, because ranks 1–8 have now been used up.

Therefore, we add these ranks together:

$$9 + 10 = 19$$

and divide this by the number of d values which have the same value of 3 (i.e. 2 d values of 3) which is:

$$19 ÷ 2 = 9.5$$

So, both the d values of 3 are given the rank of 9.5.

Now there are only two remaining d values, each of which is 4. These d values occupy the next two ranks, i.e. 11 and 12, because ranks 1–10 have now been used up. Therefore we add these ranks together

$$11 + 12 = 23$$

and divide this by the number of d values which have the same value of 4 (i.e. 2 d values of 4): = 11.5.

$$23 ÷ 2 = 11.5$$

Thus, the d values of 4 are each given the rank of 11.5.

Many people get very irritated by this ranking procedure, especially when calculating tied ranks, because a slip of just one figure can throw everything out. To avoid this, you may wish to write out all the ranks you will be using (which will be the same as the number of differences to be ranked) and cross them off as you use them. Here, then, we would write out the following ranks: 1, 2, 3, 4, 5, 6, 7, 8, 9, 10, 11, 12, and strike them off as we go along.

Remember, the highest rank should be the same as the number of differences between scores you are ranking. Here we are ranking 12 d values, so the highest rank will be 12.

**6.** Now write in by each rank the plus or minus sign of the corresponding d value. Therefore, the first rank of 5.5 is given a plus sign because it has a corresponding d value of + 2.

**7.** Put all the ranks with a + sign into column 5, 'Rank of + differences'. Put all the ranks with a – sign into column 6, 'Rank of minus differences'.

**8.** Add up the ranks for the column 5 'Rank of + differences' to give the total ($\Sigma$) for the + ranks, i.e. + 68.5. Add up the ranks for the column 6 'Rank of – differences' to give the total ($\Sigma$) for the – ranks, i.e. –9.5.

**9.** Take the smaller of the two rank totals, ignoring the plus or minus sign, as your value of $T$ (i.e. $T$ = 9.5).

**10.** Find $N$ by counting up the number of subjects (or in the case of matched groups, pairs of Ss) omitting those who had d values of 0, i.e. 15 – 3 = 12.

### Looking up the value of T for significance

To see whether this $T$ value of 9.5 represents a significant difference in the confidence levels experienced with uniformed and non-uniformed physiotherapists, it must be looked up in the probability tables for the Wilcoxon test (Table A2.2, p. 210).

Down the left-hand column you will see values of $N$, while across the top you will see 'Levels of significance' for one- and two-tailed tests. Under each of these are columns of figures which are called critical values of $T$.

To find out whether our T value is significant at one of the levels indicated, we must first locate our $N$ value of 12 down the left-hand column. To the right of this you will see four numbers which represent the critical values of $T$ for this number of Ss. These values are:

$$17 \quad 14 \quad 10 \quad 7$$

Each of these figures is associated with the corresponding $p$ value indicated at the top of the column.

For example, a critical value of 14 is associated with a probability of 0.05 for a two-tailed test, and 0.025 for a one-tailed test.

In order for your $T$ value to be significant at a given level, it has to be *equal to or smaller than* one of these four figures. So, taking our T value

of 9.5, look at the first figure to the right of $N$ = 12, i.e. 17. Our T value is smaller than 17, so look at the next figure: 14. Our $T$ value is smaller than 14, so look at the next figure: 10. Our T value is smaller than 10, so look at the next figure: 7. Our $T$ value is larger than 7. Therefore our $T$ value comes somewhere between the critical values of 7 and 10 in the table.

Because we have a one-tailed hypothesis (more confidence with uniforms) this means our results are significant between the 0.01 and 0.005 (or 1–2%) levels. Now, to be significant at a given level, the $T$ value must be equal to or smaller than the critical value of $T$. Because it is smaller than 10 but larger than 7, we must comply with convention and select the value of 10, which is associated with a significance level of 1%. Had our $T$ value equalled 10 exactly, we would say that our results are signficant at $p$ equals 0.01. However, our $T$ value is smaller than 10, which means that its significance is actually less than 0.01. Therefore we express this as:

$$p < 0.01 \; (< \text{means 'less than'})$$

This means that the probability of our results being due to random error is less than 1%.

### Interpreting the results

Our $T$ value is associated with a $p$ value of < 0.01 level (i.e. <1% level) which means that there is less than a 1% chance that our results are due to random error. If you remember, we said a good rule of thumb for claiming support for your hypothesis is a probability of 5% (or 0.05) or less. Because our $T$ has a smaller $p$ value than 5%, we can say that our results are significant. But, it is very important to note that you must check the averages for each set of data (A = 4, B = 2.533) to see whether the results are in the direction you predicted (i.e. larger on the uniform condition), since occasionally, you may get significant results which are actually the reverse of what you predicted and therefore would not support your hypothesis.

Here, the results are in the direction you predicted and therefore, we can say that your hypothesis has been supported (i.e. we can reject the null hypothesis).

We can state this in the following way:

Using a Wilcoxon test on the data ($T = 9.5$, $N = 12$), the results were found to be significant at $p < 0.01$ level for a one-tailed test. This suggests that long-stay patients experience greater degrees of confidence when being treated by a uniformed physiotherapist than by a non-uniformed physiotherapist.

(At what level would the results have been significant had the hypothesis been two-tailed?)

**Activity 13.2** (Answers on pages 232)

1. To practise ranking, rank order the results in Table 13.5 using the guidelines above. Remember to rank from smallest to biggest, omitting any zero scores, ignoring the plus and minus signs of the $d$ values, and giving the average rank for tied $d$ values.

**Table 13.5**

| Subject | Condition A | Condition B | d | Rank |
|---|---|---|---|---|
| 1 | 10 | 9 | + 1 | |
| 2 | 8 | 9 | − 1 | |
| 3 | 9 | 7 | + 2 | |
| 4 | 6 | 7 | − 1 | |
| 5 | 5 | 4 | + 1 | |
| 6 | 8 | 3 | + 5 | |
| 7 | 7 | 6 | + 1 | |
| 8 | 9 | 9 | 0 | |
| 9 | 9 | 6 | + 3 | |
| 10 | 5 | 6 | − 1 | |
| 11 | 7 | 3 | + 4 | |
| 12 | 8 | 4 | + 4 | |

2 To practise looking up $T$ values, look up the following and say whether you would classify them as significant
(i) $T = 7$ $N = 9$ one-tailed
(ii) $T = 7$ $N = 15$ two-tailed
(iii) $T = 15$ $N = 13$ one-tailed
(iv) $T = 20$ $N = 16$ one-tailed
(v) $T = 16$ $N = 12$ two-tailed
(vi) $T = 32$ $N = 16$ one-tailed
(vii) $T = 7$ $N = 12$ two-tailed
(viii) $T = 12$ $N = 13$ one-tailed

3 Calculate a Wilcoxon on the following data:
  $H_1$ Traction is more effective than surgical collars for patients with cervical spondylosis.
  Is this a one or two-tailed hypothesis?
  Brief method: Select two groups of 12 cervical spondylosis patients, matched on sex, age, length and severity of condition, and previous treatments, and treat Group 1 with traction and Group 2 with surgical collars. After 3 weeks, compare the movement regained on a 7-point scale (1 = no improvement, 7 greatly improved). Table 13.6 shows some possible results.

**Table 13.6**

| Subject pair | Condition A Traction | Condition B Collar |
|---|---|---|
| 1 | 3 | 3 |
| 2 | 4 | 3 |
| 3 | 5 | 4 |
| 4 | 4 | 3 |
| 5 | 7 | 3 |
| 6 | 4 | 4 |
| 7 | 4 | 4 |
| 8 | 6 | 5 |
| 9 | 5 | 3 |
| 10 | 3 | 2 |
| 11 | 6 | 3 |
| 12 | 4 | 3 |

Write down the $T$ value
  $N$ value
  $p$ value
and state whether or not your results are significant, using the format of the paragraph on this page.

# NON-PARAMETRIC TESTS: SAME- AND MATCHED-SUBJECT DESIGNS, THREE OR MORE CONDITIONS AND ORDINAL OR INTERVAL/RATIO DATA

## 1. Friedman test

This test is similar to the Wilcoxon in that it is used for related and matched-subject designs. However, the Friedman is used when either

a. *one group* of subjects is tested under *three or more conditions;* the results from the conditions are compared for differences.
  or

b. *three or more groups* of *matched subjects* are each tested in *one condition;* the results from the groups are compared for differences.

You would use this test if you had either design 1b or 2b on page 120 and ordinal or interval/ratio data.

However, the Friedman test only tells you whether the results from each condition differ and not whether the results from one condition are better. For this reason, any hypothesis which relates to the Friedman must predict general differences and not a specific direction to the results. In other words, it must be *two–tailed.*

When calculating this test, you end up with a numerical value $\chi r^2$, which you then look up in the probability tables associated with the Friedman test to see whether this represents a significant difference between your conditions.

### Example

To illustrate this, let's suppose that you are a teacher in a large school of physiotherapy. You've noticed that over the last two or three years students seem to do consistently worse on the geriatric and neurology clinical placements, than on orthopaedic and cardiothoracic placements. This may be due to a number of factors, such as the quality of the theoretical preparation or clinical supervision. However, before moving on to find the cause, you must first establish whether or not your observation is correct. Your hypothesis is:

$H_1$    Third-year physiotherapy students perform differently in various clinical settings.

This is a two-tailed hypothesis, as it predicts no direction to the differences.

To test this hypothesis, you randomly select 17 students in the final year of their training and compare their marks (on a 10-point scale; 1 = disastrous, 10 = excellent) in four clinical settings: geriatric, neurology, orthopaedics and cardiothoracic.

Your design, then, looks like Figure 13.9.

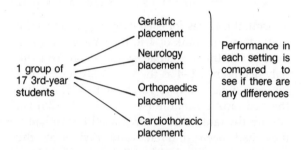

**Figure 13.9** Design to test whether physiotherapy students perform differently in various clinical settings.

Your data is as shown in Table 13.7.

**Table 13.7**

| Subject | Condition A Geriatric | | Condition B Neurology | | Condition C Orthopaedics | | Condtion D Cardiothoracic | |
|---|---|---|---|---|---|---|---|---|
| | Score | Rank | Score | Rank | Score | Rank | Score | Rank |
| 1 | 5 | 1 | 6 | 2 | 8 | 4 | 7 | 3 |
| 2 | 6 | 2.5 | 6 | 2.5 | 7 | 4 | 5 | 1 |
| 3 | 3 | 1 | 7 | 3.5 | 7 | 3.5 | 6 | 2 |
| 4 | 8 | 2 | 9 | 3 | 10 | 4 | 7 | 1 |
| 5 | 7 | 1.5 | 9 | 3.5 | 9 | 3.5 | 7 | 1.5 |
| 6 | 6 | 1.5 | 8 | 3 | 9 | 4 | 6 | 1.5 |
| 7 | 5 | 1 | 8 | 3 | 9 | 4 | 7 | 2 |
| 8 | 5 | 1 | 8 | 2.5 | 10 | 4 | 8 | 2.5 |
| 9 | 4 | 1 | 6 | 2 | 8 | 3 | 9 | 4 |
| 10 | 3 | 1 | 5 | 2 | 8 | 4 | 7 | 3 |
| 11 | 6 | 2 | 5 | 1 | 8 | 4 | 7 | 3 |
| 12 | 6 | 2.5 | 4 | 1 | 7 | 4 | 6 | 2.5 |
| 13 | 7 | 2 | 5 | 1 | 9 | 4 | 8 | 3 |
| 14 | 3 | 1 | 7 | 3 | 8 | 4 | 6 | 2 |
| 15 | 2 | 1 | 5 | 2 | 7 | 3.5 | 7 | 3.5 |
| 16 | 5 | 1 | 6 | 2.5 | 7 | 4 | 6 | 2.5 |
| 17 | 4 | 1 | 6 | 2 | 7 | 3.5 | 7 | 3.5 |
| | $\Sigma = 85$ | $T_C = 24$ | $\Sigma = 110$ | $T_C = 39.5$ | $\Sigma = 138$ | $T_C = 65$ | $\Sigma = 116$ | $T_C = 41.5$ |
| | $\bar{x} = 5$ | | $\bar{x} = 6.471$ | | $\bar{x} = 8.118$ | | $\bar{x} = 6.824$ | |

## Calculating the Friedman test

In order to calculate the Friedman you must take the following steps.

**1.** Firstly, add up the scores for each condition, i.e.

$$\Sigma A = 85 \quad \Sigma B = 110 \quad \Sigma C = 138 \quad \Sigma D = 116$$

2. Find out the means for each condition

$$\bar{x}A = 5 \quad \bar{x}B = 6.471 \quad \bar{x}C = 8.118 \quad \bar{x}D = 6.824$$

**3.** Rank the scores for each subject (i.e. *across* the row) giving the rank of 1 to the smallest score, a rank of 2 to the next smallest and so on. You will only need ranks 1–4 as there are only four scores for each subject. Where you have tied scores, use the tied rank procedure (see pages 125–126) i.e. add up the ranks these scores would have had if they had been different, and divide by the number of scores which are the same. Therefore, if we look at subject 2, she scored 5 in cardiothoracic, 6 in geriatric, 6 in neurology and 7 in orthopaedics. Thus 5 gets a rank of 1; the two 6s, had they been different would have had ranks of 2 and 3 (because rank 1 has now been used up); so we add 2 and 3 to get 5, and divide this by the total number of scores which are the same (i.e. 2, because there are 2 scores of 6), giving 2.5. This, then is the rank we give the 6s. The score of 7 in orthopaedics gets a rank of 4 because ranks 1–3 have been used up.

**4.** Now add up the ranks for each condition (i.e. for each clinical setting). This is called $T_C$.

$$T_C \text{ for A} = 24 \quad T_C \text{ for B} = 39.5$$
$$T_C \text{ for C} = 65 \quad T_C \text{ for D} = 41.5$$

**5.** You now have to find the value of $\chi r^2$ from the following formula:

$$\chi r^2 = \left[\left(\frac{12}{NC(C+1)}\right)(\Sigma T_C^2)\right] - 3N(C+1)$$

where   $N$   = number of Ss in the group (or in the case of matched designs, the number of sets of subjects) i.e. 17

        $C$   = number of conditions i.e. 4

        $T_C$   = total of the ranks for each condition

$T_C$ for condition A = 24
$T_C$ for condition B = 39.5
$T_C$ for condition C = 65
$T_C$ for condition D = 41.5

$T_C^2$   = each rank total squared
     i.e: $24^2$; $39.5^2$; $65^2$; $41.5^2$
     = 576; 1560.25; 4225; 1722.25

$\Sigma$   = sum or total of all the calculations following it

$\Sigma T_C^2$ = the sum of the squared ranks for each condition i.e.,
     576 + 1560.25 + 4225 + 1722.25
     = 8083.5

Remember! Do all the calculations in brackets first, starting with divisions and multiplications and finally additions and subtractions.

Thus, if we substitute some values in the formula, then:

$$\chi r^2 = \left[\left(\frac{12}{17 \times 4(4+1)}\right) \times 8083.5\right] - 3 \times 17(4+1)$$

$$= \left[\left(\frac{12}{68 \times 5}\right) \times 8083.5\right] - 255$$

$$[0.035 \times 8083.5] - 255$$

$$= 282.923 - 255$$

$$\chi r^2 = 27.923$$

## Looking up the value of $\chi r^2$

To look up $\chi r^2$ in the tables, you also need the degrees of freedom value. This is the number of conditions minus 1, i.e. 4 – 1 = 3. As you will see, there are three main tables for the Friedman test: Tables A2.3a, A2.3b (pages 211, 212) and A2.1 (page 209). Table A2.3a is used where there are three conditions and only 2–9 subjects in each condition; Table A2.3b is for four conditions, with 2–4 Ss in each, and Table A2.1 is for anything larger, i.e. more conditions or more subjects.

Because we have four conditions and 17 subjects, we must use Table A2.1. (This table is also for use with the $\chi^2$ test.) You will see that in the left-hand column, entitled 'df', there are various degrees of freedom values. Look down this column until you have found the df for this example, i.e. 3. You will see five numbers, called critical values, to the right:

6.25   7.82   9.84   11.34   16.27

Each of these values is associated with the level of probability shown at the top of its column, e.g. 11.34 is associated with a $p$ value of 0.01. To be significant at a given level, our $\chi r^2$ value must be *equal to* or *larger than* the values here. So, if we take the first value 6.25, our $\chi r^2$ value is larger; it is also larger than 7.82, 9.84, 11.34 and 16.27. Therefore we take the value 16.27 and look up the column to see what the associated level of significance is, i.e. 0.001 or the 0.1% level. Because our $\chi r^2$ value of 27.923 is larger than the critical value of 16.27, this means that our results are significant at less than ($<$) the 0.001 level. (Had our $\chi r^2$ value been 16.27 exactly, we would say our $p$ value equals 0.001.)

This means that there is less than a 0.1% chance that our results are due to random error.

Note that because the Friedman only allows you to predict differences and not specific directions to the results, your hypothesis must be two-tailed and so this level of significance represents the level for a two-tailed hypothesis. Because our usual cut-off point is 5% and our $p$ value is less than that, i.e. 0.1%, we can say that our results are significant at $< 0.1\%$ level.

### Interpreting the results

The results are associated with a $p$ value of less than 0.1%. This means that there is less than a 0.1% probability of our results being due to random error. As the standard cut-off point is 5%, we can reject our null hypothesis and say that our results are significant. In other words, students do perform differently in a variety of clinical settings. We can express this in the following way:

> Using a Friedman test on the data ($\chi r^2$ = 27.923, $N$ = 17), the results were found to be significant at $p < 0.001$, for a two-tailed test. This suggests that 3rd-year physiotherapy students perform significantly differently in four clinical settings, and so supports the experimental hypothesis. The null hypothesis can therefore be rejected.

Do note, however, that the Friedman only allows us to identify differences and not to say in which setting they performed better. If, however, you do expect a trend in the results of a related or matched-subject design (e.g. that students do worst in geriatrics, followed by cardiothoracic, followed by neurology and best in orthopaedics) you would need the Page's L trend test (see next section).

If you had only three conditions and fewer subjects then you would use Table A2.3a. For example, supposing you had three conditions and seven subjects, and a $\chi r^2$ value of 7.5, you would look to find your value of $N$ across the top of the table, (remember $N$ = the number of Ss or subject pairs). Under this you will see a column for the $\chi r^2$ value, and to the right the corresponding $p$ value or significance level. So taking the column for $N$ = 7, look down the $\chi r^2$ value to find 7.5. Since our $\chi r^2$ value must be equal to or larger than those given to be significant at a particular level, we find that our value of 7.5 is larger than 7.143, but smaller than 7.714. We must take the critical value of 7.143 (because our $\chi r^2$ value must be equal to or larger than the critical value given) which gives us a corresponding $p$ value of 0.027 or 2.7%.

However, because our $\chi r^2$ value of 7.5 is larger than 7.143, this means our $p$ value is even less than ($<$) 0.027. Had our $\chi r^2$ value equalled the critical value of 7.143, we would say that our $p$ value equals 0.027. So, our results have a $p$ value of $<0.027$. Using the standard cut-off of 0.05, we can say our results are significant. We can therefore reject the null hypothesis, and accept the experimental hypothesis.

Supposing, however, we had four conditions, and four subjects or pairs of subjects and a $\chi r^2$ value of 2.6, we would need to use Table A2.3b which is for use with four conditions and 2–4 Ss. Here we would find the column corresponding to our $N$ value, and look down the $\chi r^2$ values to find our own of 2.6. Because our value has to be equal to or larger than the values given to be significant at a given level, we can see that our $\chi r^2$ value of 2.6 is larger than 2.4 but smaller than 2.7. Therefore we have to take the value next smallest to our own, i.e. 2.4, which gives us a $p$ value of 0.524 or 52.4%. Because of our standard 5% cut-off point, this $p$ value cannot be classified as significant because it is larger. Therefore we would have to conclude that our results were not significant, our hypothesis was not supported and we would have to accept the null (no relationship) hypothesis.

---

**Activity 13.3** (Answers on page 232)

1 To practise looking up $\chi r^2$ values, look up the following and say whether they are significant.
  (i)   $C = 4$   $N = 3$   $\chi r^2 = 7.4$   $p$
  (ii)  $C = 4$   $N = 10$  $\chi r^2 = 9.92$  $p$
  (iii) $C = 3$   $N = 6$   $\chi r^2 = 5.72$  $p$
  (iv)  $C = 3$   $N = 12$  $\chi r^2 = 35.7$  $p$
  (v)   $C = 3$   $N = 8$   $\chi r^2 = 9.3$   $p$

2 Calculate a Friedman on the following data:
  $H_1$  The muscle tone of the quadriceps differs for Asian, Caucasian and African-Caribbean children.
  Method: Select seven children in each ethnic group, matched for age, sex, fitness, activity levels and compare their muscle tone, using a 5-point scale: 5 = very high tone and 1 = very poor tone.
    You might obtain the results shown in Table 13.8.

**Table 13.8**

| Subject | Condition A Asian | Condition B Caucasian | Condition C African-Caribbean |
|---|---|---|---|
| 1 | 3 | 4 | 5 |
| 2 | 2 | 2 | 5 |
| 3 | 2 | 3 | 4 |
| 4 | 1 | 2 | 3 |
| 5 | 3 | 2 | 2 |
| 6 | 1 | 2 | 1 |
| 7 | 3 | 3 | 3 |

Write down the $\chi r^2$ value and the $p$ value. State whether or not your results are significant, and what they mean, using the example given on page 129.

## 2. Page's *L* trend test

This test is an extension of the Friedman test, in that it is used when

a. the design is a same- or matched-subject one
b. the data is ordinal or interval/ratio
c. there are three or more conditions (i.e. one group of Ss doing three or more conditions, or three or more matched groups of Ss each doing one condition).

However, there is one salient difference: whereas the Friedman test can only be used to discover whether there are differences between the conditions without saying which condition is significantly bettter or worse than the others, the Page's *L* trend test is used when the experimenter

had predicted a *trend* in the results. For example when comparing the quality of three schools of physiotherapy, the experimenter, in the hypothesis, predicts that School A is better than School B, which in turn is better than School C. This contrasts with the sort of hypothesis which must be used with the Friedman test, which would simply predict differences in quality between the three schools. Thus we might have the following types of design with the Page's *L* trend test.

1. In a comparison of a group of students' attitudes to three types of teaching method, it is predicted that the seminar method will be most popular, followed by the lecture method, with tutorials least popular. The design in Figure 13.10 could be used.

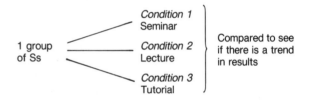

**Figure 13.10** Design for assessing popularity of teaching methods.

2. In a comparison of three types of exercise techniques following prostatectomy, it is predicted that Exercise A will be more effective than Exercise B which will be more effective than Exercise C. Three groups of patients, matched for age, duration of illness, length of postoperative time, severity of illness, etc., are given one of the exercise regimes and compared for continence after 1 month. This design shown in Figure 13.11 is used.

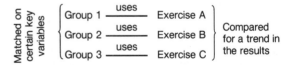

**Figure 13.11** Design for assessing effectiveness of exercise techniques.

The Page's *L* trend test then essentially assesses whether there is a significant trend in the results. When calculating it you derive the value of *L*, which is then looked up in the probability tables associated with the Page's test to see whether this value represents a significant trend in your results.

Because you are predicting a *specific direction* to the results when you use a Page's $L$ trend test, the hypothesis must be one-tailed.

### Example

Let's take the first hypothesis that in order to evaluate students' preferences for three types of teaching approach, you predict that the seminar method will be more popular than the lecture method, with the tutorial being least popular; a trend is predicted, i.e. seminar > lecture > tutorial (> means 'greater than').

You select a group of 10 students and ask them to rate the three methods on a 5-point scale (5 = most preferred, 1 = least preferred). In order to analyse the results you must set out your data such that the scores you predict will be the smallest (i.e. tutorial) are placed on the left, and the scores you predict to be the largest are placed on the right as in Table 13.9.

### Calculating the Page's L trend test

**1.** In order to calculate the value of $L$ you must take the following steps: First find the total scores for each condition:

$$\Sigma_1 = 20 \quad \Sigma_2 = 32 \quad \Sigma_3 = 38$$

Then find the mean score for each condition

$$\bar{x}_1 = 2 \quad \bar{x}_2 = 3.2 \quad \bar{x}_3 = 3.8$$

**2.** Rank the scores for each subject (or sets of matched Ss) across the row, as for the Friedman, giving the rank of 1 to the lowest score, the rank of 2 to the next lowest etc. If you have two or more scores which are the same, you must give these the average rank (see pages 125–126 on how to deal with tied scores), i.e. you add up the value of the ranks they would have obtained had they been different and divide by the number of scores that are the same. For example, S1 has two scores of 3. Had these scores been the two lowest but different scores they would have had the ranks 1 and 2. These rank values are added together (3) and divided by 2 (because there are two scores of 3) to give the average rank, 1.5, which is entered alongside the scores of 3.

**3.** Add up the ranks for each condition, i.e.

$$T_{C1} = 12 \quad T_{C2} = 22.5 \quad T_{C3} = 25.5$$

**4.** Find the value of $L$ from the formula

$$L = \Sigma(T_{C1} \times C) + \Sigma(T_{C2} \times C) + \Sigma(T_{C3} \times C)$$

where $\Sigma$ = the total or sum of any symbols that follow it

$T_C$ = total of ranks for each condition,
i.e. $T_{C1} = 12; \quad T_{C2} = 22.5; \quad T_{C3} = 25.5$

**Table 13.9**

| Subject | Condition 1 Tutorial | | Condition 2 Lecture | | Condition 3 Seminar | |
|---|---|---|---|---|---|---|
| | Score | Rank | Score | Rank | Score | Rank |
| 1 | 3 | 1.5 | 4 | 3 | 3 | 1.5 |
| 2 | 2 | 1.5 | 2 | 1.5 | 4 | 3 |
| 3 | 3 | 1.5 | 3 | 1.5 | 5 | 3 |
| 4 | 1 | 1 | 3 | 3 | 2 | 2 |
| 5 | 2 | 1.5 | 3 | 3 | 2 | 1.5 |
| 6 | 2 | 1 | 4 | 2 | 5 | 3 |
| 7 | 1 | 1 | 2 | 2 | 4 | 3 |
| 8 | 3 | 1 | 4 | 2.5 | 4 | 2.5 |
| 9 | 2 | 1 | 4 | 2 | 5 | 3 |
| 10 | 1 | 1 | 3 | 2 | 4 | 3 |
| | $\Sigma_1 = 20$ | $T_{C1} = 12$ | $\Sigma_2 = 32$ | $T_{C2} = 22.5$ | $\Sigma_3 = 38$ | $T_{C3} = 25.5$ |

$C$ = numbers allotted to the conditions from left to right
i.e. 1, 2 and 3

$(T_C \times C$ = total of the ranks for each condition multiplied by the number assigned to the condition

i.e. $T_{C1} \times 1 = 12 \times 1$
$T_{C2} \times 2 = 22.5 \times 2$
$T_{C3} \times 3 = 25.5 \times 3$

Substituting some values in the formula:

$L = (12 \times 1) + (22.5 \times 2) + (25.5 \times 3)$
$= 12 + 45 + 76.5$
$= 133.5$

**5.** To look up your value of $L$, you also need two further values: $C$, the number of conditions, i.e. 3; and $N$, the number of Ss in the group or the number of sets of matched Ss, i.e. 10.

### Looking up the value of L for significance

Turn to Table A2.4 (page 213). Across the top you will see values of $C$ (i.e. number of conditions) from 3 to 6, and down the left-hand column, values of $N$ (i.e. number of Ss or sets of matched Ss) from 2 to 12. Look across the $C$ values to find our value of $C$ = 3 and down the $N$ values to find our $N$ = 10 value.

At their intersection point you will see three numbers:

134
131
128

These are called critical values of $L$. If you look across these rows to the right-hand column, you will see that 134 represents a $p$ value of 0.001; 131 represents a $p$ value of 0.01 and 128 represents a $p$ value of 0.05. To be significant at one of these levels, your $L$ value must be *equal to* or *larger than* one of the numbers 134, 131 and 128. The obtained value of $L$ in our example is 133.5. This is larger than 131, but smaller than 134. Therefore we must take the value of 131, which represents a significance level of 0.01 or 1%. But because our $L$ value is larger than the critical value of 131, this means that the corresponding $p$ value is less than (<) 0.01. This is expressed as $p<0.01$. This means that there is less than a 1%

chance of the results being caused by random error. Because you must be predicting a specific direction to your results in order to be using a trend test, your hypothesis, by definition, must be one-tailed. Therefore, all the values in this table are values for a one-tailed hypothesis.

Using our usual cut-off point of 5%, because the $p$ value in our study is smaller, we can conclude that our results are significant at <0.01 level. Thus we can reject the null hypothesis and conclude that there is a significant trend in results as predicted in our hypothesis.

### Interpreting the results

Our results have a probability value of <0.01 which means that there is less than a 1% chance of their being due to random error. Because this $p$ value is smaller than the usual cut-off point of 0.05, we can say that our results are significant. This means we can reject the null hypothesis and accept the experimental hypothesis.

This can be expressed in the following way:

Using a Page's $L$ trend test on the data ($L$ = 133.5, $N$ = 10, $C$ = 3), the results were found to be significant at $p < 0.01$ for a one-tailed hypothesis. This suggests that the experimental hypothesis has been supported, and that students prefer seminar teaching methods to lectures, with tutorials being the least preferred approach. The null hypothesis can therefore be rejected.

**Activity 13.4** (Answers on page 232)

1 To practise looking up $L$ values, look up the following and decide at what level (if any) they are significant:
   (i)   $N = 5$   $C = 4$   $L = 142.5$   $p$
   (ii)  $N = 8$   $C = 5$   $L = 384$     $p$
   (iii) $N = 7$   $C = 3$   $L = 92$      $p$
   (iv)  $N = 12$  $C = 6$   $L = 971$     $p$
   (v)   $N = 10$  $C = 5$   $L = 455.5$   $p$

2 Calculate a Page's $L$ trend test on the following data:
   $H_1$  It is hypothesised that hydrotherapy is more effective than exercise which in turn is more effective than massage for mobilising lower limbs paralysed following a stroke.
   Method: Take three groups, each of eight subjects, matched for severity of paralysis, age, sex, previous health, length of time since stroke and other treatments, and give each group one of the three treatment procedures. After 1 month compare the percentage range of movement regained. The results are as shown in Table 13.10.

**Table 13.10**

| Subject trio | Condition 1 Hydrotherapy | | Condition 2 Massage | | Condition 3 Exercise | |
|---|---|---|---|---|---|---|
| | Score | Rank | Score | Rank | Score | Rank |
| 1 | 40 | | 25 | | 30 | |
| 2 | 55 | | 30 | | 40 | |
| 3 | 35 | | 35 | | 45 | |
| 4 | 20 | | 30 | | 40 | |
| 5 | 30 | | 20 | | 30 | |
| 6 | 50 | | 45 | | 50 | |
| 7 | 55 | | 45 | | 55 | |
| 8 | 60 | | 50 | | 60 | |

State your $L$ and $p$ values, using the sample format given on page 132.

Remember! Put the scores which are predicted to be the lowest in the left-hand column and those predicted to be the highest in the right-hand column. In other words, you will need to rearrange the table.

Remember, too, that the data in this example is of an interval/ratio type, which can be used with both non-parametric and parametric tests.

# Parametric tests for same- and matched-subject designs

## INTRODUCTION

All the statistical tests described in this chapter, like those in the previous one, are used to analyse the results from same-subject or matched-subject designs; in other words, those designs which either use one group of subjects for all the conditions, or alternatively, two or more groups of matched subjects who do one condition each (see pages 67–69 for the designs).

There is one major difference, however; all the tests in this chapter are parametric, which means that they require certain conditions to be fulfilled before they can be used, in particular that the data must be of an interval/ratio level. This requirement concerning the level of data can never, ever be violated. Parametric tests are also rather more difficult to calculate than non-parametric tests. You should always remember that for any given design, the relevant parametric and non-parametric tests do the same job: they assess whether there are significant differences (or in the case of correlations, similarities) between the conditions, but the parametric tests are more sensitive to these differences.

The designs we are interested in then are as follows:

**1. Same-subject design:** One group of subjects used in all the conditions (same-subject design)
   a. Two conditions only (Fig. 14.1).

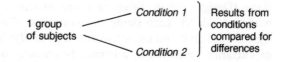

**Figure 14.1**  One group of subject tested under two conditions.

or

b. Three or more conditions (Fig. 14.2).

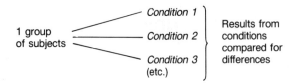

**Figure 14.2** One group of subjects tested under three or more conditions.

**2. Matched-subject design:** Two or more groups of matched subjects, each of which is used in one condition only (matched-subject designs)

a. Two matched groups only (Fig. 14.3).

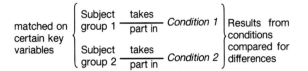

**Figure 14.3** Two groups of matched subjects each tested under one condition.

b. Three or more matched groups (Fig. 14.4).

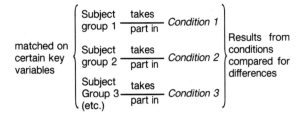

**Figure 14.4** Three or more groups of matched subjects, each tested under one condition.

Results from designs which use one group of subjects in both of two conditions (Design 1a) or two groups of matched subjects, each doing one condition (Design 2a) are analysed using the **related *t* test**.

Results from designs using one group of subjects who take part in all three (or more) conditions (Design 1b) or three or more groups of matched subjects each doing one condition (Design 2b) are analysed using the **one-way analysis of variance**, or **anova** as it is usually known, for related designs.

In addition we shall look at the **Scheffé multiple range** test which is used in conjunction with the anova (see the relevant section).

This is summarised in Table 14.1.

**Table 14.1** Parametric tests for related- and matched-subject designs

| Design | Parametric test |
|---|---|
| 1a. One group of Ss tested in two conditions | Related *t* test |
| 2a. Two groups of matched Ss, each tested in one condition only | Related *t* test |
| 1b. One group of Ss tested under three or more conditions | One-way anova for related designs, to be used with the Scheffé multiple range test |
| 2b. Three or more groups of matched Ss, each tested in one condition only | One-way anova for related designs, to be used with the Scheffé multiple range test |

It should be noted that the *t* test is sometimes referred to as 'Student's *t*' in some texts.

## PARAMETRIC TEST: ONE GROUP OF SUBJECTS AND TWO CONDITIONS, OR TWO GROUPS OF MATCHED SUBJECTS DOING ONE CONDITION EACH

### Related *t* test

Just to recap, this test is used for exactly the same designs as the Wilcoxon, in other words, where one group of subjects takes part in both of two conditions (a same-subjects design), and the results form the two conditions are then compared for differences. Alternatively, the related *t* test is used where you have two groups of matched subjects, who do one condition each (a matched-subject design) and again the results from the two conditions are compared to see if there are differences between them.

The related *t* test is especially suitable for 'before and after' type designs, for instance, when you wish to compare the effects of a treatment on one group of subjects.

When calculating the $t$ test, you find a value for '$t$', which you then look up in the probability tables for the $t$ test to see whether this value represents significant differences between the results from each condition. Remember that parametric tests are more difficult to calculate than non-parametric tests, so don't panic when you look at the formula. As long as you work through the stages systematically, you will have no difficulty.

### Example

Let's suppose you are in charge of a large physiotherapy department and it has been brought to your notice that the eight basic grade physiotherapists seem to show a distinct preference for treating young male sports injury leg fracture patients as opposed to elderly male leg fracture patients. You have challenged them about this but they deny it, so you want to produce some empirical support for your assertion.

Your experimental hypothesis, then, is:

H₁ That young male leg fracture patients receive more attention from basic grade physiotherapists than do elderly leg fracture patients.

This is a one-tailed hypothesis as it predicts a specific direction to the results.

(Note: In case this appears to be an unlikely hypothesis, there is a huge literature on the ways in which physical appearance can affect how we behave towards one another. Darbyshire (1986) and Hicks (1993) both provide overviews of some of this research as it applies to health care situations.)

To test your hypothesis, you measure the length of time each physiotherapist spends with her three sports injury fracture patients in the course of one day and total this up in minutes. You do the same for the period spent with her three elderly leg fracture patients. Because time is an interval/ratio measurement the most necessary condition for using a parametric test can be fulfilled.

Therefore you have the design shown in Figure 14.5.

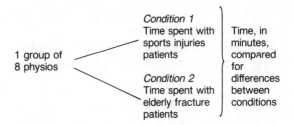

**Figure 14.5** Design of experiment to assess whether physiotherapists spend more time with sports injury patients than with elderly fracture patients.

Your results are as shown in Table 14.2.

### Calculating the related t test

To calculate the related t test, you must:

**1.** Add up the scores for each condition to give the total ($\Sigma$), i.e.:

$$\Sigma A = 461 \qquad \Sigma B = 401$$

**2.** Calculate the mean score ($\bar{x}$) for each condition, i.e.:

$$\bar{x}A = 57.625 \qquad xB = 50.125$$

**3.** Calculate the difference ($d$) between each

**Table 14.2**

| 1 Subject | Results from experiment | | Calculations* | |
| --- | --- | --- | --- | --- |
| | 2 Condition 1 Sports injury | 3 Condition 2 Elderly patients | 4 d (A – B) | 5 d² |
| 1 | 49 | 42 | + 7 | 49 |
| 2 | 57 | 45 | + 12 | 144 |
| 3 | 72 | 65 | + 7 | 49 |
| 4 | 64 | 65 | – 1 | 1 |
| 5 | 50 | 60 | – 10 | 100 |
| 6 | 45 | 35 | + 10 | 100 |
| 7 | 59 | 40 | + 19 | 361 |
| 8 | 65 | 49 | + 16 | 256 |
| $\Sigma$ | 461 | 401 | $\Sigma d = 60$ | $\Sigma d^2 = 1060$ |
| $\bar{x}$ | 57.625 | 50.125 | | |

*It does not matter which group of patients is called Condition A and which Condition B.

subject's pair of scores and enter this in column 4; i.e. for each subject take the score of Condition B away from the score of Condition A (e.g. for S1, 49 – 42 = 7). Remember to put in the plus and minus signs for each $d$ value.

**4.** Add these differences up to give $\Sigma d$, remembering to take account of the plus and minus values, i.e.:

$$\Sigma d = 60$$

**5.** Square each difference to give $d^2$, e.g. $7^2 = 49$, and enter these in column 5 $(d^2)$.

**6.** Add up the $d^2$ values to give $\Sigma d^2$, i.e.:

$$\Sigma d^2 = 1060$$

**7.** Square the total of the differences, i.e.:

$$60^2 = 3600 = (\Sigma d)^2.$$

It is important to recognise the difference in meaning between

$\Sigma d^2$ (stage 6) which means to add up all the squared differences

and $(\Sigma d)^2$ (Stage 7) which means to add up all the differences and square the total.

**8.** Find the $t$ from the following formula:

$$t = \frac{\Sigma d}{\sqrt{\dfrac{N\Sigma d^2 - (\Sigma d)^2}{N-1}}}$$

where $\Sigma d$ = the total of the differences (i.e. 60)
  $(\Sigma d)^2$ = the total of the differences, squared (i.e. 3600)
  $\Sigma d^2$ = the total of the squared differences (i.e. 1060)
  $N$ = number of subjects, or pairs of matched subjects (i.e. 8)
  $\sqrt{\phantom{x}}$ = the square root of the final calculation of everything under the square root sign.

If we substitute some values, then:

$$t = \frac{60}{\sqrt{\dfrac{8 \times 1060 - 3600}{8-1}}}$$

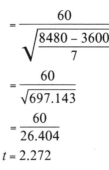

$$= \frac{60}{\sqrt{\dfrac{8480 - 3600}{7}}}$$

$$= \frac{60}{\sqrt{697.143}}$$

$$= \frac{60}{26.404}$$

$$t = 2.272$$

*Looking up the value of* t

To see whether this $t$ value is significant you need one further value, the degrees of freedom, which here is the number of subjects minus 1, i.e. 8 – 1 = 7.

Turn to Table A2.5 (page 214). You will see down the left-hand margin a number of df values. Look down the column until you find the df value of 7. To the right of that you will see six critical values of $t$ in the main body of the table:

1.415  1.895  2.365  2.998  3.499  5.405

If your value of t is equal to or larger than any of the given values, it is significant at the level indicated at the top of the column. For example, 3.499 has an associated $p$ value of 0.005 for a one-tailed test and 0.01 for a two-tailed test. So, if we look at the numbers, we can see that our $t$ value of 2.272 is larger than 1.895 but smaller than 2.365. This means that the probability associated with our $t$ value of 2.272 is somewhere between 0.05 and 0.025 for a one-tailed hypothesis. In other words the $p$ value for $t = 2.272$ must be smaller than 0.05 (or 5%) and larger than 0.025 (or 2½%).

We would therefore say that for our study and our one-tailed hypothesis, the results are significant at less than 0.05 (or 5%). Because of convention, we would never say that $p$ is greater than 0.025 and so we must focus on the value of 1.895 in the table.

We express this as: $p < 0.05$ (< means 'less than'). Had our $t$ value been exactly the same as the critical value of 1.895 in the table, we would have said that $p = 0.05$.

## Interpreting the results

Our results have an associated probability of less than 0.05, which means that the chances of random error accounting for the outcome of our experiment are less than 5 in 100. Because the usual cut-off point for claiming that the results are significant is 5%, we can conclude that our results are significant, at less than the 5% level.

However, because we have a one-tailed hypothesis we can only say that our hypothesis has been supported if the results are in the direction predicted. This means that providing the average amount of time spent with the sports injury patients is greater than the average amount of time spent with the elderly leg fracture patients, we can reject the null hypothesis and accept that our experimental hypothesis has been supported. Since the averages are 57.625 and 50.125 minutes respectively, the results are in the predicted direction and we can conclude that basic grade physiotherapists spend significantly more time with young sports injury patients than with elderly leg fracture patients. We can state this as follows:

> Using a related t test on the data (t = 2.272, N = 8), the results are significant at $p < 0.05$, for a one-tailed test. The experimental hypothesis has been supported, suggesting that young male fracture patients receive significantly more treatment time from basic grade physiotherapists, than do elderly male fracture patients. The null hypothesis can therefore be rejected.

Remember, had the average time been reversed (i.e. more time spent with the elderly patients), we could not claim that the hypothesis had been supported.

---

**Activity 14.1** (Answers on page 232)

1 To practise looking up t values, look up the following and say whether or not they are significant and at what level.
   (i)   df = 11   t = 2.406   one-tailed  p
   (ii)  df = 14   t = 1.895   two-tailed  p
   (iii) df = 19   t = 2.739   one-tailed  p
   (iv)  df = 7    t = 3.204   one-tailed  p
   (v)   df = 9    t = 2.973   two-tailed  p

2 Calculate a related t test on the following data:
   H₁ Student physiotherapists with 'A'-level physics do better on their 1st year theory exam than students without 'A'-level physics.
   Is this hypothesis one- or two-tailed?
   Method: Select two groups, each of 12 students, matched on certain key features such as overall 'A'-level points,

attendance levels, quality of teaching etc. Of these, one group has 'A'-level physics and the other does not. Compare the performance of the two groups on their 1st year theory exam. The marks are as shown in Table 14.3.

**Table 14.3**

| 1 Subject pair | Results from experiment | | Calculations | |
|---|---|---|---|---|
| | 2 Condition 1 'A'-level physics | 3 Condition 2 No 'A'-level physics | 4 d | 5 $d_2$ |
| 1 | 64 | 68 | | |
| 2 | 59 | 60 | | |
| 3 | 72 | 62 | | |
| 4 | 68 | 58 | | |
| 5 | 58 | 49 | | |
| 6 | 70 | 62 | | |
| 7 | 65 | 61 | | |
| 8 | 62 | 50 | | |
| 9 | 73 | 71 | | |
| 10 | 45 | 49 | | |
| 11 | 56 | 54 | | |
| 12 | 67 | 68 | | |

State the t value, the df value, and the p value expressed in a similar format to that on this page.

# PARAMETRIC TESTS: ONE GROUP OF SUBJECTS AND THREE OR MORE CONDITIONS, OR THREE OR MORE GROUPS OF MATCHED SUBJECTS

## One-way analysis of variance (anova) for related- and matched-subject designs

The one-way anova for related- and matched-subject designs is the parametric equivalent of the Friedman test. In others words it is used for designs which use one subject group in three or more conditions, and the results from these conditions are compared for differences between them. Alternatively, it is used where the experimenter has got three or more groups of matched subjects who do one condition each. The results from each condition are compared for differences (see Designs 1b and 2b page 138).

It is called a 'one-way' anova because it only deals with experiments which manipulate one independent variable. If you ever hypothesised a relationship between two independent variables and a DV (see Ch. 6) you would require a two-way anova, or, in extremis, a relationship between three independent variables and a DV, then you would require a three-way anova. However, these are outside the scope of this book and the reader is referred to Greene & D'Oliveira (1982) and Ferguson (1976).

Like all parametric tests, the data must be of an interval/ratio level, and the remaining three conditions should be more or less fulfilled.

When calculating an anova you find a value for 'F' which is then looked up in the probability tables for anovas to find out whether this value represents a significant difference between conditions. Like the Friedman test, the anova only tells us whether there are overall differences between conditions, and not the direction of the differences, and so the hypothesis must be two-tailed.

### Example

Because the anova is quite complicated to calculate, it may be helpful to explain its purpose beforehand. Let's imagine that you have noticed that your senior grade II physiotherapists seem to show a high degree of clinical skill but they seem less competent in their supervision of trainees and in their interpersonal skills. Obviously, if your observations are correct, you will need to do some staff development on the weaker areas. You therefore decide to make an evaluation of a group of 10 senior grade II physiotherapists in the three different aspects of their job: clinical skills, inter-personal skills and supervision skills.

Your hypothesis then is

H$_1$  Senior II physiotherapists show different levels of professional competence in three aspects of their job: clinical, supervisory and interpersonal skills.

To see if there is any difference in the competence shown in these areas you decide to compare the performance of the group on each aspect, giving marks out of 20. As this is an interval/ratio scale of measurement, we can fulfil this requirement of a parametric test.

Therefore we have the design shown in Figure 14.6.

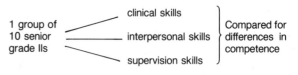

**Figure 14.6** Design for comparison of differences in various skills in physiotherapists.

Further suppose that you have collected and set out the results which look as shown in Table 14.4.

**Table 14.4**

| Subject | Condition 1 Clinical | Condition 2 Interpersonal | Condition 3 Supervisory | Total for Ss $T_S$ |
|---|---|---|---|---|
| 1 | 15 | 12 | 11 | 38 |
| 2 | 12 | 9 | 8 | 29 |
| 3 | 13 | 10 | 11 | 34 |
| 4 | 10 | 10 | 12 | 32 |
| 5 | 17 | 14 | 10 | 41 |
| 6 | 8 | 12 | 11 | 31 |
| 7 | 11 | 12 | 9 | 32 |
| 8 | 14 | 9 | 9 | 32 |
| 9 | 16 | 8 | 12 | 36 |
| 10 | 10 | 9 | 8 | 27 |
| Total $T_C$ | $T_{C1}$ = 126 | $T_{C2}$ = 105 | $T_{C3}$ = 101 | Grand total = 332 |

You are hypothesising that the performance of the group varies according to the aspect of the job, and therefore you would expect there to be significant differences or *variations* between the condition totals (126, 105 and 101). This, obviously, is one potential source of variation in the results and is called a *between–conditions* comparison.

However, because each subject is assessed on all three conditions, we can also compare the overall performances of the subjects, to see if there is any variation in competence between the physiotherapists, i.e. a comparison of all the $T_S$ totals. This comparison allows us to look at another potential source of variation in the scores: a *between–the–subjects* comparison. This is illustrated in Figure 14.7 for the example given above using the data from the first five subjects:

The solid vertical lines in Figure 14.7 indicate the comparisons which can be made between conditions, to see if there is any difference in

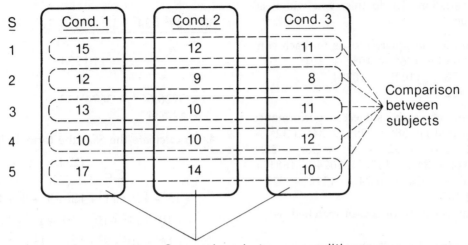

| S | Cond. 1 | Cond. 2 | Cond. 3 |
|---|---------|---------|---------|
| 1 | 15 | 12 | 11 |
| 2 | 12 | 9 | 8 |
| 3 | 13 | 10 | 11 |
| 4 | 10 | 10 | 12 |
| 5 | 17 | 14 | 10 |

Comparison between subjects

Comparison between conditions

**Figure 14.7** There is variation between the subjects and variation between the conditions.

performance on each aspect of the job, as was hypothesised. This comparison concentrates on one source of potential variation in the results: the between-conditions variation.

The dotted lines indicate the comparisons which can be made between subjects, to see if there is any difference in the overall performances among the subjects. This comparison concentrates on a second potential source of variation in the results: the between-subject variation.

There is, of course, a third source of potential variation in scores: that due to random error.

If we consider these sources of variation for a moment, it can be seen that ideally what we would hope to find from our anova is:

a. significant differences between the performance of the job tasks, i.e. a significant *between-conditions* comparison, since this was what was hypothesised, and
b. no significant differences between the subjects, since this would suggest that they were a fairly representative and similar sample.

The purpose of the one-way related anova is to find out whether any of these sources of variation are responsible for significant differences in results.

In order to do this, we need a number of values:

the sums of squares      ($SS$)
the degrees of freedom    (df)
the mean squares        ($MS$)
the F ratios            ($F$)

for each source of variation. When these have been calculated they are entered into a table the format of which is shown in Table 14.5.

**Table 14.5**

| Source of variation of scores | Sums of squares ($SS$) | Degress of freedom (df) | Mean squares ($MS$) | F ratios ($F$) |
|---|---|---|---|---|
| Variation between conditions, i.e. aspects of job | $SS_{bet}$ | $df_{bet}$ | $MS_{bet}$ | $F_{bet}$ |
| Variation between subjects' overall performance | $SS_{subj}$ | $df_{subj}$ | $MS_{subj}$ | $F_{subj}$ |
| Variation due to random error | $SS_{error}$ | $df_{error}$ | $MS_{error}$ | |
| Total | $SS_{tot}$ | $df_{tot}$ | | |

Firstly, do not panic – the calculations are surprisingly easy, if rather laborious! Follow the steps described below (the data are on page 142).

*Calculating the one-way anova*

**1.** We must first calculate the $SS$ values for each

source of variation. To do this, you will need several values:

$\Sigma T_C^2$ = sum of the squared totals for each condition i.e. $126^2 + 105^2 + 101^2$
= 15876 + 11025 + 10201
= 37102

$\Sigma T_S^2$ = sum of each subject's performance squared i.e. $38^2 + 29^2 + 34^2 + 32^2 + 41^2 + 31^2 + 32^2 + 32^2 + 36^2 + 27^2$
= 1444 + 841 + 1156 + 1024 + 1681 + 961 + 1024 + 1024 + 1296 + 729
= 11 180

$n$ = number of Ss or sets of matched Ss
= 10

$C$ = number of conditions
= 3

$N$ = total number of scores, i.e. $n \times C$
= 30

$\Sigma x$ = grand total (of scores)
= 332

$(\Sigma x)^2$ = grand total squared
= $332^2$
= 110 224

$\dfrac{(\Sigma x)^2}{N}$ = a constant to be substracted from all SS
= $\dfrac{110\ 224}{30}$
= 3674.133

$x$ = each individual score

$\Sigma x^2$ = the sum of each squared individual score
= $15^2 + 12^2 + 11^2 + 12^2 + 9^2 + 8^2 + 13^2 + 10^2$
$+ 11^2 + 10^2 + 10^2 + 12^2 + 17^2 + 14^2 + 10^2$
$+ 8^2 + 12^2 + 11^2 + 11^2 + 12^2 + 9^2 + 14^2 + 9^2$
$+ 9^2 + 16^2 + 8^2 + 12^2 + 10^2 + 9^2 + 8^2$
= 3840

2. To calculate the $SS_{bet}$ the formula is:

$$\frac{\Sigma T_C^2}{n} - \frac{(\Sigma x)^2}{N}$$

$$= \frac{126^2 + 105^2 + 101^2}{10} - \frac{110\ 224}{30}$$

= 3710.2 – 3674.133
= 36.067

3. To calculate the $SS_{subj}$ the formula is:

$$\frac{\Sigma T_s^2}{c} - \frac{(\Sigma x)^2}{N}$$

$$= \frac{38^2 + 29^2 + 34^2 + 32^2 + 41^2 + 31^2 + 32^2 + 32^2 + 36^2 + 2}{31}$$

$$= \frac{110\ 224}{30}$$

= 3726.667 – 3674.133
= 52.534

4. To calculate the $SS_{tot}$ the formula is:

$$\Sigma x^2 - \frac{(\Sigma x)^2}{N}$$

$= 15^2 + 12^2 + 11^2 + 12^2 + 9^2 + 8^2 + 13^2$
$+ 10^2 + 11^2 + 10^2 + 10^2 + 12^2 + 17^2$
$+ 14^2 + 10^2 + 8^2 + 12^2 + 11^2 + 11^2$
$+ 12^2 + 9^2 + 14^2 + 9^2 + 9^2 + 16^2 + 8^2$
$+ 12^2 + 10^2 + 9^2 + 8^2 - \dfrac{110\ 224}{30}$

= 3840 – 3674.133
= 165.867

5. To calculate the $SS_{error}$ the formula is:

$SS_{tot} - SS_{bet} - SS_{subj}$
= 165.867 – 36.067 – 52.534
= 77.266

6. To calculate the df values:

$df_{bet}$ = number of conditions – 1
= 3 – 1
= 2

$df_{subj}$ = number of Ss – 1 (or sets of matched Ss – 1)
= 10 – 1
= 9

$df_{tot}$ = N – 1
= 30 – 1
= 29

$df_{error}$ = $df_{tot} - df_{bet} - df_{subj}$
= 29 – 2 – 9
= 18

7. To calculate the $MS$ values:

$$MS_{bet} = \frac{SS_{bet}}{df_{bet}}$$

$$= \frac{36.067}{2}$$

= 18.034

$$MS_{subj} = \frac{SS_{subj}}{df_{subj}}$$

$$= \frac{52.534}{9}$$

$$= 5.837$$

$$MS_{error} = \frac{SS_{error}}{df_{error}}$$

$$= \frac{77.266}{18}$$

$$= 4.293$$

**8.** To calculate the $F$ ratios:

$F$ ratio for the between-conditions variation

$$= \frac{MS_{bet}}{MS_{error}}$$

$$= \frac{18.034}{4.293}$$

$$= 4.201$$

$F$ ratio for the between-subjects variation

$$= \frac{MS_{subj}}{MS_{error}}$$

$$= \frac{5.837}{4.293}$$

$$= 1.36$$

We can now fill in our table using these values (Table 14.6).

### Looking up the values of the F ratios

We need to look up these $F$ ratios to find out whether they represent significant differences between the conditions and/or between the subjects. Turn to Tables A2.6a–d (pages 215–218) which are the probability tables for the anova.

Table A2.6a shows the critical values of $F$ at $p < 0.05$.

Table A2.6b Shows the critical values of $F$ at $p < 0.025$.

Table A2.6c shows the critical values of $F$ at $p < 0.01$.

Table A2.6d shows the critical values of $F$ at $p < 0.001$.

Note again, that as the anova can only tell us whether there are general differences and not

**Table 14.6**

| Source of variation in scores | Sums of squares $SS$ | Degrees of freedom $df$ | Mean squares $MS$ | $F$ ratios |
|---|---|---|---|---|
| Variation in scores between conditions, i.e. aspects of job | 36.067 | 2 | 18.034 | 4.201 |
| Variation in scores between subjects | 52.534 | 9 | 5.837 | 1.36 |
| Variation in scores due to random error | 77.266 | 18 | 4.293 | |
| Total | 165.867 | 29 | | |

whether these differences are in a specific direction, these values are for a two-tailed hypothesis.

On each of these Tables you will see that there are values called $v_1$ across the top and $v_2$ down the left-hand column. These are df values. To look up the F ratio for the between-conditions comparison, we need the $df_{bet}$ value and the $df_{error}$ value. Taking Table A2.6a first, locate the $df_{bet}$ (i.e. 2) across the top row, and the $df_{error}$ (i.e. 18) down the left-hand column. Where they intersect is the critical value of $F$ for these df values. If our $F$ ratio of 4.21 is equal to or larger than the critical value, it is significant at the $p$ value stated at the top of the table. As 4.021 is larger than 3.55, we can conclude that our results have an associated probability of less than 5%.

But can we do any better? Turn to Table A2.6b and repeat the process. Because our value of 4.201 is smaller than the interesction value of 4.56 our results are not significant at the 0.025 level. Therefore, the probability that our results are due to random error is less than 0.05.

This is expressed, then, as $p < 0.05$.

To find out whether there are differences between the subjects' overall performances (i.e. whether the $F$ ratio of 1.36 is significant), we need the $df_{subj}$ value (in this case 9) and the $df_{error}$ value (in this case 18). Look across the $v_1$ values in Table A2.6a for 9, and down the left-hand column for 18. You will see that there is no $v_1$ value of 9, so you must take the next smallest. At the intersection point the critical value is 2.51. As our *F* ratio is smaller than this, the results can be said to be not significant. In other words, there is no significant difference between subjects in their overall performance.

### Interpreting the results

Our results have an associated probability level of less than 5%, which means that the chances of random error accounting for the results are less than 5 in 100. Since the usual cut-off point is 5%, we can say that our results are significant, which means that the physiotherapists perform some parts of their job better than others. However, the between-subjects *F* ratio is not significant, which suggests that the physiotherapists concerned did not differ from each other in terms of their overall job performance.

If we take these two results together we can conclude that the senior grade II physiotherapists do indeed perform differently on each aspect of their job, and since there is no significant difference in the overall quality of the physiotherapists concerned we may assume that the differences are due to some factor associated with their department, training, attitudes, etc. We can express this in the following way:

> Using a one-way anova for related subject samples on the data ($F = 4.201$, $N = 10$) it was found that the results were significant at $p < 0.05$. This suggests that there are significant differences in performance levels on the three aspects of the physiotherapist's job investigated. These differences cannot be attributed to variations in the subjects since the *F* ratio for the between-subjects calculations was not significant ($F = 1.36$, $p = $ NS). Therefore, the null hypothesis can be rejected.

It must be remembered that the anova tells you that there are significant differences between the conditions and not which condition has better or worse scores. For instance in this example, we know that senior grade IIs perform differently on three aspects of their job but we do not know whether the difference lies between:

> clinical and interpersonal
> or
> clinical and supervisory

or
interpersonal and supervisory
or
all three.

In order to find out you need to use the Scheffé multiple range test in the next section. However, the Scheffé can only be used if the results from the anova are significant.

---

**Activity 14.2** (Answers on page 232–233)

1 To practise looking up *F* ratios, look up the following and state whether or not they are significant and at what level:
   (i) *F* ratio bet $= 4.96$ $df_{bet} = 2$ $df_{error} = 10$ *p*
   (ii) *F* ratio subj $= 4.22$ $df_{subj} = 7$ $df_{error} = 15$ *p*
   (iii) *F* ratio subj $= 2.21$ $df_{subj} = 11$ $df_{error} = 20$ *p*
   (iv) *F* ratio bet $= 5.15$ $df_{bet} = 14$ $df_{error} = 8$ *p*
   (v) *F* ratio subj $= 3.14$ $df_{subj} = 9$ $df_{error} = 14$ *p*
   (vi) *F* ratio bet $= 3.98$ $df_{bet} = 10$ $df_{error} = 12$ *p*

Remember! Use all the Tables to find the smallest *p* value possible.

2 Calculate a one-way anova for related designs on the following data:
   $H_1$  There is a relationship between the type of treatment used on hip replacement patients and the distance walked after 1 week of therapy.

Brief method: Select three groups each of 6 hip replacement patients, matched on age, sex, mobility prior to operation, length of time postoperative etc. Each group is treated using one of three different types of therapy. After I week, their mobility is measured in terms of yards walked, with the results shown in Table 14.7.

**Table 14.7**

| S | Condition A Suspension | Condition B Free exercise | Condition C Hydrotherapy |
|---|---|---|---|
| 1 | 15 | 16 | 11 |
| 2 | 12 | 14 | 14 |
| 3 | 10 | 14 | 12 |
| 4 | 14 | 15 | 12 |
| 5 | 22 | 19 | 13 |
| 6 | 17 | 18 | 15 |

State your *F* ratios, df values and *p* values in the manner suggested on this page.

## Scheffé multiple range test

The analysis of variance only tells you whether there are overall differences between the conditions and not where these differences lie. As a result, it is not possible from this test alone to conclude whether the scores from one condition are significantly better or worse than those from another. If you look back to the example given, the anova only allows us to conclude that physiotherapists perform differently in aspects of their job; it does not permit us to say that their performance on one task is better than their performance on another. However, if you look at the results for each condition (p. 142) it appears that the Clinical scores are better than the Interpersonal scores, with the Supervisory scores being worst. We can find out whether the differences between these sets of results are significant by comparing each pair of mean scores using the Scheffé multiple range test. In other words, we can compare:

1. the mean Clinical score with the mean Interpersonal score
2. the mean Clinical score with the mean Supervisory score
3. the mean Interpersonal score with the mean Supervisory score

to find out if the differences in performance in each area are significant. The Scheffé test should be carried out after you have calculated the anova because it uses some of the values from the anova table. Remember, too, that it should be carried out only if the results from the anova are significant.

There are a number of other multiple range tests which perform the same function, but the Scheffé has been selected because it is considered to be the best (McNemar 1963) and also because it can be used if there are unequal numbers of subjects in each condition. Obviously this latter point does not apply in same-subject and matched-subject designs (since you will, by definition, have the same number of scores in each condition) but, since the Scheffé can also be used with a one-way anova for unrelated designs and unequal subject numbers, this feature is a useful one.

When calculating the Scheffé, you find two values. Firstly, $F$ is calculated for each comparison of means you wish to make, and secondly a figure called '$F^1$' is calculated. Each $F$ is compared with the $F^1$ value. If it is equal to or larger than the $F^1$ value, then the result is significant.

### Calculating the Scheffé

There are three possible comparisons we can make using the Scheffé on our sample data:

1. Clinical vs Interpersonal scores
2. Clinical vs Supervisory scores
3. Interpersonal vs Supervisory scores.

To make these comparisons, take the following steps:

**1.** Calculate the mean score for each condition

$$\bar{x}_1 = 12.6; \quad \bar{x}_2 = 10.5; \quad \bar{x}_3 = 10.1$$

**2.** Find the value of $F$ for the first comparison (i.e. Clinical vs Interpersonal) using the following formula:

$$F = \frac{(\bar{x}_1 - \bar{x}_2)^2}{\dfrac{MS_{error}}{n_1} + \dfrac{MS_{error}}{n_2}}$$

where $\bar{x}_1$ = mean for Condition 1
$\quad\quad$ = 12.6
$\quad\bar{x}_2$ = mean for Condition 2
$\quad\quad$ = 10.5
$MS_{error}$ = mean square value for the random error variation (from the anova calculations)
$\quad\quad$ = 4.293
$\quad n_1$ = number of subjects in Condition 1
$\quad\quad$ = 10
$\quad n_2$ = number of subjects in Condition 2
$\quad\quad$ = 10

If these values are substituted, then

$$F = \frac{(12.6 - 10.5)^2}{\dfrac{4.293}{10} + \dfrac{4.293}{10}}$$

$$= \frac{4.41}{0.858}$$

$$= 5.14$$

**3.** Repeat the calculations for the other two comparisons, using the appropriate means and $n$ values.

Thus for the comparison of the Clinical and Supervisory scores, the formula is:

$$F = \frac{(\bar{x}_1 - \bar{x}_3)^2}{\dfrac{MS_{error}}{n_1} + \dfrac{MS_{error}}{n_3}}$$

$$= \frac{(12.6 - 10.1)^2}{\dfrac{4.293}{10} + \dfrac{4.293}{10}}$$

$$= 7.284$$

and for the comparison of the Interpersonal and Supervisory scores, the formula is:

$$F = \frac{(\bar{x}_2 - \bar{x}_3)^2}{\dfrac{MS_{error}}{n_2} + \dfrac{MS_{error}}{n_3}}$$

$$= \frac{(10.5 - 10.1)^2}{\dfrac{4.293}{10} + \dfrac{4.293}{10}}$$

$$= 0.187$$

**4.** Using the $df_{bet}$ and $df_{error}$ values derived from the anova (i.e. 2 and 18 respectively), turn to Table A2.6a and locate the $df_{bet}$ value across the $v_1$ row, and the $df_{error}$ down the $v_2$ column. At the intersection point, you will find the value of 3.55. This is the critical value for $F$ at the $< 5\%$ or $< 0.05$ level of significance. The $< 5\%$ level is selected because of the extreme stringency of the Scheffé test. If a smaller $p$ value were to be selected, you would be far less likely to obtain significant results on the Scheffé. However, should you ever get any results that look as though they are considerably more significant than the 5% level, you can repeat steps 4–6 with Tables A2.6b (1%), A2.6c (2½%) and A2.6d (0.1%).

**5.** Calculate $F^1$ using the formula:

$$F^1 = (C - 1) F°$$

where $C$ = the number of conditions
        = 3
    $F°$ = the figure at the intersection point of the appropriate df values in the Table
        = 3.55
$F^1$ = (3 − 1) 3.55
        = 7.1

**6.** Compare the $F$ values derived from the calculations in steps 2 and 3 with the $F^1$ value above. If the $F$ value is equal to or larger than the $F^1$ value it is significant.

Therefore, taking our $F$ values of

     5.14
     7.284
     0.187

we can see that only one is larger than the $F^1$ value, i.e. the comparison between the Clinical and Supervisory scores.

### Interpreting the results

The results from the Scheffé test indicate that there is only one significant difference between pairs of performance scores, that is between the Clinical and Supervisory scores (at $p < 0.05$). This suggests that the main reason for the significant results of the anova is the difference between senior grade II physiotherapists in clinical and supervisory skills.

---

**Activity 14.3** (Answers on page 233)

Carry out a Scheffé test on the following results:
$H_1$   There is a difference in the efficacy of four teaching approaches used with student physiotherapists.
Method: A group of 6 student physiotherapists is given comparable information in four different ways: seminar, tutorial, lecture, and individual reading. They are tested on their understanding and receive marks out of 20. A one-way anova for related designs was computed on the scores and the following relevant results obtained:

$df_{bet}$ = 3
$df_{error}$ = 15
$MS_{error}$ = 3.87

The mean scores for each condition were

Condition 1 Seminar 11.2
Condition 2 Tutorial 13.1
Condition 3 Lecture 10.7
Condition 4 Reading  8.4

# 15

# Non-parametric tests for different- (unrelated-) subject designs

## INTRODUCTION

The statistical tests described in this chapter are used when the experimental design involves two or more than two, different unmatched groups of subjects who are compared on a certain task, activity etc. All the tests covered in this chapter are non-parametric ones, which means that they

- are less sensitive
- are easier to calculate
- can be used on nominal, ordinal or interval/ratio data.

Therefore, if you cannot fulfil the conditions required for parametric tests, you should use its non-parametric equivalent. The designs involved in this chapter, then, are for:

1. **Two different, unmatched subject groups** compared on a certain task, activity etc. (Fig. 15.1).

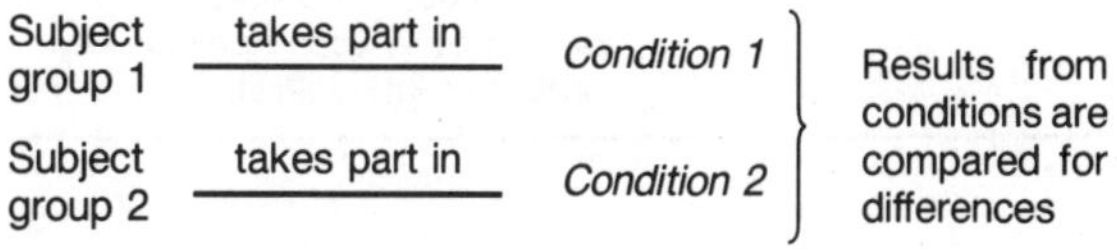

Subject group 1 —— takes part in —— *Condition 1*
Subject group 2 —— takes part in —— *Condition 2*
} Results from conditions are compared for differences

**Figure 15.1** Different-subject design: two different groups of subjects compared on a task.

or

2. **Three or more different, unmatched subject groups** compared on a certain task, activity etc. (Fig. 15.2).

**Figure 15.2** Different-subject design: three or more different, unmatched subject groups compared on a task.

Results from Design 1 are analysed using the **chi-squared** ($\chi^2$) test if the data is nominal, or the **Mann–Whitney** $U$ test if it is other than nominal (i.e. ordinal or interval/ratio).

Results from Design 2 are analysed using the **extended chi-squared** test if the data is nominal or the **Kruskal–Wallis** test if the data is other than nominal (i.e. ordinal or interval/ratio).

If a trend in the results is predicted, such that subject group 1 is expected to perform better than subject group 2, with subject group 3 performing worst, the **Jonckheere trend** test is used as long as the data is other than nominal. (Table 15.1).

**Table 15.1** Tests for different-subject designs

| Design | Non-parametric test |
|---|---|
| 1. Two different groups of subjects, compared on a task. | Chi-squared test if data is nominal Mann-Whitney $U$ test (if data is other than nominal, i.e. ordinal or interval/ratio). |
| 2. Three or more different groups of subjects, compared on a task. | Extended chi-squared test if data is nominal Kruskal–Wallis (if just a difference in results is predicted and the data is other than nominal, i.e. ordinal or interval/ratio). Jonckheere trend test (if a trend in the results is predicted and the data is other than nominal, i.e. ordinal or interval/ratio). |

# NON-PARAMETRIC TEST: TWO DIFFERENT SUBJECT GROUPS AND NOMINAL DATA

## Chi-squared ($\chi^2$) test

This test is used when you have the sort of experimental design which uses two different, unmatched groups of subjects who are compared

on a task, activity etc. The data for the $\chi^2$ (pronounced 'Kie-squared') test must be *nominal*.

To refresh your memory, the nominal level of measurement only allows you to allocate your subjects to named categories (e.g. pass/fail; good/bad; mobile/immobile); it does not allow you to measure your subjects' responses along a dimension, i.e. how well they have passed, how mobile they are. Check Chapter 4 to make sure you're happy with this concept. As you can see, a subject may only be allocated to one category, since it is impossible to be both mobile and immobile, to pass and to fail. Because of this the $\chi^2$ can only be used when different subjects are allocated to different categories, i.e. an unrelated design.

With the $\chi^2$ test you may only use two nominal categories and two subject groups. For example you may wish to find out whether there is a difference between men and women in terms of which hip (left or right) is more likely to be replaced. You have two groups: 'men' and 'women', and two nominal categories: 'left' and 'right'.

Should you ever wish to allocate two groups to more than two nominal categories you must use the *extended* $\chi^2$ (see page 162).

It should also be noted that when you use the $\chi^2$ test, you should ensure that at least 20 subjects will be in each group. While this may sound offputting, it rarely takes too much time to collect this amount of data. You do not need to use equal numbers of subjects in each group. When you calculate the $\chi^2$ test, you find a numerical value for $\chi^2$ which you then look up in the probability tables associated with the $\chi^2$ test to see if this value represents a significant difference between the result you observed and those that could be expected by chance.

### Example

Let's suppose you were interested in the effects of encouraging early weight bearing after ligamentous ankle sprain. Your hypothesis is:

$H_1$ Patients who are encouraged to bear full weight after ligamentous ankle sprains are more likely to achieve an early restoration of normal gait pattern.

This is a 1-tailed hypothesis, since it predicts a direction to the results.

Method: You select 30 sprained ankle patients and give them full weight-bearing exercises for 15 minutes each day. A further 32 sprained ankle patients are given no exercise. After 3 days, you assess the gait pattern for each group. You count up how many patients have a normal gait pattern and how many do not.

This is a nominal level of measurement because you are using two categories: 'normal gait pattern' and 'abnormal gait pattern' and are simply allocating subjects to one of these groups.

You have a design which looks like Figure 15.3

| | | | |
|---|---|---|---|
| Subject group 1 30 sprained ankle patients | takes part in | *Condition 1* Full weight-bearing exercises | Assessed as to whether they have normal gait pattern after 3 days. The results are compared. |
| Subject group 2 32 sprained ankle patients | takes part in | *Condition 2* No weight-bearing exercises | |

**Figure 15.3** Effect of exercises on gait of sprained ankle patients: experimental design.

In other words you have two groups of subjects who can be allocated to *two* nominal categories (normal gait pattern or not.)

You end up with the results shown in Figure 15.4.

| | Normal gait pattern | Abnormal gait pattern | Marginal total |
|---|---|---|---|
| Subject group 1 Exercises | *A* 21 | *B* 9 | *A*+*B* 30 |
| Subject group 2 No exercises | *C* 14 | *D* 18 | *C*+*D* 32 |
| Marginal totals | *A*+*C* 35 | *B*+*D* 27 | Grand total, *N* 62 |

**Figure 15.4** Format of data when calculating the $\chi^2$ test.

## *Calculating the $\chi^2$ test*

**1.** The first step you must always take is to set your data out in a 2 × 2 table as shown in Figure 15.4. The subject groups should go down the side and the nominal categories across the top, although it doesn't matter which category is on the left, nor which subject group is at the top. Label your cells A, B, C, and D in the same way as above (i.e. from left to right).

**2.** You must now add up the marginal totals for each row and each column, i.e.:

$$A + B = 21 + 9 = 30$$
$$C + D = 14 + 18 = 32$$
$$A + C = 21 + 14 = 35$$
$$B + D = 9 + 18 = 27$$

**3.** Calculate the grand total $N$ either by adding up the vertical marginal totals, i.e.

$$30 + 32 = 62$$

or by adding up the horizontal marginal totals, i.e.

$$35 + 27 = 62$$

(The answer will be the same.)

**4.** Find $\chi^2$ from the formula:

$$\chi^2 = \frac{N\left[(AD - BC) - \frac{N}{2}\right]^2}{(A+B)(C+D)(A+C)(B+D)}$$

where $N$ = the grand total, i.e. 62

$AD$ = Cell A × Cell D = 21 × 18 = 378

$BC$ = Cell B × Cell C = 9 × 14 = 126

The values under the division line are all the marginal totals:

$$A + B = 30$$
$$C + D = 32$$
$$A + C = 35$$
$$B + D = 27$$

Therefore, if we substitute these values in the formula:

$$\chi^2 = \frac{62\left[(378 - 126^*) - \frac{62}{2}\right]^2}{30 \times 32 \times 35 \times 27}$$

$$= \frac{3\,028\,142}{907\,200}$$

$$\chi^2 = 3.338$$

(*If you get a minus number from the calculations in the inner brackets, ignore the minus sign)

**5.** Before this $\chi^2$ value can be looked up in the probability tables to see if it represents a significant difference, the df value is required. Use the df formula of:

$$(r - 1)(c - 1)$$

where   $r$ = the number of rows
         $c$ = the number of columns

$$= (2 - 1)(2 - 1)$$
$$= 1$$

Obviously, in a 2 × 2 table like this, the df will always equal 1.

### Looking up the value of $\chi^2$ for significance

To find out whether the $\chi^2$ value of 3.338 represents a significant difference in gait pattern between patients who have done full weight-bearing exercise and those who have not, it must be looked up in the probability tables associated with the $\chi^2$ test (Table A2.1).

Down the left-hand column you will see df values from 1–30. Look down this column until you find the df value of 1. To the right of this are five numbers, called critical values of $\chi^2$:

$$2.71 \quad 3.84 \quad 5.41 \quad 6.64 \quad 10.83.$$

Each of these critical values is associated with the probability level at the top of its column, e.g. the critical value of 5.41 is associated with 0.02 for a two-tailed test. You will see that the $p$ values in the table are only associated with two-tailed hypotheses. If you have a one-tailed hypothesis, as we have here, simply look up your $\chi^2$ value as described, find the two-tailed $p$ value and halve it (see pages 89–90).

In order for our $\chi^2$ value of 3.338 to be significant at one of these levels, it has to be equal to or larger than one of these numbers. Our value is larger than 2.71 but smaller than 3.84. Therefore, the probability associated with our obtained $\chi^2$ value must be less than 0.05 (or 5%) but larger than 0.025 (or 2½%) for a one-tailed hypothesis. (Remember we have had to halve the $p$ values in the table which are for two-tailed hypotheses). The convention is that we say that $p$ is less than

0.05 (or 5%) rather than greater than 0.025 (or 2½%). This is expressed as $p < 0.05$.

This means that the probability of our results being due to random error is less than 5%.

### Interpreting the results

Our $\chi^2$ value has an associated probability level of less than 0.05 or 5%, which means that the chance of random error being responsible for the results is less than 5%. Because a 5% cut-off point is usually used to claim that the results support the experimental hypothesis, we can say that our results are significant.

However, before we can finally conclude that the hypothesis has been supported, just go back to the 2 × 2 table and check the results are in the predicted direction, because it is quite possible sometimes to obtain significant results which are opposite to those predicted in the hypothesis and so would not support the hypothesis.

Here we find that more of the exercise group have a normal gait pattern (21 vs 14) and more of the non-exercise group have an abnormal gait pattern (18 vs 9). Therefore the results are as predicted. We can reject the null (no difference) hypothesis on this basis. This can be expressed in the following way:

Using a $\chi^2$ test on the data ($\chi^2$ = 3.338, df = 1) the results were found to be significant at $p <$ 0.05, for a one-tailed test. This suggests that the null hypothesis can be rejected and that patients who are encouraged to bear full weight after ligamentous ankle sprain are more likely to achieve an early restoration of normal gait pattern.

**Activity 15.1** (Answers on page 233)

1 In order to practise looking up $\chi^2$ values, look up the following and say what the associated $p$ value is and whether or not it is significant.
   (i) $\chi^2$ = 4.02     one-tailed     df = 1     $p$
   (ii) $\chi^2$ = 5.91     two-tailed     df = 1     $p$
   (iii) $\chi^2$ = 3.84     two-tailed     df = 1     $p$
   (iv) $\chi^2$ = 2.62     two-tailed     df = 1     $p$
   (v) $\chi^2$ = 6.95     one-tailed     df = 1     $p$

2 Calculate a $\chi^2$ test on the following.
   $H_1$   Teachers of physiotherapy are more likely to study in Open University degree courses than clinically-based physiotherapists of comparable years of experience since qualifying. (Is this a one- or two-tailed hypothesis?)
   Method: You randomly select 35 teachers of physiotherapy

and 42 clinically-based physiotherapists and ask them whether or not they have ever undertaken an OU degree course.

The results are as shown in Figure 15.5.

|                                     | OU course | No OU course |
|-------------------------------------|-----------|--------------|
| Teachers of physiotherapy           | 25        | 10           |
| Clinically-based physiotherapists   | 15        | 27           |

**Figure 15.5**  Are teachers of physiotherapy more likely than clinically-based physiotherapists to undertake an OU degree course?

State your $\chi^2$ value, $p$ value, using the sample format given on page 152.

## NON-PARAMETRIC TEST: TWO DIFFERENT, UNMATCHED SUBJECT GROUPS AND ORDINAL OR INTERVAL/RATIO DATA

### Mann–Whitney $U$ test

This test is used to analyse results from experiments which have compared two different unmatched groups of subjects on a task (see Design 1, page 149). The Mann–Whitney $U$ test simply compares the results from each group to see if they differ significantly. This test can only be used with ordinal or interval/ratio data. It cannot be used with nominal data.

When calculating this test, you end up with a numerical value, '$U$' which you look up in the probability tables associated with the Mann–Whitney test, to see if the $U$ value does, in fact, represent a significant difference between the groups.

### Example

Suppose you were interested in testing the hypothesis that there is a difference in the rate of healing of non-infected bedsores among bedridden elderly care patients when treated by infra-red or ice-cube massage.

Your hypothesis would be:

$H_1$  There is a difference in the healing rates of non-infected bedsores of bedridden elderly care patients when treated by infra-red as opposed to ice-cube massage.

This is a two-tailed hypothesis as it does not predict a direction to the results.

In order to do this, you select a group of 28 elderly care patients, all of whom have non-infected bedsores. (Assume constant errors have been eliminated, e.g. length of time bedridden.) Randomly allocate 15 patients to infra-red and 13 to ice-cube massage.

Therefore, we have the design shown in Figure 15.6.

Group 1
15 elderly patients — treated by — *Condition 1* Infra-red

Group 2
13 elderly patients — treated by — *Condition 2* Ice-cube massage

The two groups are compared for extent of healing (e.g. on a 9-point scale where 9 = totally healed, 1 = not at all healed).

**Figure 15.6**  Design of experiment to test whether there is a difference in healing rates of bedsores depending on type of treatment.

Essentially, you would administer different treatments to each group and compare the extent of the healing after a given period of time, e.g. 7 days. (Note that because we don't have to match the subjects, you can use different numbers in each group.) You might end up with the results shown in Table 15.2.

**Table 15.2**

| Subject | *Condition 1* Infra-red | Rank | Subject | *Condition 2* Ice-cube massage | Rank |
|---------|-------------------------|------|---------|-------------------------------|------|
| 1       | 6                       | 18   | 1       | 7                             | 22.5 |
| 2       | 5                       | 12.5 | 2       | 9                             | 27.5 |
| 3       | 7                       | 22.5 | 3       | 6                             | 18   |
| 4       | 3                       | 2.5  | 4       | 5                             | 12.5 |
| 5       | 5                       | 12.5 | 5       | 6                             | 18   |
| 6       | 4                       | 7    | 6       | 7                             | 22.5 |
| 7       | 4                       | 7    | 7       | 7                             | 22.5 |
| 8       | 3                       | 2.5  | 8       | 8                             | 25.5 |
| 9       | 8                       | 25.5 | 9       | 9                             | 27.5 |
| 10      | 6                       | 18   | 10      | 6                             | 18   |
| 11      | 5                       | 12.5 | 11      | 5                             | 12.5 |
| 12      | 4                       | 7    | 12      | 4                             | 7    |
| 13      | 3                       | 2.5  | 13      | 5                             | 12.5 |
| 14      | 3                       | 2.5  |         |                               |      |
| 15      | 4                       | 7    |         |                               |      |
| Total   | 70                      | 159.5|         | 84                            | 246.5|
| Mean    | 4.667                   |      |         | 6.462                         |      |

### Calculating the Mann–Whitney U test

To calculate the Mann–Whitney, take the following steps:

**1.** First calculate the totals ($\Sigma$) and means for each condition; i.e.:

| Condition 1 | Total: | 70 |
| | Mean: | 4.667 |
| Condition 2 | Total: | 84 |
| | Mean: | 6.462 |

**2.** Taking the *whole set of scores together* (i.e. all 28 scores) rank them giving the rank of 1 to the lowest, 2 to the next lowest and so on. Where there are two or more scores the same, use the tied rank procedure (see pages 125–126), i.e. add up the ranks the scores would have obtained had they been different and divide this number by the number of scores that are the same. Thus 3 is the lowest score, but there are four scores of 3. Therefore add up the ranks 1, 2, 3 and 4 (the ranks they would have obtained had they been different) and divide by 4 because there are four scores of 3:

$$\frac{1 + 2 + 3 + 4}{4} = 2.5$$

Assign the rank of 2.5 to all the scores of 3. (See columns labelled 'Rank'.) Remember! Put the scores from both conditions together, as though they were just one set of scores, when you do the ranking. Many students forget to do this.

**3.** Add the rank totals for each condition separately:

$$\text{Rank total 1} = 159.5$$
$$\text{Rank total 2} = 246.5$$

**4.** Select the larger rank total, i.e. 246.5 to use in the formula below.

**5.** Find $U$ from the formula:

$$U = n_1 n_2 + \frac{n_x(n_x + 1)}{2} - T_x$$

where $n_1$ = the number of subjects in Condition 1 (i.e. 15)

$n_2$ = the number of subjects in Condition 2 (i.e. 13)

$T_x$ = the larger rank total (i.e. 246.5)

$n_x$ = the number of Ss in the condition with the larger rank total (i.e. Condition 2 = 13)

Therefore if we substitute these values:

$$U = 15 \times 13 + \frac{13(13 + 1)}{2} - 246.5$$

$$= 195 + 91 - 246.5$$

$$= 39.5$$

**6.** Because there are unequal numbers in each condition, it is necessary to repeat the calculations for the smaller rank total (i.e. 159.5) as well.

Here $T_x$ becomes the smaller rank total (159.5), and $n_x$ becomes the number of subjects in the condition with the smaller rank total (i.e. Condition 1 = 15 subjects).

$$U_2 = 15 \times 13 + \frac{15(15 + 1)}{2} - 159.5$$

$$= 195 + 120 - 159.5$$

$$= 155.5$$

We now have two values of $U$:

$$U = 39.5$$
$$U_2 = 155.5$$

We need to look up the *smaller* of these two $U$ values in the appropriate table (Table A2.7a–d, pages 219–220).

*Note:* If you use equal numbers of subjects in each condition, you only need to carry out the first calculation of $U$, using the larger rank total and the appropriate $n$ value. If you use unequal numbers you will have to find both $U$ values and select the smaller one.

*Looking up the value of U for significance*

In order to find out whether our $U$ value of 39.5 represents a significant difference in healing rates, you have to look up this value in Tables A2.7a–d. There are four probability tables for the Mann–Whitney, each one representing different $p$ values (see headings). Table A2.7a represents the smallest (most significant) $p$ values, while Table A2.7d represents the largest (least significant) $p$ value. To look up your $U$ value you also need the:

$$n_1 \text{ value (15)}$$
$$n_2 \text{ value (13)}$$

Starting with Table A2.7a, look across the top row until you find your $n_1$ value of 15, and down the left-hand column for your $n_2$ value of 13. Where these two points intersect is the number 42. In order to be significant at a given level, your $U$ value must be equal to or smaller than the value at the intersection point. As 39.5 is smaller than 42, our results are significant at either 0.005 for a one-tailed test or 0.01 for a two-tailed test. As we only predicted a general difference in healing rates in our hypothesis without specifying which treatment would be better, we have a two-tailed hypothesis. Therefore, our results are significant at the 0.01 or 1% probability level.

But, if you notice, our $U$ value of 39.5 is actually smaller than the value of 42 at the intersection point. This means our results are even more significant than the 1% level. This is expressed as:

$$p < 0.01 \text{ or } < 1\%$$

Had our $U$ value been the same as the value at the intersection point, the results would have been significant at exactly the 0.01 or 1% level. This would have been expressed as:

$$p = 0.01 \text{ (or } 1\%)$$

However, our results have a probability of less than 1% which means that the chance of random error accounting for our results is less than 1%.

Supposing, however, our $U$ value had been 52.5, with our $n$ values the same. Using A2.7a, we would find that the intersection value is 42. Because our $U$ of 52.5 is larger than this value, it would not be significant at the probability levels of 0.005 and 0.01 given in the heading. Therefore, we would move on to Table A2.7b. At this intersection point, for $n_1 = 15$, $n_2 = 13$, the value is 47. Our $U$ value is larger than this and so cannot be classified as significant at this level either. Turn on to Table A2.7c. The intersection value here is 54. Our $U$ value is smaller and so would be significant at the $< 0.05$ level for a two-tailed test.

If you ever find your $U$ value is larger than the relevant intersection values in Table A2.7d, your results would not be significant.

## Interpreting the results

Our $U$ value has an associated probability level of less than 1% which means that there is less than a 1% chance of random error causing the results. If you remember, it was said that a good cut-off point for claiming that your results were significant and supported your hypothesis was the 5% level or less. Since our $p$ value is less than 5% we can claim our results are significant; our null (no relationship) hypothesis can therefore be rejected and the experimental hypothesis supported.

Although the hypothesis did not predict which of the two treatments would be better, it is useful to compare the means from each condition to see which method was, in fact, more successful. Here the mean scores are 4.667 and 6.462 for infra-red and ice-cube massage respectively, which means that ice-cube massage was more effective. This can be stated in the following way:

Using a Mann–Whitney $U$ test to analyse the data ($U = 39.5$, $n_1 = 15$, $n_2 = 13$), the results were found to be significant at $p < 0.01$ for a two-tailed hypothesis. This means that infra-red treatment and ice-cube massage differ significantly in their effectiveness in treating non-infected bedsores in elderly bedridden patients. Further inspection of the results suggests that ice-cube massage produces better results.

---

**Activity 15.2** (Answers on page 233)

1 To practise looking up $U$ values, look up the following and state whether or not they're significant and at what level.

| | | | | |
|---|---|---|---|---|
| (i) $n_1 = 12$ | $n_2 = 12$ | $U = 33.5$ | two-tailed | $p$ |
| (ii) $n_1 = 10$ | $n_2 = 10$ | $U = 27$ | one-tailed | $p$ |
| (iii) $n_1 = 14$ | $n_2 = 12$ | $U = 37.5$ | one-tailed | $p$ |
| (iv) $n_1 = 20$ | $n_2 = 18$ | $U = 87.5$ | one-tailed | $p$ |
| (v) $n_1 = 15$ | $n_2 = 15$ | $U = 70.5$ | one-tailed | $p$ |
| (vi) $n_1 = 18$ | $n_2 = 15$ | $U = 92.5$ | two-tailed | $p$ |

2 Calculate a Mann–Whitney $U$ test on the following:

$H_1$  Paraffin wax is more effective than a hot soak as a preparation for mobilising exercises for post-fracture patients.

Is this a 1- or 2-tailed hypothesis?

Method: Randomly select 28 patients all of whom are within 1 week post removal of plaster following forearm fracture. Randomly allocate 14 to paraffin wax treatment and the other 14 to a hot soak. Rate the ease of movement of the wrist joint, following 30 minutes of mobilising exercises, on a 7-point scale (7 = extremely easy to move, 1 = very difficult to move).

The results might be as shown in Table 15.3.

**Table 15.3**

| Subject | Condition 1<br>Paraffin<br>wax | Rank | Subject | Condition 2<br>Hot soak | Rank |
|---|---|---|---|---|---|
| 1 | 5 | | 1 | 3 | |
| 2 | 4 | | 2 | 3 | |
| 3 | 5 | | 3 | 5 | |
| 4 | 6 | | 4 | 4 | |
| 5 | 3 | | 5 | 2 | |
| 6 | 3 | | 6 | 1 | |
| 7 | 4 | | 7 | 3 | |
| 8 | 5 | | 8 | 4 | |
| 9 | 6 | | 9 | 5 | |
| 10 | 5 | | 10 | 5 | |
| 11 | 6 | | 11 | 3 | |
| 12 | 6 | | 12 | 3 | |
| 13 | 4 | | 13 | 4 | |
| 14 | 3 | | 14 | 2 | |

State the $U$ value and the $p$ value in a format similar to that suggested earlier.

## NON-PARAMETRIC TESTS: THREE OR MORE DIFFERENT, UNMATCHED SUBJECT GROUPS AND ORDINAL OR INTERVAL/RATIO DATA

### 1. Kruskal–Wallis test

This test is simply an extension of the Mann–Whitney test, in that it is used:

- when different subject groups are involved
- when the data is ordinal, or interval/ratio
- when the conditions for its parametric equivalent cannot be fulfilled.

However, while the Mann–Whitney can only be used to analyse the results from designs with two different groups of subjects, the Kruskal–Wallis is used with designs employing three or more different groups of subjects (Fig. 15.7).

| Subject<br>group 1 | takes part in | Condition 1 | |
|---|---|---|---|
| Subject<br>group 2 | takes part in | Condition 2 | Compare results<br>from the groups to<br>see if there are<br>differences<br>between them |
| Subject<br>group 3<br>(etc.) | takes part in | Condition 3 | |

**Figure 15.7** A different-subject design with three or more groups of subjects. The Kruskal–Wallis test is used to analyse the results.

The Kruskal–Wallis, however, only tells you whether there are differences between these groups and not which results are better or worse than the others. Therefore, the associated hypothesis must be two-tailed (i.e. just predicting differences in the results with no specific direction to them). Should you ever predict a trend in your results (e.g. that Group 1 will perform better than Group 2, which in turn will perform better than Group 3 etc.) with this sort of unrelated design, you would use a **Jonckheere trend** test to analyse your results.

However, with the Kruskal–Wallis, you calculate a value called '$H$', which you then look up in the probability tables associated with the Kruskal–Wallis test, to find out whether the $H$ value represents significant differences between the groups.

### Example

Let's suppose you are working with stroke patients and are trying to help them regain the use of paralysed limbs. You always give the patients some preparatory warm-up exercises, but would be interested to see whether some of these preparations are more effective than others. So you decide to compare the effectiveness of three preparatory procedures on the contraction of the biceps.

Your hypothesis, then, is:

$H_1$  There is difference in the strength of muscle contraction in the biceps, according to whether it is preceded by 2 minutes infrared radiation, 2 minutes specific warm-up or 2 minutes general warm-up.

In order to test this out, you select 30 stroke patients and randomly allocate them to one of the three groups. Following the 2 minutes selected preparation you rate the strength of their biceps contraction on a 5-point scale (5 = very strong, 1 = very weak).

Your design looks like Figure 15.8., and your results look like Table 15.4.

**Table 15.4**

| Subject* | Condition 1 Infrared | Rank | Subject | Condition 2 Specific | Rank | Subject | Condition 3 General | Rank |
|---|---|---|---|---|---|---|---|---|
| 1 | 3 | 16 | 1 | 4 | 24 | 1 | 2 | 8 |
| 2 | 4 | 24 | 2 | 5 | 29 | 2 | 3 | 16 |
| 3 | 2 | 8 | 3 | 5 | 29 | 3 | 3 | 16 |
| 4 | 2 | 8 | 4 | 4 | 24 | 4 | 4 | 24 |
| 5 | 1 | 2.5 | 5 | 4 | 24 | 5 | 1 | 2.5 |
| 6 | 3 | 16 | 6 | 3 | 16 | 6 | 3 | 16 |
| 7 | 4 | 24 | 7 | 2 | 8 | 7 | 2 | 8 |
| 8 | 1 | 2.5 | 8 | 3 | 16 | 8 | 1 | 2.5 |
| 9 | 2 | 8 | 9 | 5 | 29 | 9 | 3 | 16 |
| 10 | 2 | 8 | 10 | 4 | 24 | 10 | 3 | 16 |
| Total | 24 | 117.0 | | 39 | 223 | | 25 | 125.0 |
| Mean | 2.4 | | | 3.9 | | | 2.5 | |

\* Because this is a different-, unmatched-subject design, you do not have to have equal numbers of subjects in each group, although it is easier if you do.

| Subject group 1 (10 stroke patients) | takes part in | Condition 1 Infra-red |
|---|---|---|
| Subject group 2 (10 stroke patients | takes part in | Condition 2 Specific warm-up |
| Subject group 3 (10 stroke patients) | takes part in | Condition 3 General warm-up |

Groups compared for differences in muscle contraction

**Figure 15.8** Do differing preparatory procedures have different effects on the strength of muscle contraction?

## Calculating the Kruskal–Wallis test

**1.** Calculate the totals and mean scores for each condition:

Condition 1 Total = 24 $\bar{x}$ = 2.4
Condition 2 Total = 39 $\bar{x}$ = 3.9
Condition 3 Total = 25 $x$ = 2.5.

**2.** Taking *all* the scores together, as though they were a single set of 30 scores, rank the scores, giving a rank of 1 to the lowest score, a rank of 2 to the next lowest etc. Where 2 or more scores are the same, apply the average ranks procedure (see pages 125–126); i.e. add up the ranks the scores would have obtained had they been different and divide this number by the total number of scores that are the same. Thus, in the example, 1 is the lowest score, but there are 4 scores of 1. Had these been different, they would have been ranked 1, 2, 3 and 4. So add these ranks up (10) and divide by 4 because there were four scores of 1, giving 2.5. Give the rank of 2.5 to all the scores of 1. Remember that you have now used up ranks 1–4, so you must start with 5 next.

Remember! Rank all the scores together, as though they were just one set of 30 scores.

**3.** Add the rank total for each condition separately to give $T$:

$$T_{C1} = 117.0$$
$$T_{C2} = 223$$
$$T_{C3} = 125.0$$

**4.** Find the value of $H$ from the following formula:

$$H = \left[ \frac{12}{N(N+1)} \left( \sum \frac{T_C^2}{n_C} \right) \right] - 3(N+1)$$

where $N$ = total number of subjects (i.e. 30)
$n_C$ = number of subjects in each group (i.e. $n_1$ = 10; $n_2$ = 10; $n_3$ = 10)
$T_C$ = rank totals for each condition (i.e. $T_{C1}$ = 117; $T_{C2}$ = 223; $T_{C3}$ = 125)
$T_C^2$ = rank total for each condition *squared* (i.e. $117^2$; $223^2$; $125^2$)
$\Sigma$ = total of any calculations following

$\sum \dfrac{T_C^2}{n_C}$ = each rank total squared and divided by the number of subjects in that condition

i.e. $\dfrac{117^2}{10} + \dfrac{223^2}{10} + \dfrac{125^2}{10}$

Substituting these values:

$$H = \left[ \dfrac{12}{30(30+1)} \times \left( \dfrac{117^2}{10} + \dfrac{223^2}{10} + \dfrac{125^2}{10} \right) \right]$$
$$- 3 \times 31$$

$$= \left[ \dfrac{12}{930} \times (1368.9 + 4972.9 + 1562.5) \right] - 93$$

$$= (0.013 \times 7904.3) - 93$$

$$= 102.756 - 93$$

$$= 9.756$$

### Looking up the H value for significance

To find out whether $H$ = 9.756 represents significant differences between the results from each group, you will also need the df value. This is the number of conditions minus 1, i.e. 3 – 1 = 2. Turn to Tables A2.1 and A2.8 (pages 209 and 222). Table A2.8 covers the probability levels for experiments using three groups of subjects, with 1–5 subjects in each group, while Table A2.1 covers the probability levels for experiments with more subjects and more conditions. (This is also the chi-squared table.)

Because we have 10 subjects in each condition we use Table A2.1. Down the left-hand column you will see various df values. Look down the column until you find our df of 2. To the right of this are 5 numbers:

$$4.60 \quad 5.99 \quad 7.82 \quad 9.21 \quad 13.82$$

These are called critical values and each one is associated with the probability level indicated at the top of the column, e.g. 7.82 has a $p$ value of 0.02. To be significant at a given level, our $H$ value has to be *equal to* or *larger than* one of these numbers. So, with our $H$ of 9.756, we can see that it is larger than 9.21, but smaller than 13.82. This means that for our two-tailed hypothesis,

the probability associated with the obtained $H$ value of 9.756 must be somewhat less than 0.01 (or 1%) but somewhat greater than 0.001 (or 1%). To comply with convention, we would say that $p$ is less than 0.01 (or 1%). (Remember with the Kruskal–Wallis, we can only predict general differences in our results, therefore any hypothesis must be two-tailed). This is expressed as $p < 0.01$ or <1%. This means that there is less than a 1% chance that our results are due to random error. (Had our $H$ value been equal to the critical value, $p$ would have been 0.01 exactly. This would have been expressed as $p$ = 0.01 or 1%.)

### Interpreting the results

Our $H$ value of 9.756 has a probability of <0.01 (or <1%) which means that the probability of random error accounting for the results is less than 1%. As you will remember, it was noted earlier that the usual cut-off point for assuming support for the experimental hypothesis is the 5% level or less. As our $p$ value is less than 1%, it is smaller than the cut-off point of 5% and therefore we can say that our results are significant. This means we can reject the null hypothesis and accept the experimental hypothesis. This can be expressed in the following way:

> Using a Kruskal–Wallis test on the data ($H$ = 9.756, $N$ = 30) the results were found to be significant at $p < 0.01$. This suggests that there is a significant difference in the strength of muscle contractions with different preparation techniques among stroke patients. This means that the experimental hypothesis has been supported.

Remember that the Kruskal–Wallis will only tell you that there are differences between your conditions and not which preparation is most effective. If you had hypothesised a trend in the results, e.g.

specific warm-up is better than general warm-up which in turn is better than infra-red

and had used the same unmatched design, you would have used a Jonckheere trend test to analyse your results (see p. 159).

Because we used more than 5 Ss in our experiment, we had to use Table A2.1 to look up our $H$ value. Suppose, however, that we had used instead, 5 Ss in condition 1, 4 in condition 2 and 3 in condition 3, and had obtained an $H$ value of 5.438. We would now need to use Table A2.8. You will see that there is a heading 'Size of groups', under which there is every permutation of $n$ values. Your $n$ values are $n_1 = 5$, $n_2 = 4$ and $n_3 = 3$. Therefore you need to find these $n$ values (in any order) in the columns and to the right of these you will see six values of $H$:

7.4449
7.3949
5.6564
5.6308
4.5487
4.5231

and to their right, the relevant $p$ values. (You do not need the df value here.)

To be significant at a given level, our $H$ value must be *equal to* or *larger than* the critical values here. Our $H$ value of 5.438 is larger than 4.5487 but smaller than 5.6308. These values are associated with probabilities of 0.050 and 0.099, and so our obtained $H$ value must have a probability of less than 0.099 but greater than 0.050. Because of convention, we would say that our $H$ of 5.438 has a probability of less than 0.099. Because our cut-off point is 0.05, we must accept the null (no relationship) hypothesis, i.e. our results would not be significant.

**Activity 15.3** (Answers on page 233)

1 To practise looking up $H$ values, look up the following and state whether or not they are significant and at what level.
   (i) $n_1 = 3$    $n_2 = 4$    $n_3 = 3$    $H = 5.801$    $p$
   (ii) $n_1 = 5$    $n_2 = 5$    $n_3 = 4$    $H = 5.893$    $p$
   (iii) $n_1 = 12$    $n_2 = 10$    $n_3 = 10$    $n_4 = 10$
      df = 3    $H = 8.5$    $p$
   (iv) $n_1 = 3$    $n_2 = 3$    $n_3 = 5$    $H = 7.0234$    $p$
   (v) $n_1 = 10$    $n_2 = 12$    $n_3 = 14$    $n_4 = 14$    $n_5 = 14$
      df = 4    $H = 15.23$    $p$
   (vi) $n_1 = = 10$    $n_2 = 10$    $n_3 = 8$    $n_4 = 10$
      df = 3    $H = = 6.86$    $p$
2 Calculate a Kruskal–Wallis on the following data:
   $H_1$    Compliance with postnatal exercise instructions varies according to whether the instructions are (a) oral, (b) written by the physiotherapist, or (c) written by the patient herself.
   Method: Select 15 women within 1 week of parturition and randomly allocate 5 to oral instruction, 5 to physiotherapist-written instructions and 5 to self-written instructions. After 1 week compare their self-reported compliance (on a 5-point scale where 5 = did every exercise daily, 1 = did no exercises at all). The results are as shown in Table 15.5.

**Table 15.5**

| Sub-ject | Condi-tion 1 Oral | Rank | Sub-ject | Condi-tion 2 Physio. | Rank | Sub-ject | Condi-tion 3 Self | Rank |
|---|---|---|---|---|---|---|---|---|
| 1 | 3 | | 1 | 3 | | 1 | 4 | |
| 2 | 2 | | 2 | 3 | | 2 | 3 | |
| 3 | 2 | | 3 | 3 | | 3 | 4 | |
| 4 | 3 | | 4 | 2 | | 4 | 3 | |
| 5 | 1 | | 5 | 3 | | 5 | 5 | |

State the $H$ and $p$ values in the format recommended earlier.

## 2. Jonckheere trend test

This test is used with the same experimental designs as the Kruskal–Wallis, i.e.

- three or more different- (unmatched-) subject groups are being compared
- the data is ordinal or interval/ratio
- the conditions required for a parametric test cannot be fulfilled (see p. 150 for the design).

However, the one major difference which determines whether you use a Kruskal–Wallis or Jonckheere trend test relates to your hypothesis. If you simply predict that there will be differences between the groups, without specifying which group will perform best or worst then you use the Kruskal–Wallis. However, if you predict a trend in your results, e.g.

Group A will do better than Group B who in turn will do better than Group C

then you are predicting a definite direction to your results and you should use the Jonckheere to analyse them. Therefore any hypothesis associated with the Jonckheere must be one-tailed.

When calculating the Jonckheere, you end up with a numerical value called 'S', which you look up in the probability tables associated with the Jonckheere test, to see whether this value represents a significant trend in the results.

It should be stressed here that you must have the *same numbers of subjects in each group* for the Jonckheere. This is not necessary for the Kruskal-–Wallis, but it is an essential here.

*Example*

If we look back at the example given on page 156,

i.e. that there will be a difference in the strength of muscle contraction in the biceps of stroke patients according to the type of preparation used, we can see that because we only predicted a difference in efficacy without specifying which preparation would be best, we used a Kruskal–Wallis. However, if we restated that hypothesis to predict a specific direction to the results:

$H_1$ There is a difference in the strength of the biceps muscle contraction in stroke patients according to the type of preparation used, *with 2 minutes' specific warm-up being more effective than 2 minutes' general warm-up which in turn is more effective than 2 minutes' infra-red.*

we are predicting a specific directional trend to the results which would require the Jonckheere trend test to analyse them. We would therefore have the design shown in Figure 15.9.

| | | | |
|---|---|---|---|
| Subject group 1 (10 stroke patients) | takes part in | *Condition 1* Specific warm-up | Groups are compared on strength of muscle contraction, predicting that Group 1 will do better than Group 2 who, in turn, will do better than Group 3. |
| Subject group 2 (10 stroke patients | takes part in | *Condition 2* General warm-up | |
| Subject group 3 (10 stroke patients) | takes part in | *Condition 3* Infra-red | |

**Figure 15.9** Specific warm-up exercises are more effective than general warm-up which is, in turn, more effective than infrared. The Jonckheere trend test is used to analyse the results.

If we use the previous data, we can see whether or not there was a definite trend in results. These results are as in Table 15.6.

**Table 15.6**

| Subject | *Condition 1* Infrared | Subject | *Condition 2* Specific | Subject | *Condition 3* General |
|---|---|---|---|---|---|
| 1 | 3 | 1 | 4 | 1 | 2 |
| 2 | 4 | 2 | 5 | 2 | 3 |
| 3 | 2 | 3 | 5 | 3 | 3 |
| 4 | 2 | 4 | 4 | 4 | 4 |
| 5 | 1 | 5 | 4 | 5 | 1 |
| 6 | 3 | 6 | 3 | 6 | 3 |
| 7 | 4 | 7 | 2 | 7 | 2 |
| 8 | 1 | 8 | 3 | 8 | 1 |
| 9 | 2 | 9 | 5 | 9 | 3 |
| 10 | 2 | 10 | 4 | 10 | 3 |

### *Calculating the Jonckheere trend test*

So, taking the data from the previous example, we first have to set out the conditions such that the condition expected to obtain the lowest scores is on the left, and the condition expected to obtain the highest scores is on the right, the remaining condition in the middle. In other words, the conditions must be ordered from lowest on the left, to highest on the right, with any intermediary conditions ordered accordingly.

Therefore, because we have predicted that the infra-red group will do worst, followed by the general warm-up group, with the specific warm-up group doing best, we must re-order the above data to put the infra-red group on the left, the general warm-up in the middle and the specific warm-up on the right as in Table 15.7.

**Table 15.7**

| Subject | *Condition 1* Infrared | Subject | *Condition 2* General | Subject | *Condition 3* Specific |
|---|---|---|---|---|---|
| 1 | 3 (8) | 1 | 2 (9) | 1 | 4 |
| 2 | 4 (3) | 2 | 3 (7) | 2 | 5 |
| 3 | 2 (15) | 3 | 3 (7) | 3 | 5 |
| 4 | 2 (15) | 4 | 4 (3) | 4 | 4 |
| 5 | 1 (18) | 5 | 1 (10) | 5 | 4 |
| 6 | 3 (8) | 6 | 3 (7) | 6 | 3 |
| 7 | 4 (3) | 7 | 2 (9) | 7 | 2 |
| 8 | 1 (18) | 8 | 1 (10) | 8 | 3 |
| 9 | 2 (15) | 9 | 3 (7) | 9 | 5 |
| 10 | 2 (15) | 10 | 3 (7) | 10 | 4 |
| $\bar{x}$ | 2.4 | | 2.5 | | 3.9 |

To calculate the Jonckheere:

**1.** First calculate the mean score for each condition (Condition 1 = 2.4, Condition 2 = 2.5 and Condition 3 = 3.9).

**2.** Starting with the extreme left-hand condition and the first score (i.e. 3) count up all the scores to the right of Condition 1 (i.e. in Conditions 2 and 3) which are larger than this score. Do not count any scores which are the same.

Therefore, in Condition 2, only Subject 4 with a score of 4 achieved a higher score, while in Condition 3, Subjects 1, 2, 3, 4, 5, 9 and 10 all obtained higher scores. This means that in total, 8 scores in Conditions 2 and 3 are higher than the score of 3. This number is put in brackets by Subject 1, Condition 1's score.

Do exactly the same for the second score (4) in Condition 1. There are no scores in Condition 2 which are larger and 3 scores in Condition 3 which are larger. Thus the total of 3 is put in brackets by Subject 2, Condition 1. Continue in this way for the rest of the scores in Condition 1.

Do the same for each score in Condition 2, although, of course, you will only be comparing these with Condition 3 since it is only these scores which are to the right of Condition 2.

Because Condition 3 has no scores to the right the procedure terminates with the last subject in Condition 2.

**2.** Before we can calculate $S$, we need two more values: $A$ and $B$. To find $A$: add up *all* scores in brackets to give the value $A$, i.e.

$$A = 8 + 3 + 15 + 15 + 18 + 8 + 3 + 18 + 15 + 15$$
$$+ 9 + 7 + 7 + 3 + 10 + 7 + 9 + 10 + 7 + 7$$
$$\therefore A = 194$$

**3.** In order to find out $B$, which is the maximum value $A$ could have been, had all the scores in Conditions 2 and 3 been bigger than those in Condition 1 and all the scores in Condition 3 been bigger than those in Condition 2, we use the formula:

$$B = \frac{C(C-1)}{2} \times n^2$$

where $n$ = number of Ss in each condition
$C$ = number of conditions

Therefore $n = 10$
$C = 3$
$$B = \frac{3(3-1)}{2} \times 10^2$$
$$= 300$$

**4.** Calculate $S$ using the following formula:

$$S = (2 \times A) - B$$
$$= (2 \times 194) - 300$$
$$S = 88$$

## Looking up the value of S for significance

To look up $S = 88$, turn to Table A2.9 (page 223) where you will see two tables: the top one is for significance levels of <5% and the lower one for levels of <1%. Both are for one-tailed hypotheses because a specific direction to the results must be predicted in order to use the Jonckheere test.

Start with the top table first. In order to look up your $S$ value, you need the number of conditions and the number of subjects in each condition (i.e. 3 and 10 respectively). Look across the top row for the appropriate value of $n$ and down the left-hand column for the appropriate value of $C$. At the intersection point you will find the figure 88. If our $S$ value is *equal to* or *larger than* this figure, then the results are significant at the level stated in the heading of the table. As our $S$ value is exactly 88, our results are significant at the <0.05 or <5% level. This means that there is less than a 5% probability that our results are due to random error.

Had our $S$ value been larger than the intersection figure of 88 (say 131), we would move down to the second table which is associated with a probability level of <0.01 and repeat the process. The intersection figure is 124, which means the result is larger than this value and the probability of our results being due to random error is less than 0.01 or 1%.

## Interpreting the results

Because our usual cut-off point is 5%, and our results have a probability level of <5% the results can be classified as significant and we can reject the null (no relationship) hypothesis. There is less than a 5% chance that random error is responsible for our results. This means that there is a significant trend in our results with specific warm-up being better than general warm-up which in turn is better than infra-red in aiding the strength of muscle contraction. This can be expressed thus:

Using a Jonckheere trend test on the data ($S = 88$, $n = 10$), the results were found to be significant at <5% level. This means that there is a significant trend in the effectiveness of different preparation techniques for muscle contraction, with specific warm-ups being more effective than general warm-ups, and infra-red being the least effective. The null hypothesis can be rejected.

**Activity 15.4** (Answers on page 234)

1 To practise looking up *S* values, look up the following and state whether or not they are significant and at what level.
   (i) *C* = 3  *n* = 6  *S* = 61  *p*
   (ii) *C* = 5  *n* = 5  *S* = 68  *p*
   (iii) *C* = 5  *n* = 8  *S* = 151  *p*
   (iv) *C* = 3  *n* = 10  *S* = 124  *p*
   (v) *C* = 3  *n* = 7  *S* = 55  *p*
   (vi) *C* = 4  *n* = 5  *S* = 48  *p*

2 Calculate a Jonckheere trend test on the following data:
   $H_1$  There is a difference in the number of appointments kept at an out-patients' clinic according to the social class to which the patients belong, with social class 3 being better than social class 2, who in turn are better than social class 4.
   Method: Randomly select 8 patients belonging to each of the social classes and calculate the percentage of kept appointments. The data are as shown in Table 15.8.

**Table 15.8**

| Sub-ject | Condition 1 Social class 3 | Sub-ject | Condition 2 Social class 2 | Sub-ject | Condition 3 Social class 4 |
|---|---|---|---|---|---|
| 1 | 100 | 1 | 100 | 1 | 75 |
| 2 | 90 | 2 | 100 | 2 | 70 |
| 3 | 100 | 3 | 80 | 3 | 50 |
| 4 | 75 | 4 | 75 | 4 | 30 |
| 5 | 75 | 5 | 60 | 5 | 60 |
| 6 | 80 | 6 | 80 | 6 | 80 |
| 7 | 90 | 7 | 50 | 7 | 70 |
| 8 | 70 | 8 | 50 | 8 | 75 |

Remember! You must arrange your data such that the condition expected to have the lowest results is on the left, while the condition expected to have the highest results is on the right.
   State the values of *A, B, S* and *p*; express the results in the format given earlier in the section.

# NON-PARAMETRIC TEST: THREE OR MORE DIFFERENT SUBJECT GROUPS AND NOMINAL DATA

## Extended chi-squared ($\chi^2$) test

As the name implies this test is an extension of the $\chi^2$ test described earlier in the chapter. Like the earlier test it is used:

- with different subject groups
- with nominal data (re-read Ch. 4 if you need to

refresh your memory on levels of measurement)
- when the remaining conditions required for a parametric test cannot be fulfilled.
   (See p. 150 for the design.)

However, there is an important point which relates to the extended $\chi^2$ test. The ordinary $\chi^2$ test only allows you to use two groups of subjects which you can allocate to two nominal categories. This means you arrange your data in a 2 × 2 table as in Figure 15.10.

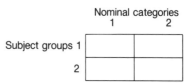

**Figure 15.10**  A 2 × 2 table for calculating the $\chi^2$ test.

However, the extended $\chi^2$ allows you to use

- Two groups of subjects and three (or more) nominal categories.
This means you arrange your data in a 2 × 3 table as in Figure 15.11.

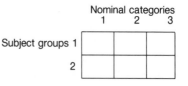

**Figure 15.11**  A 2 × 3 table for calculating the extended $\chi^2$ test, with two subject groups and three nominal categories.

- Three (or more) groups of subjects and two nominal categories:
This means you arrange your data in a 3 × 2 table, as in Figure 15.12.

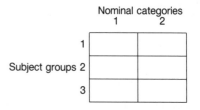

**Figure 15.12**  A 3 × 2 table for calculating the extended $\chi^2$ test, with three subject groups and two nominal categories.

• Three (or more) groups of subject and three (or more) nominal categories:

This means you arrange your data in a 3 × 3 table as in Figure 15.13.

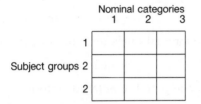

**Figure 15.13** A 3 × 3 table for calculating the extended $\chi^2$ test with three subject groups and three nominal categories.

So you may wish to ask the opinions of senior grade II physiotherapists and superintendent physiotherapists (two groups) on the issue of skill mix – 'approve', 'disapprove' and 'don't know' (three nominal categories). This would be a 2 × 3 table. You would need to use the extended $\chi^2$ test to analyse the results.

(By the way, I recognise that the heading of this subsection may be confusing, in that it implies the extended $\chi^2$ can only be used with three or more subject groups, whereas it can be used with two groups as long as they are being allocated to more than two nominal categories. I apologise for this, but as you can see, a clear, succinct title was difficult to achieve.)

The extended $\chi^2$ test only tells you whether there are overall differences between the groups and not where these differences lie. As a result any hypothesis associated with the extended $\chi^2$ must be two-tailed, in that it cannot predict a specific direction to the results.

The data you obtained in your experiment are called the 'observed' data. The main point of the $\chi^2$ test is to compare your observed data with the data you would have expected had your results been due to totally random distributions. In other words you are comparing the results obtained from your experimental hypothesis (observed data) with those predicted by your null (no relationship) hypothesis (expected data). Obviously, the greater the discrepancies between the observed and the expected data, the more likely your results are to be significant. Always ensure that you have tested sufficient subjects to obtain

expected frequencies of more than 5. The easiest way to do this is by using at least 20 subjects in each group. You do not need to use equal numbers of subjects in each group.

When calculating the extended $\chi^2$, the value of $\chi^2$ is found and this is then looked up in the probability tables associated with the test to find out whether this value represents significant differences between the observed and expected frequencies.

*Example*

Suppose in the course of your work you had to treat a very large number of patients presenting with back pain. Over the years, a pattern seems to emerge, which makes you wonder whether the stress levels associated with some jobs predispose people to generalised rather than localised back pain. You decide to find out whether your hunch is correct, by selecting three groups representing different occupational stress levels and assessing whether they had specific low back pain or general back pain. Your hypothesis is:

$H_1$  Occupations associated with different levels of stress vary with respect to the type of back pain they experience (specific low back pain vs general back pain.

You might then go into two or three back schools and select three groups of patients (with at least 20 subjects in each group) representing the occupational groups: 'High stress', 'Medium stress' and 'Low stress'. You might then simply count up how many patients in each group had been referred either for low back pain or for other forms of back pain (two nominal categories). Thus you would have:

Subject group 1
High stress jobs
Subject group 2
Medium stress jobs
Subject group 3
Low stress jobs

} Compared for differences in location of back pain (specific/general)

There are, then, three unrelated groups of subjects. Each subject's response is allocated to one of two categories (low back pain/other back pain) and the relative numbers in each category are compared using the extended $\chi^2$.

Imagine that you have carried out some research to test the hypothesis just quoted and you have obtained the following data:

| High stress jobs | low back pain | 9 |
| | other back pain | 21 |
| Medium stress jobs | low back pain | 22 |
| | other back pain | 13 |
| Low stress jobs | low back pain | 25 |
| | other back pain | 28 |

This data is then set out as in Figure 15.14.

| | Low back pain | Other back pain | Marginal totals of patients |
|---|---|---|---|
| Group 1<br>High stress | Cell 1<br>9<br>E = 14.237 | Cell 2<br>21<br>E = 15.763 | 30 |
| Group 2<br>Medium stress | Cell 3<br>22<br>E = 16.61 | Cell 4<br>13<br>E = 18.39 | 35 |
| Group 3<br>Low stress | Cell 5<br>25<br>E = 25.153 | Cell 6<br>28<br>E = 27.848 | 53 |
| Marginal totals of types of pain | 56 | 62 | Grand total (N)<br>118 |

**Figure 15.14** An example of data for the extended $\chi^2$ test, with three subject groups and two nominal categories.

You should ensure that the cells are numbered as shown in Figure 15.14, i.e. from left to right. Make sure your subject groups are down the left-hand side, and the nominal categories across the top, although the order in each case is irrelevant.

## Calculating the extended $\chi^2$ test

So, to calculate the $\chi^2$ test, take the following steps:

**1.** Add up the numbers in each row to give the marginal total for

| High stress jobs | i.e. $9 + 21 = 30$ |
| Medium stress jobs | i.e. $22 + 13 = 35$ |
| Low stress jobs | i.e. $25 + 28 = 53$. |

**2.** Add up the numbers in each column to give the marginal totals for

low back pain     i.e. $9 + 22 + 25 = 56$
other back pain    i.e. $21 + 13 + 28 = 62$

**3.** Add up either the marginal totals for patients, i.e.

$$30 + 35 + 53 = 118$$

or the marginal totals for types of pain, i.e.

$$56 + 62 = 118$$

to give the grand total ($N$) therefore:

$$N = 118$$

**4.** Calculate the expected frequency ($E$) for each cell by multiplying the two relevant marginal totals together and dividing by $N$.

$$\text{Cell 1 E} = \frac{30 \times 56}{118}$$
$$= 14.237$$

$$\text{Cell 2 E} = \frac{30 \times 62}{118}$$
$$= 15.763$$

$$\text{Cell 3 E} = \frac{35 \times 56}{118}$$
$$= 16.61$$

$$\text{Cell 4 E} = \frac{35 \times 62}{118}$$
$$= 18.39$$

$$\text{Cell 5 E} = \frac{53 \times 56}{118}$$
$$= 25.153$$

$$\text{Cell 6 E} = \frac{53 \times 62}{118}$$
$$= 27.848$$

Enter each expected frequency in the lower right-hand corner of the appropriate cell.

**5.** Calculate the following formula for $\chi_2$

$$\chi^2 = \sum \frac{(O - E)^2}{E}$$

where    $O$ = observed frequencies for each cell (i.e. your actual data)
         $E$ = expected frequencies for each cell
         $\Sigma$ = sum or total of all calculations to the right of the sign.

$$\text{Cell 1} = \frac{(9 - 14.237)^2}{14.237}$$
$$= 1.926$$

$$\text{Cell 2} = \frac{(21 - 15.763)^2}{15.763}$$
$$= 1.74$$

$$\text{Cell 3} = \frac{(22 - 16.61)^2}{16.61}$$
$$= 1.75$$

$$\text{Cell 4} = \frac{(13 - 18.39)^2}{18.39}$$
$$= 1.58$$

$$\text{Cell 5} = \frac{(25 - 25.153)^2}{25.153}$$
$$= 0$$

$$\text{Cell 6} = \frac{(28 - 27.848)^2}{27.848}$$
$$= 0$$

**6.** All these values are added together to give $\chi^2$:

$$\chi^2 = \sum \frac{(O - E)^2}{E}$$

i.e.

$$\chi^2 = 1.926 + 1.74 + 1.75 + 1.58 + 0 + 0$$
$$= 6.996$$
$$\chi^2 = 6.996$$

**7.** To look up the value $\chi^2$ 6.996, you will also need the degrees of freedom (df) value, i.e.

$$(r - 1) \times (c - 1)$$

where $r$ = number of rows (3)
$c$ = number of columns (2)

Therefore:

$$df = (3 - 1) \times (2 - 1) = 2$$

### Looking up the value of $\chi^2$ for significance

Turn to Table A2.1 (page 209). You will see down the left-hand column, different df values. Find our df = 2 value. To the right of this are 5 numbers, called critical values of $\chi^2$:

4.60   5.99   7.82   9.21   13.82

Each critical value is associated with the $p$ value at the top of its column, e.g. 9.21 has a $p$ value of 0.01. To be significant at a particular level, our $\chi^2$ values must be *equal to* or *larger than* one of these critical values. (Remember that the extended $\chi^2$ can only determine whether there are overall differences in the results, so the associated hypothesis must be two-tailed.)

Our $\chi^2$ value of 6.996 is larger than 5.99 but smaller than 7.82. This means that our results are not good enough to be significant at 0.02, but they are slightly better than the 0.05 level. Therefore, by convention we express this as $p < 0.05$ (less than 0.05). Had our $\chi^2$ value been 5.99 exactly we would have expressed this as $p = 0.05$. This means that our $\chi^2$ value is significant at the $< 0.05$ level or $< 5\%$ level. In other words, the chances of our results being due to random error are less than 5%.

### Interpreting the results

Our $\chi^2$ value has an associated probability value of $< 0.05$. This means that there is less than a 5% chance that our results could be accounted for by random error. As the usual cut-off point of 5% or less is used to claim support for the experimental hypothesis and our results have a probability of less than 5%, we can say they are significant. The null hypothesis can be rejected and the experimental hypothesis accepted. This means that there is a significant relationship between job stress and type of back pain.

This can be expressed in the following way:

Using the extended $\chi^2$ on the data ($\chi^2 = 6.996$, df = 2) the results were found to be significant at $p < 0.05$ for a two-tailed test. This suggests that occupational stress levels (Low, Medium and High) are significantly associated with type of back pain (low back pain or general back pain).

**Activity 15.5** (Answers on page 234)

1 To practise looking up $\chi^2$ values, look up the following and state whether or not they are significant.
  (i)   $\chi^2 = 3.45$    df = 2    $p$
  (ii)  $\chi^2 = 8.91$    df = 3    $p$
  (iii) $\chi^2 = 6.77$    df = 2    $p$
  (iv) $\chi^2 = 9.42$    df = 4    $p$
  (v)  $\chi^2 = 7.95$    df = 2    $p$

2 Calculate an extended $\chi^2$ on the following data.
    You are concerned about the missed appointments at the outpatients' clinic and think it may be to do with the

ease of getting to the clinic by public transport. Your hypothesis, then, is:

$H_1$  Keeping an outpatient appointment is related to the ease of access to the hospital, when using public transport.

So you select 25 patients who have a single bus journey with no changes, 30 who have to make one change of bus and 29 who have to make more than one change of bus. You simply note whether or not they missed their next appointment. You obtain the data in Figure 15.15.

Calculate an extended $\chi^2$ on these data, and state what the $\chi^2$ value is and the $p$ value. Present your results in the format suggested earlier.

|  |  | Attended | Missed |
|---|---|---|---|
|  | 1<br>No change of<br>bus | 20 | 5 |
| Subject<br>group | 2<br>One change of<br>bus | 17 | 13 |
|  | 3<br>More than one<br>change of bus | 15 | 14 |

**Figure 15.15**  Is keeping outpatient appointments related to the ease of getting to the clinic? What are the $\chi^2$ and $p$ values for these data?

CHAPTER CONTENTS



# 16

# Parametric tests for different- (unrelated-) subject designs

## INTRODUCTION

The statistical tests described in the previous chapter are used to analyse results from unrelated designs, i.e. any design which uses two or more than two groups of different, unmatched subjects. They are also used when the conditions necessary for a parametric test (see Ch. 9) cannot be fulfilled. The tests covered in this chapter are the parametric equivalent to those in the previous chapter, in other words they are used when:

- two or more than two different (unmatched) groups of subjects are used in the research and the results from each are compared for differences.
- when the conditions essential for a parametric test can be fulfilled (especially the interval/ratio level of measurement).

Therefore, the sorts of designs involved are:
**1. Two different, unmatched subject groups,** compared on a task (Fig. 16.1).

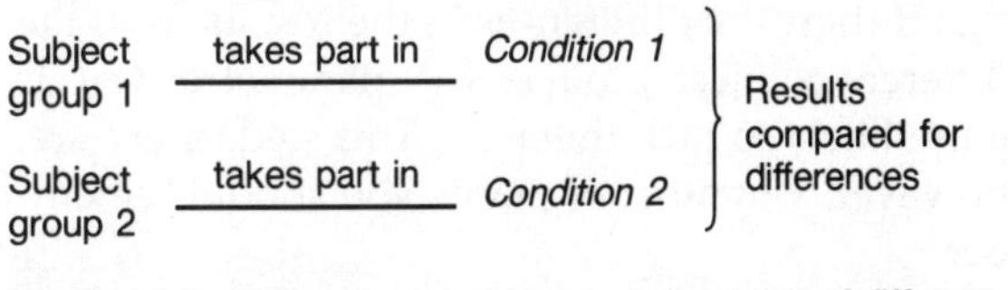


**Figure 16.1** Different-subject design: two groups of different, unmatched subjects each taking part in one condition.

**2. Three or more different, unmatched subject groups,** compared on a task (Fig. 16.2).

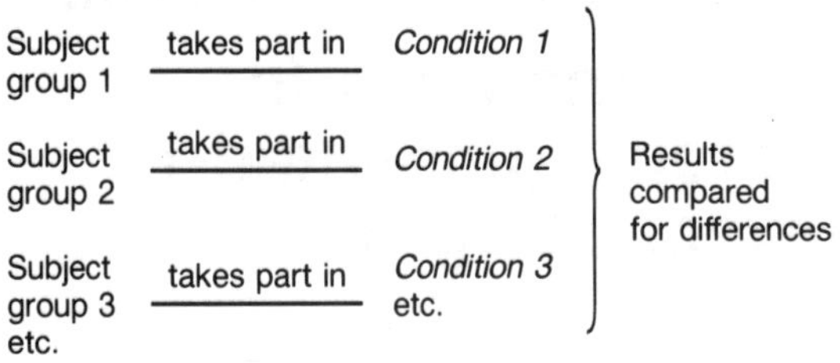

| Subject group 1 | takes part in | *Condition 1* | |
| Subject group 2 | takes part in | *Condition 2* | Results compared for differences |
| Subject group 3 etc. | takes part in | *Condition 3* etc. | |

**Figure 16.2** Different-subject design: three, or more, groups of different, unmatched subjects each taking part in one condition.

Results from experiments using Design 1 (two unmatched groups) are analysed by the unrelated *t* test, while results derived from experiments using Design 2 (three or more unmatched groups) are analysed by the one-way analysis of variance (anova) for unrelated designs. In addition, the Scheffé multiple range test can be used in conjunction with the anova for further analysis of the results. This will be explained later in the chapter (Table 16.1).

**Table 16.1** Parametric tests for different- (unrelated-) subject designs

| Design | Parametric test |
| --- | --- |
| 1. Two groups of different, unmatched subjects, each taking part in one condition. Results from conditions compared for differences. | Unrelated *t* test |
| 2. Three or more groups of different, unmatched subjects, each taking part in one condition. Results from conditions compared for differences. | One-way analysis of variance (anova) for unrelated designs, and Scheffé multiple range test |

Remember that a parametric test is much more powerful than the non-parametric equivalent, in that if there are differences in the results from the different subject groups, the parametric test is more likely to pick them up. This said, there are, however, a number of points you should remember:

1. The parametric test and its non-parametric equivalent do essentially the same job in that they compare results from the subject groups to find out whether any differences between them are significant.
2. In order to use a parametric test you must

ensure that you fulfil the necessary conditions. (see page 83).
3. If you are in any doubt as to whether a parametric test should be used, always use the non-parametric equivalent.
4. Parametric tests, although more sensitive, are more difficult to calculate.

## PARAMETRIC TEST: TWO GROUPS OF DIFFERENT SUBJECTS

### Unrelated *t* test

This test is used when the experimental design compares two separate or different unmatched groups of subjects participating in different conditions (see Design 1, page 167). It is the parametric equivalent of the Mann–Whitney *U* test. The fact that it is parametric means, principally, that you must have *interval/ratio data*. Do note that you do not need to have equal numbers in each group.

When calculating the unrelated *t* test, you find the value called '*t*', which you then look up in the probability tables associated with the *t* test to find out whether the *t* value represents a significant difference between the results from your two groups.

#### Example

In order to rehabilitate meniscectomy patients more efficiently, you wish to compare two treatments commonly in use in your department: audiobiofeedback and muscle stimulation, to see which one producess greater movement in the knee joint. Your hypothesis, then, is:

H₁  Meniscectomy patients who have lost some movement improve more quickly when treated by audiobiofeedback than by muscle stimulation.

This is a one-tailed hypothesis because it is predicting a specific direction to the results.

You might select 20 meniscectomy patients, all within 48 postoperative hours, and randomly allocate 10 patients to audiobiofeedback and 10 to muscle stimulation. After five treatment sessions, you might compare percentage range of movement for each group. Therefore, you would have the design shown in Fig. 16.3.

Group 1
10 meniscectomy — *Condition 1*
patients, within 48   Audiobio feedback
hours postoperative

Group 2
10 meniscectomy — *Condition 2*
patients, within 48   Muscle stimulation
hours postoperative

Compare percentage range of movement for each group to see if there are any differences

**Figure 16.3** Is audiobio feedback more effective than muscle stimulation for rehabilitation for meniscectomy patients?

In other words you are comparing the results of two different groups of subjects; a design and type of measurement which requires an unrelated *t* test.

You obtain the results shown in Table 16.2.

### Calculating the unrelated t test

In order to calculate *t*, you should take the following steps (the unrelated *t* test formula looks very formidable, but please don't panic! As long as you work through the following stages systematically, you shouldn't have too much difficulty).

**1.** Find the total ($\Sigma$) of the scores for each condition:

Condition 1 = 345
Condition 2 = 285

**2.** Find the average score ($\bar{x}$) for each condition, i.e.:

$\bar{x}$ for Condition 1 = 34.5
$\bar{x}$ for Condition 2 = 28.5.

**3.** Square every individual score and enter the results in the columns headed $X_1^2$ and $X_2^2$, e.g. Subject 1, Group 1, scored 40, which when squared becomes 1600.

**4.** Add up the squared scores for each condition separately to give $\Sigma X^2$, i.e.:

$$\Sigma X_1^2 = 12325$$
$$\Sigma X_2^2 = 8725$$

**5.** Take the total for each condition separately, and square it, to give $(\Sigma X)^2$, i.e:

$$(\Sigma X_1)^2 = 345^2$$
$$= 119025$$
$$(\Sigma X_2)^2 = 285^2$$
$$= 81225$$

Do make a note of the difference between the symbol '$\Sigma X^2$' which means: 'square each individual score and then add up all the squared scores', and $(\Sigma X)^2$ which means: 'add up all the individual scores for the condition and then square the result'.

**Table 16.2**

| | Group 1*, audiobiofeedback | | | Group 2, muscle stimulation | | |
|---|---|---|---|---|---|---|
| Subject | Scores ($X_1$) | | $X_1^2$ | Subject | Scores ($X_2$) | $X_2^2$ |
| 1 | 40 | | 1600 | 1 | 20 | 400 |
| 2 | 30 | | 900 | 2 | 25 | 625 |
| 3 | 35 | | 1225 | 3 | 30 | 900 |
| 4 | 25 | | 625 | 4 | 25 | 625 |
| 5 | 30 | | 900 | 5 | 15 | 225 |
| 6 | 40 | | 1600 | 6 | 40 | 1600 |
| 7 | 45 | | 2025 | 7 | 35 | 1225 |
| 8 | 35 | | 1225 | 8 | 40 | 1600 |
| 9 | 25 | | 625 | 9 | 25 | 625 |
| 10 | 40 | | 1600 | 10 | 30 | 900 |
| $\Sigma X_1 =$ | 345 | $\Sigma X_1^2 =$ | 12325 | $\Sigma X_2 =$ | 285 $\quad \Sigma X_2^2 =$ | 8725 |
| $\bar{x}_1 =$ | 34.5 | | | $\bar{x}_2 =$ | 28.5 | |

*It does not matter whether audiobiofeedback is Condition 1 or 2.

**6.** Now (take a deep breath!) calculate $t$ from the formula:

$$t = \frac{\bar{x}_1 - \bar{x}_2}{\sqrt{\dfrac{\left(\Sigma X_1^2 - \dfrac{(\Sigma X_1)^2}{n_1}\right) + \left(\Sigma X_2^2 - \dfrac{(\Sigma X_2)^2}{n_2}\right)}{(n_1 - 1) + (n_2 - 1)}} \times \sqrt{\left(\dfrac{1}{n_1} + \dfrac{1}{n_2}\right)}}$$

where  $\bar{x}_1$ = mean of scores from Condition 1
  = 34.5
 $\bar{x}_2$ = mean of scores from Condition 2
  = 28.5
 $\Sigma X_1^2$ = the square of each individual score from Condition 1 totalled
  = 12 325
 $\Sigma X_2^2$ = the square of each individual score from Condition 2 totalled
  = 8725
 $(\Sigma X_1)^2$ = the total of the individual scores from Condition 1 squared
  = $345^2$
  = 119 025
 $(\Sigma X_2)^2$ = the total of the individual scores from Condition 2 squared
  = $285^2$
  = 81 225
 $n_1$ = number of Ss in Condition 1
  = 10
 $n_2$ = number of Ss in Condition 2
  = 10

If we substitute these values in the formula:

$$t = \frac{34.5 - 28.5}{\sqrt{\dfrac{\left(12\,325 - \dfrac{119\,025}{10}\right) + \left(8\,725 - \dfrac{81\,225}{10}\right)}{(10 - 1) + (10 - 1)}} \times \sqrt{\left(\dfrac{1}{10} + \dfrac{1}{10}\right)}}$$

$$= \frac{6}{\sqrt{\dfrac{422.5 - 602.5}{18} \times \dfrac{1}{5}}}$$

$$= \frac{6}{\sqrt{56.944 \times 0.2}}$$

$$= \frac{6}{3.375}$$

$$t = 1.778*$$

*(Note: it does not matter if your $t$ value is + or −, because you ignore the sign anyway.)

**7.** Calculate the degrees of freedom from the formula:

$$\begin{aligned} \text{df} &= (n_1 - 1) + (n_2 - 1) \\ &= (10 - 1) + (10 - 1) \\ &= 18 \end{aligned}$$

*Looking up the value of* t *for significance*

To look up the value $t = 1.778$, with df = 18, turn to Table A2.5 (page 214). Down the left-hand column, you will find values of df. Look down the column until you find df = 18. To the right of this, you will see six numbers, called critical values of $t$:

  1.330  1.734  2.101  2.552  2.878  3.922

Each critical value represents a different level of probability as indicated by the bold type at the top of the table. Therefore, 2.552, for example, is associated with a probability of 0.01 for a one-tailed test and 0.02 for a two-tailed test. To be significant at one of these levels, our $t$ value must be *equal to* or *larger than* the associated critical $t$ value in the table.

Our $t$ value is larger than 1.734, but smaller than 2.101. This means that for our one-tailed hypothesis, the probability associated with our $t$ value of 1.778 comes somewhere between 0.05 (5%) and 0.025 (2½%). In other words the probability for $t = 1.778$ is less than 5%, but greater than 2½%. According to convention, we always say that $p$ is less than a given level, and so here the $p$ value for $t = 1.778$ is less than 5% (or 0.05). This is expressed as:

$$p < 0.05 \text{ (or 5\%)}$$

as < means 'less than'.

This means that the chances of random error accounting for our results are less than 5%.

Had our *t* value been 1.734 exactly, the associated probability level would have equalled 0.05. This would be expressed as $p = 0.05$.

### Interpreting the results

Our *t* value of 1.778 has an associated probability level of less than 5%, which means that the possibility of random error being responsible for the outcome of our experiment is less than 5 in 100. As the usual cut-off point for claiming support for the experimental hypothesis is 5% we can say that our results are significant. However, because we predicted a specific direction to the results (i.e. a one-tailed hypothesis), we must check that the results are in the predicted direction (i.e. audiobiofeedback being more effective than muscle stimulation); sometimes significant results are obtained which are in the opposite direction to the hypothesis and therefore do not support it.

Here, if we look at the mean scores for each condition, we can see that the average score for the audiobiofeedback condition is larger (34.5 as opposed to 28.5). Therefore, the experimental hypothesis has been supported. This can be stated in the following way:

Using an unrelated *t* test on the data (*t* = 1.778, df = 18) the results were found to be significant (*p* < 0.05 for a one-tailed hypothesis). The null hypothesis can therefore be rejected. This means that audiobiofeedback is more effective than muscle stimulation for developing movement in meniscectomy patients.

**Activity 16.1** (Answers on page 234)

1 To practise looking up *t* values, look up the following and state whether or not they are significant and at what level:
   (i)   *t* = 2.149  df = 10   one-tailed  *p*
   (ii)  *t* = 2.596  df = 16   two-tailed  *p*
   (iii) *t* = 3.055  df = 12   two-tailed  *p*
   (iv) *t* = 1.499  df = 15   one-tailed  *p*
   (v)  *t* = 3.204  df = 18   two-tailed  *p*

2 Calculate an unrelated *t* test on the following data

   H₁ Absenteeism is greater among basic grade physiotherapists than among senior grade IIs.
   Method: Randomly select 15 basic grade physiotherapists and 12 senior grade II physiotherapists, and count up the number of days each subject was absent during the previous 12 months. The results are as shown in Table 16.3.

**Table 16.3**

| Condition 1, basic grade | | Condition 2, senior grade II | |
|---|---|---|---|
| Subject | Score | Subject | Score |
| 1 | 18 | 1 | 17 |
| 2 | 22 | 2 | 12 |
| 3 | 10 | 3 | 15 |
| 4 | 14 | 4 | 10 |
| 5 | 25 | 5 | 19 |
| 6 | 19 | 6 | 8 |
| 7 | 17 | 7 | 5 |
| 8 | 28 | 8 | 14 |
| 9 | 18 | 9 | 18 |
| 10 | 14 | 10 | 21 |
| 11 | 15 | 11 | 20 |
| 12 | 22 | 12 | 16 |
| 13 | 23 | | |
| 14 | 19 | | |
| 15 | 24 | | |

State the *t*, df and *p* values, using the format outlined earlier.

## PARAMETRIC TEST: THREE OR MORE GROUPS OF DIFFERENT SUBJECTS

### One-way analysis of variance (anova) for unrelated- (different-)subject designs

The one-way anova for unrelated designs is the parametric equivalent of the Kruskal–Wallis test, i.e. it is used to compare results from three or more conditions, with different, unmatched subject groups in each condition, as shown in Figure 16.2 (page 168).

It is used when the prerequisite conditions for a parametric test can be fulfilled, the most important of which is that the data is of an interval/ratio level.

The one-way anova is so-called because it analyses results from experiments where only one independent variable (IV) is manipulated. (All the statistical tests and designs covered in this book relate solely to the manipulation of one IV). More complex designs which manipulate two IVs simultaneously are analysed using a two-way anova; those which manipulate three IVs simultaneously require a three-way anova. (Refresh your memory by re-reading Chapter 6.) All this is outside the domain of this book, but the reader is referred to Ferguson (1976) for more information on this topic.

The anova only tells you whether there are general, non-specified differences in the results from the different conditions; it does not tell you which group is better than the others. (To find this out, once you have calculated your anova, you will need to use the Scheffé test, but more of that later.) Because of this, any hypothesis associated with the anova must, of necessity, be two-tailed.

Essentially, what the one-way unrelated anova does is to tell you whether the differences in scores from each condition are sufficiently large to be classified as significant. But if you look back to the outline design on page 168 you will see that different subject groups are doing different conditions. Therefore, any variation between the scores from the conditions must also reflect the variations between the subject groups.

This source of variation is called *between-conditions variance*. However, because different subjects are involved in each condition, it is conceivable that any outcome in the results is due not to differences between conditions, but to individual differences amongst the subjects, of inherent variations in personality, ability reactions to the study etc., i.e. the result of random error. Thus, this is another source of potential variation in the results and is known as *error variance*.

Obviously, you would wish your results to be the outcome of the different conditions and not random error. Thus, the degree of between-condition variance should be much larger than the error variance. What the one-way unrelated anova does is to tell you whether your results are due to real differences between the experimental conditions or alternatively to random error in the form of individual differences.

*Example*

An actual example might clarify all this. If we go back to the hypothesis quoted for the unrelated *t* test, i.e. meniscectomy patients who have lost some movement inprove more quickly when treated by audiobiofeedback than by muscle stimulation. Suppose we add a further treatment group of ice-packs to this, such that our hypothesis becomes:

$H_1$  There is a difference in the degree of movement of the knee joint among meniscectomy patients according to whether they have been treated with audio biofeedback, muscle stimulation or ice-packs.

(Note the inevitable change to a two-tailed hypothesis in the latter example.)

Obviously, what you are predicting here are differences in percentage range of movement between the groups as a result of different treatments. Therefore, you are anticipating a significant degree of between-group variation. However, suppose you picked your subjects badly, such that all the most motivated were accidentally put in the audiobiofeedback group. Almost inevitably, this type of treatment would produce the best results, not because of the nature of the treatment, but because of the idiosyncrasies of the subjects. In other words random error would account for your results. Obviously, the sort of situation which has all the most motivated subjects inadvertently allocated to one group is very unlikely to occur, particularly if you randomly allocate your subjects to conditions, but the point is this: your results could be due to genuine differences in terms of treatment, or to some quirks of your subjects. Obviously, you want your results to be due to the former and what the one-way unrelated anova does is to tell you how probable it is that your results are due to the IV and not to random error.

Thus, when you calculate the one-way unrelated anova, you have to find out the degree of variation in the scores due to the differences between experimental conditions (between-conditions variance) and that due to random error (error variance). This will give you an '$F$ ratio' which you then look up in the probability tables associated with the anova to see if it represents a significant result. Please note, however, that the following formula is only appropriate for designs with *equal numbers of subjects* in each group.

Let's suppose, then, that we added this third treatment group to our earlier experiment, such that we were now comparing the degrees of movement in three groups of meniscectomy patients following different kinds of treatment: audiobiofeedback, muscle stimulation and ice-packs. Thus we have the sort of design shown in Figure 16.4.

Group 1
10 meniscectomy receive
patients
— Condition 1
Audio-
bio feedback

Group 2
10 meniscectomy receive
patients
— Condition 2
Muscle
stimulation

Group 3
10 meniscectomy receive
patients
— Condition 3
Ice-packs

Compared after treatment for percentage range of movement

**Figure 16.4** Comparison of three different rehabilitation procedures for meniscectomy patients.

When we calculate the one-way unrelated anova we need to set out a table for the sources of variance in scores, like Table 16.4.

**Table 16.4**

| Source of variance | Sums of squares (SS) | Degrees of freedom (df) | Mean squares (MS) | F ratio |
|---|---|---|---|---|
| Variation in results due to treatment (between conditions) | $SS_{bet}$ | $df_{bet}$ | $MS_{bet}$ | $F_{bet}$ |
| Variation in results due to random error | $SS_{error}$ | $df_{error}$ | $MS_{error}$ | |
| Total | $SS_{tot}$ | $df_{tot}$ | | |

So, using the scores from the unrelated $t$ test, together with some new data for the ice-pack group, we have the scores shown is Table 16.5.

### Calculating the one-way anova for unrelated designs

To calculate the sums of squares (SS) for each source of variation, take the following steps:

**1.** Calculate the value $\Sigma T_C^2$, which is the sum of the squared total for each condition, i.e.:

$$T_1^2 = 345^2$$
$$= 119025$$
$$T_2^2 = 285^2$$
$$= 81225$$

**Table 16.5**

| Condition 1 Audiobiofeedback | | Condition 2 Muscle stimulation | | Condition 3 Ice-packs | |
|---|---|---|---|---|---|
| Subject | Score | Subject | Score | Subject | Score |
| 1 | 40 | 1 | 20 | 1 | 25 |
| 2 | 30 | 2 | 25 | 2 | 30 |
| 3 | 35 | 3 | 30 | 3 | 40 |
| 4 | 25 | 4 | 25 | 4 | 35 |
| 5 | 30 | 5 | 15 | 5 | 25 |
| 6 | 40 | 6 | 40 | 6 | 25 |
| 7 | 45 | 7 | 35 | 7 | 20 |
| 8 | 35 | 8 | 40 | 8 | 30 |
| 9 | 25 | 9 | 25 | 9 | 35 |
| 10 | 40 | 10 | 30 | 10 | 35 |
| $\Sigma T_1$ = 345 | | $\Sigma T_2$ = 285 | | $\Sigma T_3$ = 300 | |

$$T_3^2 = 300^2$$
$$= 90000$$

Therefore:

$$\Sigma T_C^2 = 119025 + 81225 + 90000$$
$$= 290250$$

**2.** Find the value of $n$, which is the number of subjects in each condition

$$n = 10$$

**3.** Calculate the value of $N$, which is the total number of scores, i.e.:

$$N = 10 + 10 + 10$$
$$= 30$$

**4.** Calculate $(\Sigma x)^2$ which is the grand total of all the scores, squared, i.e.:

$$(\Sigma x)^2 = (345 + 285 + 300)^2$$
$$= 930^2$$
$$= 864900$$

**5.** Calculate the value of $\dfrac{(\Sigma x)^2}{N}$ (this value is subtracted from all calculations), i.e.:

$$\frac{(\Sigma x)^2}{N} = \frac{(930)^2}{30}$$
$$= \frac{864900}{30}$$
$$= 28830$$

**6.** Thus to calculate the $SS_{bet}$ use the formula:

$$\frac{\Sigma T_C^2}{n} - \frac{(\Sigma x)^2}{N} = \frac{345^2 + 285^2 + 300^2}{10} - \frac{864\,900}{30}$$

$$= \frac{119025 + 81225 + 90000}{10} - 28830$$

$$= 195$$

**7.** Calculate $SS_{tot}$ from the following formula:

$$\Sigma x^2 - \frac{(\Sigma x)^2}{N}$$

where $\Sigma x^2 = $ the square of each individual score, all added together:

$$\begin{aligned}
\Sigma x^2 &= 40^2 + 30^2 + 35^2 + 25^2 + 30^2 + 40^2 + 45^2 + 35^2 \\
&\quad + 25^2 + 40^2 + 20^2 + 25^2 + 30^2 + 25^2 + 15^2 \\
&\quad + 40^2 + 35^2 + 40^2 + 25^2 + 30^2 + 25^2 + 30^2 \\
&\quad + 40^2 + 35^2 + 25^2 + 25^2 + 20^2 + 30^2 + 35^2 \\
&\quad + 35^2 \\
&= 30400
\end{aligned}$$

Therefore

$$\begin{aligned}
SS_{tot} &= 30400 - 28830 \\
&= 1570
\end{aligned}$$

**8.** Calculate $SS_{error}$ from the formula $SS_{tot} - SS_{bet}$

$$\begin{aligned}
SS_{error} &= 1570 - 195 \\
&= 1375
\end{aligned}$$

**9.** Calculate the df values:

$$\begin{aligned}
df_{bet} &= \text{number of conditions} - 1 \\
&= 3 - 1 \\
&= 2 \\
df_{tot} &= N - 1 \\
&= 30 - 1 \\
&= 29 \\
df_{error} &= df_{tot} - df_{bet} \\
&= 29 - 2 \\
&= 27
\end{aligned}$$

**10.** Divide each $SS$ value by its own df value to obtain the MS value, i.e.:

$$\begin{aligned}
MS_{bet} &= \frac{SS_{bet}}{df_{bet}} \\
&= \frac{195}{2} \\
&= 97.5
\end{aligned}$$

$$\begin{aligned}
MS_{error} &= \frac{SS_{error}}{df_{error}} \\
&= \frac{1375}{27} \\
&= 50.926
\end{aligned}$$

**11.** Calculate the $F$ ratio by using

$$\frac{MS_{bet}}{MS_{error}}$$

$$= \frac{97.5}{50.926}$$

$$= 1.915$$

Insert all these values into the appropriate slots in your anova table (see p. 173), as in Table 16.6.

**Table 16.6**

| Source of variance | SS | df | MS | F ratio |
|---|---|---|---|---|
| Variation due to treatment, i.e. between-conditions | 195 | 2 | 97.5 | 1.915 |
| Variation due to random error | 1375 | 27 | 50.926 | |
| Total | 1570 | 29 | | |

To look the $F$ ratio up in Tables A2.6a–d, you also need the df values for each source of variation, i.e. 2 and 27. If you turn to Tables A2.6a–d you will see that they each deal with critical values of $F$ for different significance levels:

Table A2.6a = $p < 0.05$
Table A2.6b = $p < 0.025$
Table A2.6c = $p < 0.01$
Table A2.6d = $p < 0.001$

Starting with Table A2.6a which represents the largest and therefore least significant probabilities ($p < 0.05$) you will see various numbers associated with $v_1$, which are the $df_{bet}$ values across the top, and $v_2$ values down the left-hand side which are the $df_{error}$ values. Therefore, locate your $df_{bet}$ of 2 along the top and the $df_{error}$ of 27 down the left-hand column. Where these two lines intersect you will see the number 3.35. To be significant at the $p < 0.05$ level, our $F$ value has to be *equal to* or *larger than* the given value of 3.35. Since $F = 1.915$ is smaller, we must conclude our results are not significant.

### Interpreting the results

Because our $F$ value of 1.915 is smaller than the number observed at the appropriate intersection point on Table A2.6a, we have to conclude that our results are not significant at $<0.05$, and that the probability of our results being due to random error is greater than 5%. Since the normal cut-off level for claiming support for the experimental hypothesis is 5% or less, we have to accept the null (no relationship) hypothesis. This means that there is no relationship between type of treatment for meniscectomy patients (audio-biofeedback, muscle stimulation or ice-packs) and percentage movement of the knee joint. This can be expressed as:

Using a one-way anova for unrelated designs ($F = 1.915$, $df_{bet} = 2$, $df_{error} = 27$) the results were not significant (p is greater than 5% for a two-tailed hypothesis). Therefore the null hypothesis must be accepted. This indicates that there is no relationship between type of treatment given to meniscectomy patients (audiobiofeedback, muscle stimulation and ice-packs) and subsequent degree of movement of the knee joint.

Had our $F$ value been larger, say 5.234, it would obviously have been significant on Table A2.6a's probabilities. But could we do any better? Turn to Table A2.6b ($p < 0.025$) and repeat the process. The value at the intersection point using df values of 2 and 27 is 4.24. Our $F$ value is larger than this and so is significant at the $<0.025$ level. Repeat the process with Table A2.6c ($p < 0.01$). The value at the intersection point is 5.49. Our $F$ ratio is smaller and so is not significant at this level. Therefore, in this case we would conclude that the $F$ value of 5.234 is significant at the $p < 0.025$ level.

Remember that because an anova only tells us whether there are differences and not in which direction these difference lie, the p values are for a two-tailed hypothesis. Had you obtained significant results and you wanted to find out which

group did significantly better than the others, youwould need to use the Scheffé (see next section). However, it must be stressed that you should only use the Scheffé if you obtained significant results from your anova.

**Activity 16.2** (Answers on page 234)

1 To practise looking up $F$ ratios, look up the following and state whether or not they are significant and at what level.
   (i)   df = 3   df = 12   $F = 6.103$   p
   (ii)  df = 2   df = 10   $F = 15.76$   p
   (iii) df = 3   df = 15   $F = 4.01$   p
   (iv)  df = 3   df = 12   $F = 5.95$   p

2 Calculate a one-way unrelated anova on the following data:
   $H_1$ Clapping has a differential effect on cystic fibrosis patients of different ages.
   Method: Select seven cystic fibrosis patients aged 3–5 years: seven aged 6–8, and seven aged 9–11. Measure their vital capacity prior to treatment and convert it to a percentage of the normal age-related average. Following 1 month of treatment, measure the vital capacity of each subject in the same way. Compare the differences in percentage capacity. Results are shown in Table 16.7.

**Table 16.7**

|   | 3–5 years | 6–8 years | 9–11 years |
|---|-----------|-----------|------------|
| 1 | 25 | 15 | 10 |
| 2 | 35 | 30 | 20 |
| 3 | 30 | 20 | 20 |
| 4 | 20 | 15 | 25 |
| 5 | 20 | 25 | 15 |
| 6 | 25 | 30 | 10 |
| 7 | 15 | 15 | 20 |

**State your** $F$ ratio and p value in a format similar to that suggested. Also, present your values in an anova table.

## Scheffé multiple range test for use with one-way anovas for unrelated designs

The analysis of variance only tells us whether there are significant differences between the results from each condition. It does not tell us which group(s) did better or worse than the others. For example, let's take the hypothetical case given in Activity 16.2 that clapping is differentially effective with cystic fibrosis patients of different ages. Further, let's imagine that the results were significant. These results only tell us that clapping has more effect on some age groups than others, but it doesn't tell us whether one group benefits significantly more or less. In other words, we can't tell from the results of the anova alone whether there are significant differences between:

> 3–5-year-olds and 6–8-year-olds
> and/or
> 3–5-year-olds and 9–11-year-olds
> and/or
> 6–8-year-olds and 9–11-year-olds.

If we want to find this out, we must use a Scheffé multiple range test.

There are three important points which relate to the use of the Scheffé:

- The Scheffé can only be used if the results from the anova are significant.
- The formula for the Scheffé has already been presented in conjunction with the one-way anova for related samples. The formula for the Scheffé for use with the anova for unrelated samples is the same, but is presented again here for ease and clarity.
- The Scheffé can only be carried out after an anova has been performed. It cannot be used independently.

Essentially what the Scheffé does is to compare the mean scores from each condition to see if the difference between them is significant.

When calculating the Scheffé you have to find two values: $F$ is computed first for *each* comparison of means you wish to make. This is then compared with a second value: $F^1$. If any $F$ is equal to or larger than $F^1$ then the difference between the two relevant means is significant.

*Example*

Let's take the example given in Activity 16.2 i.e. that there is a relationship between the effect of clapping and the age of the cystic fibrosis patient. Suppose you repeated the experiment, with six subjects in each group this time and you obtained the data shown in Table 16.8.

**Table 16.8**

| Subject | Condition 1 | Condition 2 | Condition 3 |
|---|---|---|---|
| | 3–5 years | 6–8 years | 9–11 years |
| 1 | 35 | 20 | 10 |
| 2 | 30 | 25 | 15 |
| 3 | 33 | 30 | 15 |
| 4 | 30 | 20 | 20 |
| 5 | 25 | 25 | 20 |
| 6 | 25 | 15 | 10 |
| $\Sigma$ | 178 | 135 | 90 |
| $\bar{X}$ | 29.667 | 22.5 | 15.0 |

You can perform a one-way anova for unrelated designs on the data. The outcome looks like Table 16.9.

**Table 16.9**

| Source of variance | SS | df | MS | F ratio |
|---|---|---|---|---|
| Variation due to treatment, i.e. between-conditions | 645.445 | 2 | 322.723 | 15.088 |
| Variation due to random error | 320.833 | 15 | 21.389 | |
| Total | 966.278 | 17 | | |

$F = 15.088$ is significant at $p < 0.001$.

This means that there are significant differences in before/after vital capacities between the three groups of cystic fibrosis patient. However, in order to find out whether one group does significantly better than another as a result of clapping we need to compare:

1. 3–5-year-olds and 6–8-year-olds
2. 3–5-year-olds and 9–11-year-olds
3. 6–8-year-olds and 9–11-year-olds

using the Scheffé multiple range test.

*Calculating the Scheffé multiple range test*

**1.** Calculate the mean score for each group i.e.

Condition 1 3–5-year-olds = 29.667 ($\bar{x}_1$)
Condition 2 6–8-year-olds = 22.5 ($\bar{x}_2$)
Condition 3 9–11-year-olds = 15.0 ($\bar{x}_3$)

**2.** Find the value of $F$ for the first comparison you wish to make, i.e: 3–5-year-olds vs 6–8-year-olds, using the following formula:

$$F = \frac{(\bar{x}_1 - \bar{x}_2)^2}{\dfrac{MS_{error}}{n_1} + \dfrac{MS_{error}}{n_2}}$$

where $\bar{x}_1$ = mean for Condition 1
= 29.667
$\bar{x}_2$ = mean for Condition 2
= 22.5
$MS_{error}$ = the $MS_{error}$ value from the anova table
= 21.389
$n_1$ = the number of subjects in Condition 1
= 6
$n_2$ = the number of subjects in Condition 2
= 6

Substituting these values:

$$F = \frac{(29.667 - 22.5)^2}{\dfrac{21.389}{6} + \dfrac{21.389}{6}}$$

$$= \frac{(7.167)^2}{3.565 + 3.565}$$

$$= \frac{51.366}{7.13}$$

$$= 7.204$$

**3.** Repeat the calculations for the second comparison, i.e. 3–5-year-olds vs 9–11-year-olds. Substitute the appropriate means and $n$ values:

$$F = \frac{(\bar{x}_1 - \bar{x}_3)^2}{\dfrac{MS_{error}}{n_1} + \dfrac{MS_{error}}{n_3}}$$

$$= \frac{(29.667 - 15)^2}{\dfrac{21.389}{6} + \dfrac{21.389}{6}}$$

$$= 30.171$$

**4.** Repeat the calculations for the third comparison, i.e. 6–8-year-olds vs 9–11-year-olds.

Substitute the appropriate means and $n$ values:

$$F = \frac{(\bar{x}_2 - \bar{x}_3)^2}{\dfrac{MS_{error}}{n_2} + \dfrac{MS_{error}}{n_3}}$$

$$= \frac{(22.5 - 15)^2}{\dfrac{21.389}{6} + \dfrac{21.389}{6}}$$

$$= 7.889$$

**5.** To calculate $F^1$, use the $df_{bet}$, and the $df_{error}$ values derived from the anova table (i.e. 2 and 15 respectively). Turn to Table A2.6a: critical values of $F$ at $p < 0.05$. Locate $df_{bet}$ (2) across the top row and $df_{error}$ (15) down the left-hand column. At their intersection point, you will see the figure '3.68' ($F°$).

Find the $F^1$ from the formula:

$$F^1 = (C - 1) \, F°$$

where $F°$ is the figure at the intersection point
= 3.68
$C$ is the number of conditions = 3
Therefore:

$$F^1 = (3 - 1) \, 3.68$$
$$= 7.36$$

6. Compare each $F$ value derived from the comparison of pairs of means with the $F^1$ value above. If the $F$ value is *equal to* or *larger than* $F^1$, then the result is significant at $p < 0.05$ (because we used the $p < 0.05$ table to calculate $F^1$).

If we take our $F$ values:

1. 7.204
2. 30.171
3. 7.889

we can see that only comparison (1) is not significant (3–5-year-olds vs 6–8-year-olds).

This means that the differences between 3–5-year-olds and 9–11-year-olds, and 6–8-year-olds and 9-11-year-olds are significant and that there is less than a 5% probability that the results are due to random error.

It is important to point out that to derive $F^1$ we used the $p < 0.05$ table. The reason for this relates to the extreme stringency of the Scheffé; if we were to derive $F^1$ from the smaller $p$ value tables, we would rarely get significant results using this test.

However, should you ever obtain results from the Scheffé which look as though they might be significant at a lower $p$ value, just re-calculate $F^1$ using Tables A2.6a–d. Here, the $F$ value of 30.71 (comparison 2) above seems to be significant at a smaller probability level. If we recalculate $F^1$ using Table A2.6d ($p < 0.001$) we get

$$F^1 = (3 - 1)11.34$$
$$= 22.68$$

The $F$ value of 30.171 is larger than this and so this comparison (3–5-year-olds vs 9–11-year-olds) is significant at $p < 0.001$.

### Interpreting the results

We have obtained the following results:

1. The comparison between the 3–5- and 6–8-year-olds was not significant. This means that any differences between these two groups could be explained by random error. Therefore there is no significant difference in improvement in vital capacity between these groups as a result of clapping.

2. The comparison between the 3–5- and 9–11-year-olds is significant at $p < 0.001$. This means that there is less than a 0.1% chance that the differences between these groups are attributable to random error. Therefore, we can conclude that the 3–5 year group benefits from clapping significantly more than the 9–11 year group (mean scores 29.667 and 15.0 respectively).

3. The comparison between the 6–8- and 9–11-year-olds is significant at $p < 0.05$. There-fore, there is less than a 5% probability that random error could account for the differences between these groups. The 6–8-year-old group benefits significantly more from clapping than does the 9–11-year-old group.

These results might be expressed in the following way:

Having calculated a one-way anova for unrelated designs on the data and obtained significant results ($F = 15.088$, $p < 0.001$), comparisons of means were performed using the Scheffé multiple range test. The results indicated that: (a) there was no significant difference between the 3–5- and 6–8-year-olds ($F = 7.204$); (b) the comparison between the 3–5- and 9–11-year-olds was significant at $p < 0.001$ ($F = 30.171$) with the 3–5 year age group benefiting more from treatment; (c) the comparison between the 6–8- and 9–11-year-olds was significant at $p < 0.05$ ($F = 7.889$) with the 6–8-year-olds benefiting more from treatment.

**Activity 16.3** (Answers on page 234)

Carry out a Scheffé on the following results:
$H_1$  There is a difference in the 'A'-level standards of students accepted at a school of physiotherapy over the last decade.
Method: Randomly select 10 students who were accepted for training in 1975, 10 who were accepted in 1980 and 10 who were accepted in 1985. For each student, count up their total 'A'-level points (Grade A = 5 marks, Grade E = 1). Perform a one-way anova for unrelated subject designs on the data. You obtain the following figures:
$F = 6.01$; $p < 0.01$
$df_{bet} = 2$
$df_{error} = 27$
$MS_{error} = 2.11$
$\bar{x}_1$ (1975 'A'-level results) = 6.3
$\bar{x}_2$ (1980 'A'-level results) = 7.75
$\bar{x}_3$ (1965 'A'-level results) = 10.15

# 17

# Non-parametric and parametric tests for correlational designs

## INTRODUCTION

All the tests described in this chapter are for use with correlational designs rather than experimental designs. Let's recap on the characteristics of correlational designs.

Firstly, while the experimental design is concerned with finding differences between sets of scores, the correlational design looks for the degree of *association* between them. Furthermore, with a correlational design neither of the two variables in the hypothesis is manipulated. Therefore, there is no IV or DV. As a result, a correlational design cannot ascertain which variable is having an effect on the other and thus, no cause and effect can be determined. All that can be concluded is whether or not there is any association in the scores for the two variables. Although this failure to ascribe cause and effect in correlational designs means that the researcher ends up with less precise information than would be obtained from experimental designs, it should also be pointed out that correlational designs are more acceptable if any ethical considerations are involved, because the researcher is not manipulating anything. Therefore, correlational designs are frequently used in medical research.

The way in which this association between sets of scores is assessed involves using the appropriate statistical test, which calculates a **correlation coefficient** between the sets of scores. This will result in a figure somewhere between $-1$ and $+1$. The closer the figure is to $-1$, the stronger the negative correlation between the scores. This means that large scores on one variable are associated with small scores on the other. The closer the figure is to $+1$, the stronger the positive correlation between the scores. In other words, high scores on one variable are associated with high scores on the other (and by definition, low scores on one variable are associated with low scores on the other). The closer the correlation coefficient is to 0, the weaker the relationship is between the scores.

To carry out a correlational design, you would usually select just one group of subjects. These subjects would represent a whole range of scores on one of the variables in the hypothesis. The implication of this is that in order to cover a range of numbers, the data must be ordinal or interval/ratio. (It is possible to carry out a correlational study with non-dimensional nominal data, but the analyses possible are not very powerful and so such correlations are not often carried out.) You would then measure each subject on the other variable to find out if there was a relationship between them.

For instance, if we take the example, that the greater the number of cigarettes smoked, the greater the incidence of bronchitis, we could select a group of subjects who vary in terms of the number of cigarettes they smoked, i.e. represented a whole range of scores on the smoking variables as in Table 17.1.

**Table 17.1**

| Subject | No. of cigarettes |
|---------|-------------------|
| 1 | 0 |
| 2 | 15 |
| 3 | 10 |
| 4 | 20 |
| 5 | 30 |
| 6 | 0 |
| 7 | 5 |
| 8 | 25 |
| 9 | 40 |
| 10 | 20 |

We would then collect information on their incidence of bronchitis over the last few years.

We would expect that the subject who smoked fewest cigarettes would have the lowest incidence of bronchitis, while the one who smoked most would have the highest incidence, with the other subjects ranging in between accordingly (see Table 17.2).

**Table 17.2**

| Subject | Cigarettes | Bronchitis |
|---------|------------|------------|
| 1 | 0 | 0 |
| 2 | 15 | 2 |
| 3 | 10 | 2 |
| 4 | 20 | 4 |
| 5 | 30 | 5 |
| 6 | 0 | 0 |
| 7 | 5 | 1 |
| 8 | 25 | 4 |
| 9 | 40 | 6 |
| 10 | 20 | 4 |

By computing the appropriate statistical test, we could find out whether there is a correlation between the scores shown in Table 17.2. Such a design differs from an experimental design in that although the experimental design would also predict a relationship between smoking and lung disease, it would have to manipulate the smoking variable in order to assess its effects on bronchitis. This would be done by selecting two groups of subjects, smokers and non-smokers, measuring the incidence of bronchitis for each and comparing the results to see if there are differences between the groups.

Obviously, whether you use an experimental or a correlational design depends on what you are predicting and the sort of research area you are involved in. If you're still unsure about the differences in assumptions and approach between experimental and correlational designs, re-read Chapter 6. When you have done this, plan out a correlational and an experimental design for the hypothesis in Activity 17.1.

**Activity 17.1** (Answers on page 234)
H$_1$ There is a relationship between age of patient and vital capacity.

## Statistical tests for correlational designs

The tests that are covered in this chapter are appropriate for two sorts of correlational design:

**1.** Those that compare *two* sets of scores to see if there is a correlation between them. In addition, a further test will be provided in this section, which allows you to *predict* scores on one variable, if you know the scores on the other.

**2.** Those that compare *three or more* sets of scores to see if there is a correlation between them.

Therefore, the tests shown in Table 17.3 are included in this chapter. These are both non-parametric and parametric. Each will be outlined separately.

**Table 17.3**

| Design | Non-parametric test | Parametric test |
|--------|---------------------|-----------------|
| One group of subjects; *two* sets of scores compared for the degree of association between them | Spearman rank order correlation coefficient If you wish to predict scores on one variable from your knowledge of scores on the other, use a linear regression equation | Pearson product moment correlation coefficient If you wish to predict scores on one variable from your knowledge of scores on the other, use a linear regression equation |
| One group of subjects; *three or more* sets of scores compared for the degree of association between them | Kendall's coefficient of concordance | — |

## Statistical tests which compare two sets of scores

Within this section, we shall look at two statistical tests, each of which can be used to assess the correlation betwen two sets of scores. In other words, you would typically take a group of subjects who represented a whole range of scores

on one variable, and you would compare these with just one set of scores on the other variable, to see if they were associated in some way. Like the statistical tests for experimental designs, you can use either a non-parametric test to analyse your results, or, as long as you can fulfil the necessary conditions, (see page 83) a parametric test. The most important of these conditions is the sort of data you have. In order to use a parametric test, you must have interval/ratio data.

The tests are:

1. Non-parametric: Spearman rank order correlation coefficient if the data are at least ordinal or interval/ratio.
2. Parametric: Pearson product movement correlation coefficient if the data are interval/ratio.

## NON-PARAMETRIC TEST: CORRELATIONAL DESIGNS WHICH COMPARE TWO SETS OF SCORES

### Spearman rank order correlation coefficient test

*Example*

Let's suppose you were interested in the hypothesis:

$H_1$  There is a correlation between the length of rest in support splints and the degree of pain experienced by rheumatoid arthritis patients, such that the longer the time in splints, the lower the degree of pain (i.e. a negative correlation). (This is a one-tailed hypothesis as it is predicting the type of correlation anticipated i.e. negative).

You would select a number of patients who had been in support splints for varying periods and assess the intensity of the pain experienced (say on a 7-point scale: 7 = intense, 1 = none). You anticipate that if your hypothesis is correct, the patients who had been in splints the longest would have least pain, while the patients who had been in splints the shortest time would have the most pain.

Your results might look like Table 17.4.

Because one set of scores (the pain measure) is only ordinal, we cannot fulfil the conditions necessary for a parametric test and so the Spearman must be used. It should be remembered that it does not matter at all that one variable is of an interval/ratio type (number of days in splints) and that the other is of an ordinal type, since all this correlational test does is to tell you whether the highest scores on one variable are associated with the highest or lowest scores on the other, irrespective of the nature of the scores. Therefore, as long as your data is not nominal, you can compare anything using the Spearman: weight with height, percentage range of movement with pain etc.

When calculating the Spearman you will find a correlation coefficient called '$r_s$' or 'rho', which you then look up in the probability tables associated with the Spearman test to see whether this value represents a significant correlation between the two variables.

### Calculating the Spearman test

To calculate the Spearman test, take the following steps:

**1.** Rank order the scores on Variable $A$, giving the rank of 1 to the smallest score, the rank of 2

to the next smallest and so on. Enter these ranks in the column 'Rank $A$'. Repeat the procedure for the scores in variable $B$ and enter the ranks in the column 'Rank $B$'.

If some scores are the same, follow the procedure for tied ranks (see pages 125–126). In other words add up the ranks these scores would have had if they had been different and divide this total by the number of scores that are the same. For example, in Variable $B$, the lowest score is 1, but subjects 3, 6 and 7 all had this score. Thus, had these scores been different they would have had the ranks 1, 2 and 3. Therefore, add these ranks up, and divide by 3 (because there are three scores of 1), i.e.

$$\frac{1 + 2 + 3}{3} = 2$$

Assign the average rank of 2 to each score of 1.

**2.** For each subject take the Rank $B$ score from the Rank $A$ score to give $d$.

Enter these differences in the column entitled '$d$ ($A - B$)', i.e:

$$\text{subject 1, Rank } A - \text{Rank } B = 2 - 7.5$$
$$= -5.5$$

**3.** Square each $d$ to give $d^2$, and enter this in the appropriate column, entitled '$d^2$', i.e.

$$-5.5^2 = 30.25$$

**Table 17.4**

| Subject | Results from the experiment | | Calculations from the statistical test | | | |
|---------|-----------------------------|---|----------------------------------------|---|---|---|
| | Variable $A$*<br>No. of days<br>in splints | Variable $B$<br>Pain felt on a<br>7-point scale | Rank $A$ | Rank $B$ | $d$<br>($A$-$B$) | $d^2$<br>($A$-$B$)$^2$ |
| 1 | 4 | 5 | 2 | 7.5 | $-5.5$ | 30.25 |
| 2 | 10 | 3 | 5 | 4.5 | $+0.5$ | 0.25 |
| 3 | 15 | 1 | 8 | 2 | $+6$ | 36 |
| 4 | 7 | 3 | 3 | 4.5 | $-1.5$ | 2.25 |
| 5 | 2 | 6 | 1 | 9 | $-8$ | 64 |
| 6 | 21 | 1 | 9 | 2 | $+7$ | 49 |
| 7 | 14 | 1 | 7 | 2 | $+5$ | 25 |
| 8 | 12 | 4 | 6 | 6 | 0 | 0 |
| 9 | 8 | 5 | 4 | 7.5 | $-3.5$ | 12.25 |
| | | | | | $\Sigma d^2 = 219$ | |

*It does not matter which is Variable $A$ and which is $B$

**4.** Add up all the $d^2$ figures to give $\Sigma d^2$. ($\Sigma$ means 'sum or total of').

$$\Sigma d^2 = 219$$

**5.** Find $r_s$ from the following formula:

$$r_s = 1 - \frac{6\,\Sigma d^2}{N(N^2 - 1)}$$

where $\Sigma d^2$ = the total of all the $d^2$ values
= 219
$N$ = the number of subjects or pairs of scores
= 9

If we substitute these values then

$$r_s = 1 - \frac{6 \times 219}{9(81 - 1)}$$

$$= 1 - \frac{1314}{720}$$

$$= 1 - 1.825$$

$$r_s = -0.825$$

(Do not forget to put in the + or - sign in front of the $r_s$ figure, since this indicates a positive or negative correlation respectively.)

### Looking up the value of $r_s$,

Turn to Table A2.10 (page 223). Down the left-hand column you will find values of $N$, while across the top you will see levels of significance for a one-tailed test and for a two-tailed test. Firstly, find your value of $N$ down the left-hand column. To the right you will see four numbers, called critical values of $r_s$:

$$0.600 \quad 0.683 \quad 0.783 \quad 0.833$$

Each of these values is associated with the level of significance indicated at the top of the column, e.g. 0.600 is associated with 0.05 for a one-tailed test and 0.10 for a two-tailed test.

If your $r_s$ value is *equal* to or *larger than* one of these four critical values, then your results are associated with the probability level indicated at the top of the appropriate column.

Our $r_s$ value of -0.825 (ignore the minus sign for the time being) is larger than 0.783, but smaller than 0.833. This means that for our

one-tailed hypothesis, the probability associated with our $r_s$ value of 0.825 must be less than 0.01 (or 1%) but greater than 0.005 (or ½%). Convention dictates that we say that our $p$ value is less than 0.01 (rather than saying it is greater than 0.005). In other words the probability of our results being due to random error is even less than 0.01 or 1%. This is expressed as:

$$p < 0.01 \text{ (or } < 1\%) \text{ (} < \text{ means 'less than')}$$

Had our $r_s$ value been equal to the critical value of 0.783 the associated probability level would be exactly 0.01. This would be expressed as:

$$p = 0.01 \text{ (or } 1\%).$$

### Interpreting the results

Our $r_s$ value of $-0.825$ is associated with a probability level of less than 1%. This means that the chance of random error accounting for our results is less than 1 in 100. Now, given that the usual cut-off point for claiming results as significant is 5% or less, we can say that the results obtained in this experiment are significant.

As we had a one-tailed hypothesis we must check that the results are in the predicted direction before claiming that our hypothesis has been supported. We have an $r_s$ value of *minus* 0.825. This means that the two variables are negatively correlated; in other words, the longer the time in support splints, the *less* the pain. This is exactly what was predicted and so we can safely reject the null hypothesis and accept the experimental hypothesis. This can be expressed in the following way:

Using a Spearman test on the data ($r_s = -0.825$, $N = 9$) the results were found to be significant ($p < 0.01$ for a one-tailed test). This means that there is a negative correlation between the variables, such that the longer the time spent in support splints, the less the degree of pain experienced. The null hypothesis can therefore be rejected.

**Activity 17.2** (Answers on pages 235)

1. To practise looking up $r_s$ values, look up the following and state whether or not they are significant and at what level.
   (i) $r = 0.784$  $N = 10$  one-tailed  $p$
   (ii) $r = 0.812$  $N = 6$  two-tailed  $p$
   (iii) $r = 0.601$  $N = 16$  two-tailed  $p$

(iv)  $r = 0.506$    $N = 12$  two-tailed    $p$
(v)  $r = 0.631$    $N = 18$  one-tailed    $p$

2 Calculate a Spearman on the following data:
   H$_1$  There is a relationship between the length of
         lunch-break taken (in minutes) by basic grade
         physiotherapists and their degree of clinical
         competence (on a 7-point scale, 7 = excellent, 1 =
         very poor).
   Method: You select a group of 10 basic grade physiotherapists who take varying lunch-break times and assess
   their clinical competence. The data are as shown in Table
   17.5.

**Table 17.5**

| S | Condition A Lunch-break time | Condition B Clinical competence |
|---|---|---|
| 1 | 45 | 4 |
| 2 | 65 | 3 |
| 3 | 50 | 5 |
| 4 | 30 | 5 |
| 5 | 75 | 2 |
| 6 | 40 | 6 |
| 7 | 55 | 5 |
| 8 | 80 | 2 |
| 9 | 35 | 6 |
| 10 | 70 | 3 |

State your $r_s$ and $p$ values in a format similar to the one outlined earlier.

# PARAMETRIC TEST: CORRELATIONAL DESIGNS WHICH COMPARE TWO SETS OF SCORES

## Pearson product moment correlation coefficient

As was noted earlier, the Pearson is the parametric equivalent of the Spearman test, in that it is used for correlational designs which compare two sets of data for their degree of association. It may be used when the prerequisite conditions for a parametric test can be fulfilled, in particular interval/ratio data (see page 83).

As long as the data are of an interval/ratio level, it does not matter if one variable is measured in yards, feet etc. and the other in kilos, percentages, minutes. The Pearson formula can accommodate different sorts of measurement as long as they are of an interval/ratio level.

### Example

Let's suppose you were interested in finding out whether there is a correlation between body weight and range of movement in the hip among osteoarthritis patients. Your hypothesis is:

H$_1$  There is a negative correlation between body weight and range of movement of the hip in osteoarthritis patients (i.e. high body weights are associated with low ranges of movement).

This is a one-tailed hypothesis as it is predicting the type of correlation expected, i.e. negative.

In order to test your hypothesis, you select 10 40–50-year-old female osteoarthritis patients who represent a range of body weights, and each of whom has suffered from the condition for between 36–42 months. You measure the percentage range of movement in their hip joints, and take the average of these scores. The results are as shown in Table 17.6.

### Calculating the Pearson test

The Pearson formula involves some rather large numbers, as you will see. These may look very off-putting initially, but you should be all right as long as you have a calculator.

**1.** Add up all the scores on variable $A$ to give $\Sigma A$, i.e.:

$$\Sigma A = 1471$$

**2.** Add up all the scores on variable $B$ to give $\Sigma B$, i.e.:

$$\Sigma B = 365$$

**3.** Multiply each subject's variable $A$ score by their variable $B$ score, i.e.

$$\text{Subject 1} = 140 \times 40$$
$$= 5600$$
$$\text{Subject 2} = 128 \times 45$$
$$= 5760$$

Enter each result in Column '$A \times B$'

**4.** Add up all the scores in Column $A \times B$ to give $\Sigma(A \times B)$, i.e.:

$$\Sigma(A \times B) = 52\ 910$$

**5.** Square each subject's variable $A$ score and enter the result in column '$A^2$', e.g:

$$\text{for Subject 1} = 140^2$$
$$= 19\ 600$$

**Table 17.6**

| Subject | Results from the experiment | | Calculations | | |
| --- | --- | --- | --- | --- | --- |
| | Variable $A$ Weight in lbs | Variable $B$ Range of move- ment | $A \times B$ | $A_2$ | $B_2$ |
| 1 | 140 | 40 | 5600 | 19 600 | 1600 |
| 2 | 128 | 45 | 5760 | 16 384 | 2025 |
| 3 | 170 | 25 | 4250 | 28 900 | 625 |
| 4 | 132 | 40 | 5280 | 17 424 | 1600 |
| 5 | 154 | 30 | 4620 | 23 716 | 900 |
| 6 | 135 | 35 | 4725 | 18 225 | 1225 |
| 7 | 143 | 45 | 6435 | 20 449 | 2025 |
| 8 | 149 | 50 | 7450 | 22 201 | 2500 |
| 9 | 158 | 30 | 4740 | 24 964 | 900 |
| 10 | 162 | 25 | 4050 | 26 244 | 625 |
| $\Sigma$ | $\Sigma A = 1471$ | $\Sigma B = 365$ | $\Sigma(A \times B) =$ 52 910 | $\Sigma A^2 =$ 218 107 | $\Sigma B^2 =$ 14 025 |

**6.** Square each subject's variable $B$ score and enter the result in column '$B^2$', e.g.:

$$\text{for Subject 1} = 40^2$$
$$= 1600$$

**7.** Add up all the scores in column $A^2$ to give $\Sigma A^2$, i.e.:

$$\Sigma A^2 = 218\ 107$$

**8.** Add up all the scores in column $B^2$ to give $\Sigma B^2$, i.e.:

$$\Sigma B^2 = 14\ 025$$

**9.** Find the value of $r$ from the following formula:

$$r = \frac{N\Sigma(A \times B) - \Sigma A \times \Sigma B}{\sqrt{[N\Sigma A^2 - (\Sigma A)^2][N\Sigma B^2 - (\Sigma B)^2]}}$$

where $N$ = number of subjects
= 10
$\Sigma(A \times B)$ = the total of the scores in the column $A \times B$
= 52 910
$\Sigma A$ = the total of the scores in the variable $A$ column
= 1471
$\Sigma B$ = the total of the scores in the variable $B$ column
= 365

$\Sigma A^2$ = the total of the scores in the $A^2$ column
= 218 107
$\Sigma B^2$ = the total of the scores in the $B^2$ column
= 14 025
$(\Sigma A)^2$ = the total of the scores in the variable $A$ column, squared
= $1471^2$
= 2 163 841
$(\Sigma B)^2$ = the total of the scores in the variable $B$ column, squared
= $365^2$
= 133 225

Therefore, if we substitute these values in the formula:

$$r = \frac{(10 \times 52\ 910) - (1471 \times 365)}{[(10 \times 218\ 107) - 2\ 163\ 841][(10 \times 14\ 025) - 133\ 225]}$$

$$= \frac{529\ 100 - 536\ 915}{\sqrt{[2\ 181\ 070 - 2\ 163\ 841][140\ 250 - 133\ 225]}}$$

$$= \frac{-7815}{\sqrt{11\ 001.533}}$$

$$r = -0.710$$

## Looking up the value of r

To find out whether *r* is significant, you also need a df value, which here is the number of subjects minus 2 i.e:

$$df = N - 2$$
$$= 10 - 2$$
$$= 8$$

Turn to Table A2.11 (page 224). Down the left-hand column you will see a number of df values. Find our df = 8. You will see five numbers, called critical values of *r* to the right of df = 8:

0.5494  0.6319  0.7155  0.7646  0.8721

Each of these is associated with the level of significance indicated at the top of its column, e.g. 0.5494 is associated with a level of significance, for a one-tailed test of 0.05 and for a two-tailed test of 0.10.

To be significant at one of these levels, our *r* value has to be *equal to* or *larger than* the corresponding critical value. Ignoring the minus sign in front of our *r* value for the time being, we can see that our *r* of 0.71 is larger than 0.6319 but smaller than 0.7155. Since we have a one-tailed test, our *r* value has an associated probability which is *less* than 0.025 (or 2½%) but greater than 0.01 (1%). According to convention we must say that our *r* has a *p* value of less than 0.025, (rather than saying it is greater than 0.01).

This is expressed as:

$$p < 0.025 \ (< \text{ means 'less than'})$$

This means that there is less than a 2.5% chance that our results are due to random error. Had our *r* value been the same as the critical value of 0.6319 the associated probability value would have been exactly 0.025. This is expressed as:

$$p = 0.025$$

## Interpreting the results

Our *r* value has an associated probability value of <0.025, which means that the chance of random error being responsible for the results is less than 2.5 in 100.

Because the standard cut-off point for claiming results to be significant is 5% we can conclude

that the results here are significant. But before we can definitely state that they support the experimental hypothesis, we must check that the direction of the results was the one predicted. In other words did we obtain the negative correlation between the two variables that we anticipated? Our *r* value was *minus* 0.71 which means that the results do, in fact, confirm the hypothesis and that there is a negative correlation between body weight and range of movement in the hip joint of osteoarthritis patients. We can therefore reject the null hypothesis and accept the experimental hypothesis. This can be expressed in the following way:

> Using a Pearson product moment correlation test on the data (*r* = − 0.71, df = 8), the results were significant (*p* < 0.025 for a one-tailed test). This means that there is a negative correlation in osteoarthritis patients, between weight and range of movement (the higher the weight, the lower the range of movement). The null hypothesis can therefore be rejected.

**Activity 17.3** (Answers on page 235)

1 To practise looking up *r* values, look up the following and state whether or not they are significant and at what level.

|      |              |         |            |     |
|------|--------------|---------|------------|-----|
| (i)  | *r* = 0.632  | df = 6  | one-tailed | *p* |
| (ii) | *r* = 0.567  | df = 10 | two-tailed | *p* |
| (iii)| *r* = 0.779  | df = 8  | one-tailed | *p* |
| (iv) | *r* = 0.612  | df = 12 | two-tailed | *p* |
| (v)  | *r* = 0.784  | df = 13 | two-tailed | *p* |

2 Calculate a Pearson on the following data:

H₁  There is a positive correlation between students' marks on their 1st year examination and their averaged continuous assessment mark throughout the year.

Method: Randomly select 8 first year students to represent a range of examination marks. Average their continuous assessment marks for the year's assignments.

The results are as shown in Table 17.7.

**Table 17.7**

| Subject | Variable A Examination | Variable B Continuous assessment |
|---------|------------------------|----------------------------------|
| 1       | 70                     | 66                               |
| 2       | 60                     | 64                               |
| 3       | 49                     | 54                               |
| 4       | 54                     | 50                               |
| 5       | 66                     | 70                               |
| 6       | 72                     | 68                               |
| 7       | 40                     | 49                               |
| 8       | 62                     | 65                               |

**State your** *r* and *p* values in the suggested format.

## NON-PARAMETRIC TEST WHICH COMPARES THREE OR MORE SETS OF SCORES

Both the Spearman and the Pearson test are used for correlational designs which look for the degree of association between only two sets of scores, for instance, comparing the theory and practice exam marks for a group of students to see if they correlate.

However, there will be many occasions when you may want to see if three or more sets of scores are associated in some way.

For example, you may be involved in chairing an interview panel of four people which is concerned with appointing a new deputy superintendent in the department. There are six candidates for the post. You decide to ask each member of the panel to rank order these candidates in terms of their suitability for the job. Obviously, if there were consensus in terms of choice the decision would be easy, but you know that is unlikely to be the case. So, you will have to analyse the rankings in order to see whether there is *overall* agreement. In other words, you have *one* group of six candidates, each of whom is ranked by four people. You need to assess the four sets of rankings given to each candidate to see how far the opinions of the panel agree.

Therefore, in this case, rather than having two sets of scores to analyse for correlations, you have four sets. Such a design requires a test called the **Kendall coefficient of concordance**.

## Kendall coefficient of concordance

This is a non-parametric test which can only be used when the data is ordinal, i.e. when you have three or more sets of rank orderings. This does not, of course, mean that you cannot use this test when you have interval/ratio data; all you would do here is to rank order your data and use the rank orderings in the test.

A further point to remember is that this particular formula of the Kendall coefficient of concordance can only be used if the number of people or objects being ranked is seven or less. So, for instance, you might ask four therapists to rank order six patients in terms of how compliant they are. Thus there are four judges (or sets of rankings) and six objects or people being ranked. If you want to design an experiment where more than seven objects or people are being ranked, you will need another formula and you are referred to Siegel (1956). However, you should find the formula provided here sufficient for most purposes.

One other point to note about this test: both the Spearman and Pearson tests produce a correlation coefficient which may be somewhere between − 1 (negative correlation) through 0 (no correlation) to + 1 (positive correlation), whereas the Kendall coefficient of concordance only gives us a value from 0 to + 1, i.e. an indication of whether there is no correlation at all between the sets of scores (0) or a positive correlation (+ 1). It does not give a negative correlation. If we think about this a bit more, the reason for this becomes clear. Where three or more sets of rankings are being compared, they cannot all disagree completely. So in the previous example, interviewer A may produce a set of rankings which are absolutely the reverse of interviewer B's. If we only had two interviewers, we could analyse this with a Spearman and we would end up with a negative correlation between the scores. But here, if Interviewers A and B disagree so completely from each other, what about interviewers C and D? If C also disagrees with A, it means by definition they must agree with B and hence there is some measure of agreement among the rankings. If D disagrees with C, it means these rankings must agree with those of A, because C disagrees with A. Therfore, all we may conclude from the Kendall coefficient of concordance is whether there is a positive correlation between the scores or whether there is no relationship. Because the Kendall coefficient of concordance only tells us whether or not there is a positive correlation between our results our hypothesis must be one-tailed.

When calculating the Kendall coefficient of concordance, a value called 's' is found. This is then looked up in the probability table associated with the Kendall coefficient of concordance, to see whether the value of s represents a significant agreement among the rankings. Remember that because the Kendall only deals with positive correlations, any hypothesis associated with it must be one-tailed.

### Example

Let's imagine that resources in your department are going to be cut again and you are forced into changing your treatment policy for a group of six cerebral palsied children. Rather than sending them all for hydrotherapy three times a week, you will only be able to send three of them three times per week, with a once-a-week session for the others. Obviously, some children benefit more from this type of treatment and you want to identify them, so that they can maintain their normal programme. So, you decide to ask the three physiotherapists who normally work with these children to rank order them according to who would benefit most from a continuation of this treatment. Therefore, you have three judges and six people being ranked. Your hypothesis therefore, is

$H_1$   There is significant agreement between the three physiotherapists' judgements of children most likely to benefit from continued hydrotherapy.

You ask the physiotherapists to rank all the children, giving a rank of 1 to the child most likely to benefit. The results you obtain are shown in Table 17.8. (When calculating the Kendall coefficient of concordance, always set the results out such that the rank orderings from each judge go across the page.)

**Table 17.8**

|  | Child | | | | | |
|---|---|---|---|---|---|---|
|  | 1 | 2 | 3 | 4 | 5 | 6 |
| physiotherapist |  |  |  |  |  |  |
| 1 | 6 | 4 | 2 | 1 | 3 | 5 |
| 2 | 6 | 2 | 3 | 4 | 1 | 5 |
| 3 | 6 | 5 | 3 | 1 | 2 | 4 |
| Total of ranks for each child | 18 | 11 | 8 | 6 | 6 | 14 |

### Calculating the Kendall coefficient of concordance

**1.** For each child add up the total of the ranks assigned, i.e.

$$1 = 18$$
$$2 = 11$$
$$3 = 8$$
$$4 = 6$$
$$5 = 6$$
$$6 = 14$$

Obviously, if all three physiotherapists had been in perfect agreement, the child most likely to benefit from a continuation of the treatment would have been assigned three ranks of 1 (total 3), the child next most likely to benefit, three ranks of 2 (total 6), etc. right up to the child least likely to benefit who would have had three ranks of 6 (18). On the other hand, had there been no agreement whatever, every child would have ended up with a.. identical rank total, i.e. every child would have received the same rank from each physiotherapist. Therefore, we would have six tied ranks:

$$\text{Ranks} \frac{1 + 2 + 3 + 4 + 5 + 6}{6} = 3.5$$

Thus each child would have got three ratings of $3.5 = 10.5$. What the formula aims to do is to assess how far the *actual* rankings accord with the rankings for *total* agreement between the judges.

**2.** Add up all the rank totals to give $\Sigma R$, i.e:

$$\Sigma R = 18 + 11 + 8 + 6 + 6 + 14$$
$$\Sigma R = 63$$

**3.** Divide $\Sigma R$ by the number of children being ranked to obtain the average rank, $\bar{x}_R$, i.e:

$$\bar{x}_R = 63 \div 6$$
$$= 10.5$$

**4.** Take each rank total away from the average rank and square the result, i.e:

$$1. (10.5 - 18)^2 = 56.25$$
$$2. (10.5 - 11)^2 = 0.25$$
$$3. (10.5 - 8)^2 = 6.25$$
$$4. (10.5 - 6)^2 = 20.25$$
$$5. (10.5 - 6)^2 = 20.25$$
$$6. (10.5 - 14)^2 = 12.25$$

**5.** Add up all these squared differences to give $s$, i.e. 115.5.

**6.** Find $W$ from the formula:

$$W = \frac{s}{\frac{1}{12} n^2 (N^3 - N)}$$

where $s$ = the total of all the squared differences between each individual rank total and the average rank

= 115.5

$n$ = the number of judges or sets of rankings

= 3

$N$ = the number of people or objects being ranked

= 6

Substituting these values:

$$W = \frac{115.5}{\frac{1}{12} 3^2 (6^3 - 6)}$$

$$= \frac{115.5}{\frac{1}{12} 9 \times 210}$$

$$= \frac{115.5}{157.5}$$

$$W = 0.733$$

### Looking up the value of s for significance

To find out whether these results are significant you need the $s$ value, (the total of squared differences between each individual rank total and the average rank), the $n$ value (the number of judges or sets of rankings), and $N$ (the number of objects or people ranked)

$$s = 115.5$$
$$n = 3$$
$$N = 6$$

Turn to Table A2.12 (page 225). This gives critical values of $s$ associated with particular values of $p$. You will see that two tables are presented, one for $p$ values of 0.05, and one for $p$ values of 0.01. (Note again that because this test only tells you whether or not there is a positive correlation between the scores, these values are associated with one-tailed hypotheses only.

Down the left-hand column you will see values of $n$, while across the top there are values of $N$.

Taking the $p$ = 0.05 table first, locate your $n$ and $N$ values and identify the number at the intersection point, i.e. 103.9. To be significant at the 0.05 level, our $s$ value must be *equal to* or *larger than* 103.9. Our $s$ value is larger (115.5) which means that our results are associated with a probability value of 0.05.

But are they significant at the 0.01 level? Repeat the process. You will find the figure at the intersection point is 122.8. Our $s$ value is smaller than this, so the results are not significant at the 0.01 level. So, we must go back to the first table.

Now, because our $s$ value is larger than the value at the intersection point, it means that the associated probability comes between the 0.05 probability of the first table and the 0.01 probability of the second. In other words, for our $s$ of 115.5, the associated probability is less than 5% (or 0.05) but greater than 1% (or 0.01). To comply with convention we have to say that our probability is less than 0.05 or 5%. This is expressed as: '$p < 0.05$' ($<$ means 'less than').

This means that the probability of random error being responsible for the results is less than 5%. Had our $s$ value been exactly the same as the number at the intersection point, our results would have been associated with a probability value which equalled 0.05. This is stated as: '$p = 0.05$'.

### Interpreting the results

Our results have an associated probability value of $<0.05$, which means that there is less than a 5% chance that random error could account for the outcome of the experiment. If we use the usual cut-off point of 5% to claim significance, we can state that the results here are, in fact, significant, and that we can reject the null hypothesis and accept the experimental hypothesis. This can be stated thus:

Using a Kendall's coefficient of concordance on the data ($s$ = 115.5, $W$ = 0.733, $n$ = 3, $N$ = 6) the results were found to be significant ($p < 0.05$ for a one-tailed test). This means that there is significant agreement among the physiotherapists as to which cerebral palsied children would benefit most from a continuation of hydrotherapy. The null hypothesis can therefore be rejected.

Should you ever have a situation where there

are a number of tied ranks, i.e. where, for instance, a judge has ranked three objects or people equally, this will have the effect of reducing the significance of your results. Try, then, to ensure that your data do not contain too many tied ranks.

One final point. Many students ask why $W$ is calculated, since it is not used to look up the significance of the results. The answer is that $W$ is the correlation coefficient, and the researcher often finds it useful to know this value in order to assess, in absolute terms, the extent of the correlation between results. In other words, the correlation coefficient is often as meaningful as the actual probability to the experimenter.

**Activity 17.4** (Answers on page 235)

1 To practise looking up $s$ values, look up the following $s$ values and state whether or not they are significant and at what level.
   (i) $s = 96.1$   $n = 4$   $N = 5$   $p$
   (ii) $s = 117.5$   $n = 5$   $N = 6$   $p$
   (iii) $s = 124.5$   $n = 3$   $N = 6$   $p$
   (iv) $s = 103.7$   $n = 6$   $N = 4$   $p$
   (v) $s = 619.2$   $n = 10$   $N = 7$   $p$

2 Calculate a Kendall coefficient of concordance on the following data. You are concerned about the variability in measurements of joint movement when using a goniometer. You decide to put this to the test.

H$_1$ There is a significant agreement between physiotherapists' measurements of joint movement using a goniometer.
   Method: Five physiotherapists each measure the degrees of knee flexion of four patients using a goniometer. The range of movement recorded is noted.

The results are as shown in Table 17.9. (*Remember the data must be rank ordered!*)

**Table 17.9**

|  | Patient | | | |
|---|---|---|---|---|
|  | 1 | 2 | 3 | 4 |
| Physiotherapist | | | | |
| 1 | 45 | 30 | 50 | 65 |
| 2 | 45 | 40 | 55 | 70 |
| 3 | 25 | 30 | 65 | 55 |
| 4 | 50 | 55 | 30 | 60 |
| 5 | 60 | 50 | 65 | 80 |

**State your** $s$, $W$ and $p$ values in the format outlined earlier.

# LINEAR REGRESSION: PREDICTING SCORES ON ONE VARIABLE FROM SCORES ON THE OTHER

We have already seen that correlational designs are used when we want to find out whether two variables are associated with each other, that is, whether high scores on one variable are related to high scores on the other, or alternatively, whether high scores on one variable are related to low scores on the other. This is a particularly valuable sort of approach in medical research because ethical issues are rarely involved.

Correlational designs can tell us whether, for example, blood pressure and reaction to a particular drug are related, or whether traction weights and degree of improvement in back pain are associated, although they cannot say which of the two variables causes an effect on the other; all they tell us is whether or not two variables co-vary together in a related way.

Now, there will be occasions when you might be quite happy to leave your research at this point, having found out whether or not the variables are correlated. For example, in the earlier illustration, you may be content with the knowledge that blood pressure and reaction to drug A are positively correlated, i.e. that the higher the blood pressure, the more adverse the reaction to the drug. This reaction, let's say, induces drowsiness.

However, let's suppose that having completed this research, you are faced with a new patient with a blood pressure reading of, say, 170/90. Now, from the results of your correlational design, you will know that this person's reaction to drug A is likely to be adverse, since they have high blood pressure. However, let's further suppose that this person drives a public transport vehicle. It is obviously essential to establish whether the degree of drowsiness induced is likely to be a danger to him or his passengers. In other words, it would be extremely useful to you to be able to predict this man's reaction more precisely from your knowlege of his blood pressure. In other words, what you want to be able to do is to predict with some degree of accuracy the scores on one variable from your knowledge of the scores on the other. What you need, therefore, is a formula whereby you can calculate the unknown score. This formula is known as a **regression formula or equation** and is of enormous use in medical research. For example, as long as you know that the two variables are correlated, it can tell you:

- the vital capacity of a man who smokes 55 cigarettes a day.
- the heart rate of someone who regularly jogs 2 miles a day.
- the theory exam performance of a student who achieved 32% in the practical exam.

So, providing you know that two variables are related, you can make predictions about one variable from your knowledge of scores on the other, using a regression formula. The Linear Regression technique can be used in conjunction with either the Pearson or the Spearman test, but the data should be of a type which assumes equal intervals. In other words it should be interval/ratio or a point scale which implies comparable distances between the points (see pages 28–30).

The convention when using regression formulae is to call the variable whose score you are trying to predict, 'Y', and the variable whose scores you already know, 'X'. Therefore, in the above example, we are trying to predict the patient's reaction to drug A (Y) from our knowledge of his blood pressure (X).

Now, it is important to reiterate that you can only use a regression equation if the two variables you are interested in have been shown to be correlated. If you look back to page 59, you will see that there are two types of correlation, a positive correlation whereby high scores on one variable are associated with high scores on the other; and a negative correlation whereby high scores on one variable are associated with low scores on the other. If scattergrams are plotted for both of these, we find that a positive correlation is represented by an uphill slope, while a negative correlation is represented by a downhill one. Furthermore, it was pointed out that a perfect one-to-one correlation would produce an absolutely smooth, straight line. However, there are very few things in this world which produce a perfect correlation, but supposing we found that the amount of time a physiotherapist spent with

a patient produced a one-to-one correlation with the patient's reported satisfaction with the treatment (on a 9-point scale) such that the longer time spent, the greater the satisfaction. If we plotted the data from this we might end up with the scattergram shown in Figure 17.1. For the

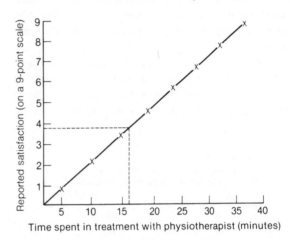

**Figure 17.1** Scattergram showing relationship between patient satisfaction and time spent with physiotherapist, supposing the correlation were perfect.

sake of the example, we shall treat this 9-point scale as though it were interval data and assume that the distances between each point are equal (see page 29).

We can draw a perfectly straight line through all the dots and it is this line which is used in your future predictions. For example, you would know from this scattergram that if you were to treat a patient for 17 minutes, the degree of reported satisfaction would be 3.6, because all you would have to do would be to locate the appropriate time along the bottom axis, and trace it vertically up to the sloping line and then move horizontally across to the satisfaction scores (see dotted line above).

You could also predict that if you treated someone for 3 minutes, their satisfaction would be 0.6; again you simply take the 3-minute time along the bottom axis, trace this up to the slope and then move left from the slope to the satisfaction scores. In other words, from your existing knowledge that these two variables are related, should you ever treat someone for a period of time which has not been incorporated in your previous calculations, you can predict how satisfied they will be.

You can see that this sloping line is obviously extremely important if you need to make this sort of prediction and therefore it has to be drawn in. However, while it is easy to draw it in when the correlation is perfect, because all the dots are lined up, it is not as easy when the correlation is imperfect and the dots are more randomly scattered.

However, as has already been pointed out very little in life conforms to a perfect correlation. It would be far more likely in the previous example that the data obtained was as shown in Table 17.10.

**Table 17.10**

| Patient | Reported satisfaction | Time spent in treatment (mins) |
| --- | --- | --- |
| 1 | 7 | 29 |
| 2 | 4 | 10 |
| 3 | 6 | 18 |
| 4 | 8 | 17 |
| 5 | 2 | 8 |
| 6 | 3 | 5 |
| 7 | 5 | 15 |
| 8 | 6 | 16 |
| 9 | 5 | 16 |
| 10 | 1 | 5 |

Statistical analysis using the Pearson test (see previous section) shows that the data are correlated ($r = 0.836$, $p < 0.005$).

If these data were plotted on a scattergram, we would find the pattern shown in Figure 17.2. There is still a general upward slope but it is far from smooth. In this case, if you had to draw a straight line through the dots, so that you could perform the same sort of prediction as before, where would you draw it? You obviously cannot connect all the dots as you would with the perfect correlation and still obtain a straight line so you need to make a decision about where to put the line so that it achieves the 'best fit'. The line of best fit is the straight sloping line which when drawn in, means that every dot is as close as possible to the line, and consequently produces

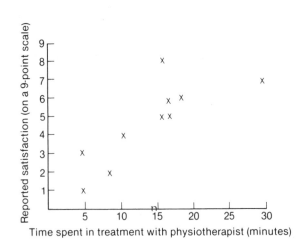

**Figure 17.2** A more likely scattergram showing the relationship between patient satisfaction and time spent with physiotherapist.

fewest errors when predicting the value of variable Y from knowledge of variable X.

Now, if you look at the last scattergram, you can see that it is almost impossible to draw in the line of best fit by eye, and if you cannot draw in this line, then how can you make predictions? For instance, if you treated someone for 12 minutes, what would this level of satisfaction be? If you only have the scattergram and no line of best fit, you can't answer this question.

What you need, then, is a regression formula such that this line of best fit can be calculated and the prediction made. This equation is:

$$Y = bX + a$$

where Y is the variable to be predicted
X is the known score
a and b are constants which have to be calculated.

(Note that the regression we are dealing with is called linear regression, because it is concerned with simple linear relationships; see the scattergram.)

*Calculating the linear regression equation*

In order to calculate these constants, take the following steps:

**1.** Calculate the Spearman or Pearson test

(whichever is appropriate) on your data to establish whether or not there is a significant correlation. If there isn't a significant correlation, don't proceed any further, since you cannot make any predictions from variables which don't correlate.

**2.** Having established that the data are correlated, make a note of whether the correlation is positive or negative. If you wish, you can plot a scattergram of the data, but it isn't essential.

**3.** Set out your data in the format shown in Table 17.11, remembering that $Y$ is the variable

**Table 17.11**

| Subject | Variable Y Satisfaction | Variable X Treatment time | X × Y | X² |
|---|---|---|---|---|
| 1 | 7 | 29 | 203 | 841 |
| 2 | 4 | 10 | 40 | 100 |
| 3 | 6 | 18 | 108 | 324 |
| 4 | 8 | 17 | 136 | 289 |
| 5 | 2 | 8 | 16 | 64 |
| 6 | 3 | 5 | 15 | 25 |
| 7 | 5 | 15 | 75 | 225 |
| 8 | 6 | 16 | 96 | 256 |
| 9 | 5 | 16 | 80 | 256 |
| 10 | 1 | 5 | 5 | 25 |
| Totals | $\Sigma Y = 47$ | $\Sigma X = 139$ | $\Sigma (X \times Y) = 774$ | $\Sigma X^2 = 2405$ |

to be predicted and $X$ is the variable from which the prediction will be made. Here, we will take the sample data already provided for the last scattergram. So, the $X \times Y$ column is: variable score $X$ multiplied by variable score $Y$, i.e.:

$$\text{for subject 1, } 7 \times 29 = 203$$

The $X^2$ column is simply the squared variable $X$ score. Therefore:

$$\text{for subject 1, } 29 \times 29 = 841$$

**4.** Add each column up to give the totals ($\Sigma$)

$$\Sigma Y = 47$$
$$\Sigma X = 139$$
$$\Sigma (X \times Y) = 774$$
$$\Sigma X^2 = 2405$$

**5.** To calculate the constants a and b, first find b from the formula:

$$b = \frac{N\Sigma(X \times Y) - (\Sigma X)(\Sigma Y)}{N\Sigma X^2 - (\Sigma X)^2}$$

where $N$ = the total number of Ss
$= 10$

$\Sigma(X \times Y)$ = the total of the $X \times Y$ column
$= 774$

$\Sigma X$ = the total of the variable $X$ column
$= 139$

$\Sigma Y$ = the total of the variable $Y$ column
$= 47$

$\Sigma X^2$ = the total of the $X^2$ column
$= 2405$

$(\Sigma X)^2$ = the total of the variable $X$ column squared
$= 139^2$
$= 19\,321$

If we substitute our values:

$$b = \frac{(10 \times 774) - (139 \times 47)}{(10 \times 2405) - 19321}$$

$$= \frac{7740 - 6533}{24\,050 - 19\,321}$$

$$= \frac{1207}{4729}$$

$$= 0.255$$

**6.** Find a from the formula:

$$a = \frac{\Sigma Y}{N} - b\frac{\Sigma X}{N}$$

where $N$ = the total number of Ss
$= 10$

$\Sigma Y$ = the total of the variable $Y$ column
$= 47$

$\Sigma X$ = the total of the variable $X$ column
$= 139$

$b$ = the result of the earlier calculation in step 5.
$= 0.255$

Substituting the values:

$$a = \frac{47}{10} - 0.255 \times \frac{139}{10}$$

$$= 4.7 - (0.255 \times 13.9)$$
$$= 4.7 - 3.545$$
$$= 1.155$$

**7.** We can now substitute the values of a and b into the regression formula

$$Y = bX + a$$

to find any value of $Y$ we require from the known value of $X$. Therefore:

$$Y = 0.255X + 1.155$$

*Interpreting the results*

Suppose, then, a patient was treated for 22 minutes (variable $X$) we can predict his level of satisfaction (variable $Y$) using the calculated values for the regression equation.

$$Y = (0.255 \times 22) + 1.155$$
$$Y = 5.61 + 1.155$$
$$= 6.765$$

Therefore, this patient's predicted level of satisfaction would be 6.765. So it is possible to calculate from any treatment time the associated degree of satisfaction.

**Activity 17.5** (Answers on page 235)

Imagine that the data in Table 17.12 were obtained from a correlational study which looked at the relationship between the amount of weight gained during pregnancy and length of labour.

**Table 17.12**

| Subject | Weight gain (in lbs) | Length of labour (in hours) |
|---|---|---|
| 1 | 17 | 8.3 |
| 2 | 35 | 16.2 |
| 3 | 28 | 12.8 |
| 4 | 21 | 9.9 |
| 5 | 20 | 10.0 |
| 6 | 30 | 15.8 |
| 7 | 24 | 14.0 |
| 8 | 32 | 17.5 |
| 9 | 20 | 11.6 |
| 10 | 26 | 12.2 |

The two variables correlate significantly, $p < 0.005$.
    Three women come in for the last antenatal visit. Their weight gains are: (a) 23 lbs (b) 16 lbs (c) 29 lbs.
    What is the estimated length of labour for each woman?

# 18

# Estimation

## INTRODUCTION

Estimation is a particularly useful statistical technique for any physiotherapist who is involved in resource management or planning. It can be thought of as a sort of statistical 'best guessing' system which, like other methods of inferential statistics, allows us to make predictions about certain characteristics of a population based on our knowledge of a small sample of that population.

However, unlike the statistical tests which we have looked at so far in this book, estimation does not involve testing a hypothesis. Instead, we collect data on the characteristics we are interested in from a sample of people, equipment or whatever, and then, using a statistical formula, we can make predictions or estimates about how far the population also possesses these characteristics. (If you are unclear about the terms it might be worth refreshing your memory by re-reading pages 63–64). The characteristics we are interested in estimating are called **parameters**.

These concepts may be best illustrated by using an example. Let's imagine you are the Principal of a School of Physiotherapy and each year you have places for 40 new students to start their training. However, over the last three years you have had at least 5–8 students drop out before the start of the course, which leaves you under the establishment figure. Clearly, if you could make an accurate estimate of potential drop-out for the forthcoming year, you could offer that number of extra places over and above the 40 students you normally take in. This means that when the new course starts, you will have the correct number of students and no resources will be wasted. However, the success of this strategy depends heavily on the accuracy of your estimates. From this example, it can be seen that formal, statistical techniques of estimation are particularly important to any planning activities, whether it be for training places, financial predictions, service delivery or whatever.

However, in order to make good and accurate estimates, the following conditions must be fulfilled:

1. You must define your area of interest clearly, avoiding vague concepts such as 'service delivery', 'patients' etc. If you mean by service delivery the treatment of frozen shoulder patients by megapulse, then you must say so. In the same way, you must also be precise about the parameters you wish to estimate. For example, if you are managing a budget for the coming year and need to consider how much must be allocated for staff development and top-up training courses, you must specify what type of course you are budgeting for. Are they local one-day events? Are they residential? Over one-week/one-month/one-term duration? The characteristics must be properly defined if estimates made about them are to have any value and precision. Therefore, the first rule of estimation is:

Define your terms and focus of interest precisely

2. The next stage involves the selection of a **random sample**, so that the estimates are based on a reasonably representative subgroup of the population in which you are interested. Random sampling was covered in Chapter 3 but essentially involves ensuring that every member of the relevant population has an equal chance of being selected. This can be achieved using random number tables, pulling names out of hats, etc. (see pages 23–24).

The sample should also be of an adequate number in relation to the population size. The concept of adequacy is difficult to define because it depends on the population being studied and the topic under investigation (see page 24).

However a good rule-of-thumb is to select as many subjects as time and budget will afford. Thus the second rule of estimation is:

Select your subjects randomly and try to ensure that the sample is of an adequate size.

3. The third stage in the estimation process is the data collection phase. Like all other forms of research, it is essential that the data collected is a valid measure of the characteristic you are interested in. Let us imagine you are interested in estimating stress levels among senior grade II physiotherapists. If you simply monitored blood pressure it would not be an adequate measure, since there may be: (a) many reasons for elevated blood pressure readings, and (b) other additional symptoms such as subjective reports of stress, all of which may be a valuable contribution to your stress indices.

Therefore, the third rule of estimation is:

Ensure the data collected is a suitable and valid measure of the characteristics being studied.

4. The last stage in the estimation process is the application of the appropriate estimation formula. There are different formulae available, and their use is determined by what it is the researcher wishes to find out. These formulae and their functions are described below. The last rule of estimation is therefore:

Apply the appropriate statistical formula for what it is you wish to estimate.

## TECHNIQUES OF ESTIMATION

The two main types of estimation procedures are 'point estimations' and 'interval estimations'.

### Point estimates

These are simply a single figure (usually a percentage or an average) which is derived from your sample and which is used as an estimate for the relevant population. For example, you might be interested in planning outpatient treatment for meniscectomy patients over the coming year. In order to do this, you select a sample of meniscectomy patients from those who have attended for treatment over the previous year, and calculate the average number of treatments required before discharge. Let's imagine that the average comes out at seven 30–minute treatments per patient (210 minutes in total). On this basis you could estimate the amount of physiotherapy time required for new meniscectomy patients as being 210 minutes. This figure is therefore a point estimate of the average treatment time for meniscectomy patients within your outpatient clinic.

What you have done here is to select a sample of meniscectomy patients (i.e. a selection from those who attended during the previous year) and you have calculated the average figure for the parameter in which you are interested (i.e. treatment time). From this you have made an estimate for that parameter for the population of meniscectomy patients who are likely to require treatment during the coming year.

However, this may not provide you with all the essential information you might need for accurate planning of resources. What you might also need to know is the proportion or percentage of the total outpatient numbers that meniscectomy patients constitute. By knowing this, you could fine-tune your provision at bit more. Consequently, then, you need to obtain a percentage point estimate of meniscectomy patients relative to the whole population of outpatients in your clinic. You might find that these patients constituted 12% of the total ourpatients for the previous 12 months and therefore you could estimate a similar percentage for the forthcoming year. This percentage point estimate of 12% coupled with the average point estimate for treatment (210 minutes per patient) would give you useful information when planning resources and finances in your unit.

I feel sure you are not too impressed by estimation thus far, since it is something that many of us do all the time at a routine and informal level, whether it be estimating our time on domestic tasks so that we know how much can be fitted into a 2-hour slot, or calculating next month's financial outgoings in order to work out whether we can afford new curtains or whatever. However, the accuracy, and thus the value, of estimation depends very largely on the quality of the random sample selected for study; in other words, how representative was the particular sample bank-balance you used when predicting next month's expenditure? A truly representative sample is almost impossible to achieve, but even if we managed it, it is still quite possible for any estimates based on the sample to be wrong, if only minutely. Where patient well-being or limited budgets are at stake, even minor inaccuracies in estimates could prove to be disastrous and consequently, it might be useful, in these circumstances, to know what degree of confidence you can place on your estimate.

## Interval estimation

The last point leads us into another variant of estimation, **interval estimation**, which involves the calculation of two figures (rather than a single one), between which we can be confident our estimate falls. So, in the example above concerning our meniscectomy outpatients, instead of saying that the estimate for average treatment time is 210 minutes, we would calculate a lower and upper limit of treatment time, for example 150 minutes to 240 minutes, and we could then estimate with a reasonable degree of confidence that the treatments for other meniscectomy patients would fall within this interval.

This procedure clearly allows a bit more leeway in our predictions but it also gives the researcher some confidence about the estimates. This concept of confidence is a crucial one in interval estimation and distinguishes interval estimates from point estimates. The amount of confidence a researcher has in their estimate is expressed as a percentage, and the higher the percentage, the more confident they are. Therefore an estimate made with 99% confidence should be more reliable than one made with 95%.

To illustrate this distinction between the point and interval estimates, suppose a researcher asks the question:

> How much treatment on average are future meniscectomy patients going to need?

A point estimate would answer:

> I don't know precisely, but my guess is an average of 210-minute sessions.

Whereas the interval estimate would reply:

I don't know precisely but I am 95% confident that average treatment needs will be between 150 minutes and 240 minutes in total.

The higher figure in this last answer (i.e. 240 minutes) is called the **upper confidence limit**, while the lower figure (i.e. 150 minutes) is called the **lower confidence limit.** The difference between these two numbers is known as the **confidence interval.** How much confidence that can be expressed in any given interval estimate depends on the formula used to calculate the estimate. These formulae are given later in the chapter.

## The theory behind interval estimates

In order to understand the theoretical basis underpinning interval estimates, it is important that you have read the sections on the normal distribution (pages 44–46) and on the standard deviation (pages 43–44).

Just to refresh your memory on the key points, a normal distribution is a frequency distribution graph, which is bell-shaped as in Figure 18.1.

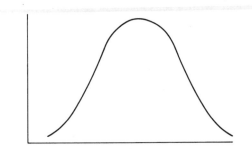

**Figure 18.1** The normal distribution curve.

This curve has a number of important properties which are essential to statistics.

The standard deviation is a number which represents how much a set of data varies, on average, from the mean of those data (see pages 43–44).

It is the relationship between the normal distribution and the standard deviation which is important to estimation. In any set of normally distributed data, a fixed percentage of that data lies within given areas on either side of the average score.

These 'given areas' are related to the standard deviations of that set of data and are as follows:

- 68% of the scores fall within one standard deviation either side of the mean
- 95% of the scores fall within two standard deviations either side of the mean
- 99.73% of the scores fall within three standard deviations either side of the mean.

These figures may be more clearly illustrated by looking back to Figure 5.16, page 46.

If you re-read the example regarding heart rate given on page 46, then the implications all this has for estimation can be explored further.

On the hypothetical basis that the average heart rate is 72 beats per minute, and the standard deviation is 5, you would know that 68% of the population have heart rates of between 67 and 77 beats per minute, 95% have heart rates between 62 and 82 beats per minute, and 99.73% have heart rates between 57 and 87 beats per minute.

These (fictitious) figures would have been calculated on a sample of people. If, for example, you wanted to make an interval estimate on heart rate for the whole population with 95% confidence in that estimate, then you need to use the mean score and add two standard deviations to it to get the upper confidence limit (i.e. 82 beats). You then take two standard deviations away from the mean to get the lower confidence limit (i.e. 62 beats). This would give us the confidence interval of 62–82 beats per minute. Because 95% of any normally distributed data lie within two standard deviations either side of the mean, you could say with 95% confidence that the heart rates of the whole population lie within that interval. This 95% figure is called the **level of confidence** and is a statement of belief that the population's heart rate will fall within the upper and lower confidence limits stated.

In the same way, you could make estimates with 68% confidence by using one standard deviation either side of the mean, or with 99.73% confidence by using three standard deviations either side of the mean. However, it is more common to use confidence levels of 90% and 99% in addition to 95% and these clearly have no direct correspondence with the standard deviations. Therefore, we need to use the appropriate estimation formulae. These are provided in the next section. These formulae also allow the researcher to make estimates form large samples (over 30) about characteristics which are not normally distributed throughout the population.

## Calculating interval estimates

There are several different formulae for calculating interval estimates and which one you use will depend on the following points:

1. Whether your sample size is greater than, equal to or less than 30.
2. Do you want to estimate the population *average* for the parameter in question (such as the average number of visits the community physiotherapist makes to elderly stroke patients), or do you require *proportions* or *percentages* (for example, the proportion of the secretarial population who sustains repetitive strain injury)?
3. The confidence level you need in your estimate. The usual level is 95%, but you may need to have more confidence (i.e. 99%) or less (90%) depending on what it is you are estimating. The more disastrous the effects of an inaccurate estimate, the more confidence you will need.

## SAMPLES LARGER THAN THIRTY

## Estimating confidence limits for the population average

If you wish to estimate population averages from data derived from samples larger than 30 the formulae contained in this section are appropriate. The first formula provided is for the most commonly used 95% confidence level. The other formulae are for the 99% and 90% levels respectively.

Supposing you were interested in the average absenteeism rate for senior grade II physiotherapists across your region. To calculate your estimate for this population, you might select a random sample of 75 senior grade IIs and work out their average absence rate over the previous

12 months. Let's say this works out at 19.0 units per annum with a standard deviation of 4.5.

What you have here is:

- a sample larger than 30
- an average or mean score for the parameter in which you are interested (i.e. absenteeism).

*The 95% confidence level*

If you need the usual 95% confidence level in your estimate, the formula is:

$$1.96 \times \frac{SD}{\sqrt{n}}$$

where 1.96 = a constant for the 95% confidence level

SD = the standard deviation of the population

n = the sample size

$\sqrt{\phantom{n}}$ = is the square root of the sample size.

It is important to note that very often the standard deviation of the population is not known. In such cases you can use the standard deviation of the sample instead.

If we now translate these figures, from the example about senior grade II physiotherapists' absenteeism rates, into the formula, we get:

$$1.96 \times \frac{4.5}{\sqrt{75}}$$

$$= 1.96 \times \frac{4.5}{8.66}$$

$$= 1.96 \times 0.52$$

$$= 1.02$$

This figure of 1.02 is then added to the average absenteeism rate of 19.0 units to give the upper confidence limit, i.e.:

$$19.0 + 1.02 = 20.02$$

It is then subtracted from the average to give the lower confidence limit, i.e.:

$$19.0 - 1.02 = 17.98$$

This gives us the confidence interval of 17.98–20.02. We can therefore say with 95% confidence that average absenteeism rates among the senior grade II population in the region will fall within these figures.

### The 99% confidence level

Should you want to make your estimates with more confidence, the formula becomes

$$2.58 \times \frac{SD}{\sqrt{n}}$$

So, using the above example, and substituting the relevant figures we get

$$2.58 \times \frac{4.5}{\sqrt{75}}$$
$$= 2.58 \times \frac{4.5}{8.66}$$
$$= 2.58 \times 0.52$$
$$= 1.34$$

The upper confidence limit is then:

$$19.0 + 1.34 = 20.34$$

and the lower confidence limit is:

$$19.0 - 1.34 = 17.66$$

So we can now say with 99% confidence that the average absenteeism will fall between 17.66 and 20.34 units.

### The 90% confidence level

If we don't need such a high level of confidence in our estimate, we can use the less stringent 90% formula:

$$1.64 \times \frac{SD}{\sqrt{n}}$$

Therefore, using the same data we get

$$1.64 \times \frac{4.5}{\sqrt{75}}$$
$$= 1.64 \times \frac{4.5}{8.66}$$
$$= 1.64 \times 0.52$$
$$= 0.85$$

The confidence interval is therefore:

$$18.15 - 19.85$$

We can estimate with 90% confidence that the average absenteeism rates for the population of senior grade II physiotherapists will be between 18.15 and 19.85 units per annum.

## Estimating confidence limits for proportions of the population

If, rather than estimating confidence limits for population averages, you wish to calculate population proportions or percentages, you will need the following formulae instead. Three formulae are provided, the first for the 95% confidence limits, the second for the 99% limits and the third for the 90% limits.

Let's imagine you are interested in the topic of carpal tunnel syndrome in pregnancy. You wish to estimate what proportion of the pregnant women population are likely to suffer this problem. You select a sample of 90 pregnant women of 35 + weeks' gestation and find that 27 of them have carpal tunnel syndrome. You therefore have a sample larger than 30 and are concerned with proportion and percentage estimates of the population.

The following formulae are therefore appropriate for this purpose.

### The 95% confidence limit

The formula for this calculation is:

$$1.96 \times \sqrt{\frac{pq}{n}}$$

where 1.96 = a constant to be used for the 95% confidence limits

$p$ = the proportion of the sample which possesses the characteristic

$q$ = the proportion of the sample which does not possess the characteristic

$n$ = the sample size

$\sqrt{\phantom{x}}$ = the square root of the calculations under this sign.

The proportion of a sample is calculated by dividing the actual number of people possessing the characteristic by the total number of people in the sample. For example, here the proportion of women with carpal tunnel syndrome would be:

$$\frac{27}{90} = 0.3$$

while the proportion of women without the syndrome is

$$\frac{63}{90} = 0.7$$

Therefore substituting these figures in the formula we get:

$$1.96 \times \sqrt{\frac{0.3 \times 0.7}{90}}$$

$$= 1.96 \times \sqrt{\frac{0.21}{90}}$$

$$= 1.96 \times \sqrt{0.0023}$$

$$= 1.96 \times 0.05$$

$$= 0.1$$

This figure of 0.1 is now added to the proportion of the sample who have carpal tunnel syndrome to get the upper confidence limit, i.e.:

$$0.1 + 0.3 = 0.4$$

It is then subtracted from the proportion of the sample who have carpal tunnel syndrome to get the lower confidence limit, i.e.:

$$0.3 - 0.1 = 0.2$$

This gives us the confidence interval of 0.2–0.4, which means that we can now estimate with 95% confidence that the proportion of the population of pregnant women who suffer carpal tunnel syndrome will lie between 0.2 and 0.4.

### The 99% confidence limit

Should you need to have greater confidence in your estimate then the following formula should be used:

$$2.58 \times \sqrt{\frac{pq}{n}}$$

If we use the example and figures above then we get

$$2.58 \times \sqrt{\frac{0.3 \times 0.7}{90}}$$

$$= 2.58 \times \sqrt{\frac{0.21}{90}}$$

$$= 2.58 \times \sqrt{0.0023}$$

$$= 2.58 \times 0.05$$

$$= 0.13$$

This number is then added to the proportion of the sample who have carpal tunnel syndrome to get the upper confidence limit, i.e.:

$$0.3 + 0.13 = 0.43$$

It is then subtracted from the proportion of the sample with carpal tunnel syndrome to get the lower confidence limit, i.e.:

$$0.3 - 0.13 = 0.17$$

Therefore, the 99% confidence interval for the proportion of the population of pregnant women with carpal tunnel syndrome is 0.17 to 0.43.

### The 90% confidence limit

If you don't need such a high level of confidence in your estimate, you can use the 90% confidence limit formula instead:

$$1.64 \times \sqrt{\frac{pq}{n}}$$

$$= 1.64 \times \sqrt{\frac{0.3 \times 0.7}{90}}$$

$$= 1.64 \times \sqrt{\frac{0.21}{90}}$$

$$= 1.64 \times \sqrt{0.0023}$$

$$= 1.64 \times 0.05$$

$$= 0.08$$

This number is now added to the proportion of

the sample with carpal tunnel syndrome to give the upper confidence limit, i.e.: 0.3 + 0.08

$$0.3 + 0.08 = 0.38$$

It is then subtracted from the proportion of the sample with carpal tunnel syndrome to give the lower confidence limit, i.e.:

$$0.3 - 0.08 = 0.22$$

Therefore, it can be predicted with 90% confidence that the proportion of the pregnant woman population who have carpal tunnel syndrome falls somewhere between 0.22 and 0.38.

## SAMPLES OF THIRTY SUBJECTS OR FEWER

Before proceeding with estimates for samples of 30 or fewer it is important to emphasise two points. Firstly, these particular calculations should only be performed if the parent population is known to be *normally distributed* on the characteristic in question. The second important point to note is that proportions of a population are not usually calculated from samples of 30 or fewer, because the estimates are likely to be unreliable. Consequently, only the formulae associated with estimating means will be provided.

Let's suppose you are interested in the promotion prospects of newly qualified physiotherapists. You select a random sample of 15 and follow them up over a 10-year period. You find that the average length of time taken to achieve a senior II grade is 4.7 years. From this sample mean you wish to calculate the population mean. Therefore, your interest is in averages and you have a sample of 30 or fewer. The following formulae are therefore appropriate.

The formula for the 99%, 95% and 90% confidence limits requires that you first calculate the standard deviation from the sample data, thus

$$SD = \sqrt{\frac{\Sigma(x - \bar{x})^2}{N - 1}}$$

where $\Sigma$ = the total
$x$ = the individual score
$\bar{x}$ = the average score

$N$ = the total number of scores in the sample
$\sqrt{\phantom{x}}$ = the square root of all the calculations under this sign

To refresh your memory on how to do this calculation, turn back to pages 43–44. Imagine for the purpose of this example that the standard deviation is 2.1 years.

The estimation calculations for the confidence limits of 99%, 95% and 90% all start off in the same way:

**1.** Calculate $N - 1$ where $N$ is the number in your sample, i.e.

$$15 - 1 = 14$$

**2.** Turn to the probability tables associated with the *t*-test (Table A2.5, page 214), where you can see that down the left-hand column are df values from 1–120. Look down this column until you find our $N - 1$ value of 14. To the right of this are the numbers

1.345  1.761  2.145  2.624  2.977  4.140

The procedures for calculating the different levels of confidence limits now change slightly, and each will be dealt with separately.

### Calculating the 95% confidence limits

We are only interested in the figure under the heading '0.05 level of significance for a two-tailed test' (see top of the Table). This terminology is explained in Chapter 9 but is of no relevance to us here. The figure at the intersection point of this column with $N - 1 = 14$, is 2.145 and is used to provide us with the 95% confidence limit, thus:

$$t \times \frac{SD}{\sqrt{N}}$$

where t = the figure derived from the probability table for t
= 2.145
SD = the standard deviation of the sample's score
= 2.1 years
$N$ = the number of subjects in the sample

= 15

$\sqrt{\phantom{x}}$ = the square root

Therefore, substituting these figures we get:

$$2.145 \times \frac{2.1}{\sqrt{15}}$$

$$= 2.145 \times \frac{2.1}{3.87}$$

$$= 2.145 \times 0.54$$

$$= 1.16$$

This figure is added to the average sample score to give the upper confidence limit, i.e.:

$$4.7 + 1.16 = 5.86$$

It is then subtracted from the average sample score to give the lower confidence limit, i.e.:

$$4.7 - 1.16 = 3.54$$

Therefore we can estimate with 95% confidence that the population of newly qualified physiotherapists will achieve a senior II grade between 3.54 and 5.86 years after qualifying.

### The 99% confidence limits

To calculate this value we need to look under the '0.01 level of significance for a two-tailed test' heading in Table A2.5 for $N$-1. Our $N$-1 value is 14 and the relevant figure at the intersection point is 2.977.

Using the formula

$$t \times \frac{SD}{\sqrt{N}}$$

and substituting our values we get

$$2.977 \times \frac{2.1}{\sqrt{15}}$$

$$= 2.977 \times \frac{2.1}{3.87}$$

$$= 2.977 \times 0.54$$

$$= 1.61$$

We now add 1.61 to the sample mean of 4.7 to get the upper confidence limit, i.e.:

$$4.7 + 1.61 = 6.31$$

We then subtract 1.61 from the sample mean of 4.7 to get the lower confidence limit, i.e.:

$$4.7 - 1.61 = 3.09$$

Therefore the 99% confidence limits are 3.09–6.31 years.

### The 90% confidence limits

To obtain the 90% confidence limits we need to select the number under the heading '0.10 level of significance for a two-tailed test' (in Table A2.5), to the right of $N$-1.

Here for our $N$-1 value of 14, the relevant figure is 1.762.

Using the formula:

$$t \times \frac{SD}{\sqrt{N}}$$

and substituting our values we get

$$1.761 \times \frac{2.1}{\sqrt{15}}$$

$$= 1.761 \times \frac{2.1}{3.87}$$

$$= 176 \times 0.54$$

$$= 0.95$$

This figure is now added to the sample mean of 4.7 to give the upper confidence limit, i.e.:

$$4.7 + 0.95 = 5.65$$

It is then subtracted from the sample mean of 4.7 to give the lower confidence limit, i.e.:

$$4.7 - 0.95 = 3.75$$

The 90% confidence limits for this example are therefore 3.75 – 5.65 years.

## KEY CONCEPTS

1. Estimation is a technique of making scientific 'best guesses' about events.
2. It is particularly useful to anyone who is involved in planning (e.g. budgets, service delivery etc).
3. The technique of estimation involves making predictions about a particular population characteristic known as a **parameter** from knowledge about a small sample of that population.
4. There are two types of estimation: **point estimates** and **interval estimates**.
5. Point estimates make a prediction of a single figure about the population parameter, whereas interval estimates make a prediction that the population parameter will fall between two figures.
6. These two figures are called **confidence limits** and the gap between them is called the **confidence interval**.
7. When using interval estimates, the predictions about the population can be made with different levels of confidence.
8. The degree of confidence is dictated by the nature of the research and the formula used to calculate the estimates.

**Activity 18.1** (Answers on page 235)

1 You are the physiotherapist in charge of an outpatients' clinic. The non-attendane levels are becoming increasingly worrying because of resource wastage and length of waiting lists. If you could make an accurate estimate of non-attendance over the next 6 months, you could double-book appointments in order to reduce wastage.

You find that the number of non-attenders of a sample of 150 patients was 57.

Estimate the confidence limits for the proportion of non-attenders in the outpatient population using the 95% confidence level.

2 You are trying to plan care activities in a new respite centre for learning disabled children. As many of these children have physical handicaps which impair their mobility and self-care activities you will need to estimate how much physiotherapy time on average, will be required per child, per week.

You select a sample of 25 learning disabled children and find that the average amount of physiotherapy time needed is 3.2 hours, with a SD of 1.7 hours.

Estimate the average amount of time that will be required by the children in this new centre, using the 99% confidence level.

3 You are responsible for the equipment budget in your district health authority. One activity involves you in estimating the mean life expectancy of your ultrasound machines over the next financial year.

You look at the life-span of a sample of 40 of these machines and find that the mean length of service is 4.3 years, with a standard deviation of 0.9 years. Using the 90% confidence level, estimate the average life expectancy of the shortwave machines in your area, so that you can get some idea of how many replacements will be needed.

# Appendix 1

# Basic mathematical principles

## BRACKETS

You will not always meet with straightforward calculations in statistical tests. Many of them have quite complex formulae and it is essential to know which part of the formula should be computed first. One way of indicating which part should be dealt with first is by using brackets. Any figures or formulae contained in brackets should be calculated before anything else, or else you will get quite incorrect results. This can be illustrated by the following examples:

$$114 - (15 + 23)$$
$$= 114 - 38$$
$$= 76$$

as opposed to:

$$(114 - 15) + 23$$
$$= 99 + 23$$
$$= 122$$

Brackets can change your answer quite dramatically. Therefore, the first principle you must remember when calculating any statistical tests is:

*all calculations contained in brackets must be carried out first.*

However, not all formulae are as convenient as this. Some have brackets within brackets, e.g.:

$$14 + [(15 \times 3) - 12]$$

In these cases, you must calculate the formula in the innermost brackets first, then go on to the formula in the next set of brackets and so on. Therefore, the above formula becomes:

$$14 + [45 - 12] = 14 + 33 = 47$$

So:

*always calculate the formula in the innermost set of brackets first and then work outwards.*

## ADDITION, SUBTRACTION, MULTIPLICATION AND DIVISION

Although any formula in brackets must always be calculated first, not all formulae have brackets.

Sometimes you will come across something like this:

$$12 + 19 - 7 - 4 + 8$$

In such cases, where you have a mixure of just additions and subtraction and no brackets, you simply start calculating from the left-hand side and work systematically across to the right. The importance of this principle can be illustrated by the following example:

$$[72 - 34 + 9]$$

If you work systematically from left to right to right, the answer 47. If, however, you do the addition first, the answer is 29 – quite different and quite incorrect. So the next principle to remember is:

*When you have a row of additions and substractions only and no brackets, start the calculations at the left–hand side and work systematically across to the right.*

Similarly, there will be occasions when you have a row of additions only, e.g.:

$$19 + 17 + 9$$

subtractions only, e.g.:

$$28 - 4 - 16$$

divisions only, e.g.:

$$45 \div 3 \div 5$$

multiplications only, e.g.:

$$7 \times 8 \times 14$$

or a mixture of multiplications and divisions, e.g.:

$$12 \times 8 \div 4$$

While it doesn't matter too much in which order these are carried out, it is easier and less confusing if you stick to the left-to-right rule.

However, quite often you will come across mixtures of addition and/or subtraction with multiplication and/or division, e.g.:

a. $71 + 9 \div 18$

or

b. $117 - 6 \times 10$

In these cases you must do the multiplication or division first, followed by the additions or subtractions. The reason for doing this can be ilustrated by the above examples. If they are calculated correctly, the answer to (a) is 71.5 and to (b) 57. If, however, you apply the left to right rule here, you end up with 4.44 and 1110 respectively. So the next rule of basic maths is that:

*multiplying and dividing are carried out before adding and subtracting.*

To recap on what has been outlined so far:
- First, carry out the calculations in brackets. If there are brackets within brackets, do the calculations in the inside brackets first.
- Second, if there are no brackets, do the multiplications and divisions first.
- Third, if there are no multiplications and divisions, just work from left to right.

Just one final point – sometimes you will see something like $9(12 - 2)$. This means $9 \times (12 - 2)$, except that the multiplication sign between the 9 and the bracket is *assumed*.

## POSITIVE AND NEGATIVE NUMBERS

It's easy to get confused over positive and negative numbers. While $40 - 20$ is simple to work out, $20 - 40$ starts to cause confusion. Perhaps the easiest way to overcome the problems of plus and minus numbers is to think of the left-hand figure as your 'bank' of money in a Monopoly® game. Obviously, you can add to your bank or you can take away from your bank, but both transactions will alter the resulting amount of money you have to play with. Suppose you started with £200 but then landed on your competitor's Mayfair property, which meant you owed them £300. You have, then £200 – £300. This means that you are £100 in the red, in other words you have –£100. Suppose now that another player landed on your Park Lane property which meant you could receive £200. Because you're already in debt to the tune of £100, half the money you're owed must go towards putting your debt right, which means that you're £100 in credit. In other words you have:

$$- £100 + £200 = £100$$

However, it's often more expensive than this in Monopoly®. Suppose that while you are £100 in debt, you land on the Strand and owe a further £50. This means you have one debt of £100 ($-£100$) plus another debt of £50 ($-£50$). This can be expressed as:

$$(-£100) + (-£50) = - £150$$

There are, of course, many occasions when you will be either multiplying or dividing plus and minus numbers, e.g.

$$(+5) \times (-10) \text{ or } (-80) \div (+8)$$

Multiplying or dividing a mixture of plus and minus numbers always gives a minus answer. So in the examples above, the answers are $-50$ and $-10$ respectively. Multiplying or dividing positive numbers *only* always results in positive answers, but multiplying or dividing minus numbers only also produces a positive number. If you think about this in terms of double negatives in speech, 'I didn't do nothing' actually means 'I did something'. Similarly, double negatives in maths also mean a positive.

We can state some further mathematical principles now:

1. Adding two negative numbers results in a negative answer, e.g.:

$$(-20) + (-10) = -30$$

2. Adding one plus number to a minus number is the same as taking the minus number from the plus number, e.g.:

$$-24 + 6 = -18$$
$$+6 - 24 = -18$$

3. Multiplying two positive numbers always results in a positive answer.
4. Multiplying one positive number by one negative number always results in a negative answer.
5. Multiplying two negative numbers always results in a positive answer.
6. Dividing two positive numbers always results in a positive answer.
7. Dividing one positive number by one negative number always results in a negative answer.
8. Dividing two negative numbers always results in a positive answer.

## SQUARES AND SQUARE ROOTS

Two common calculations you will have to carry out in the statistical tests are squares and square roots.

The **square** of a number is quite simply that number multiplied by itself and is expressed by a small 2 thus:

$$8^2$$

This means that you multiply 8 by 8. So whenever you see the small $^2$ to the top right of a number, you simply multiply that number by itself. The answer you will obtain will always be a positive number, since if you square $+8$ you multiply $+8 \times +8$ which will give you $+64$, while if you square $-8$, you multiply $-8 \times -8$ which will still give you $+64$, since multiplying two negative numbers always gives a positive number.

The **square root** of a number is actually the opposite of the square, in that the square root of any given number is a number which multiplied by itself gives the number you already have. It is expressed by the symbol $\sqrt{\ }$. Therefore $\sqrt{25} = 5$, since $5 \times 5 = 25$.

While your calculator will almost certainly have a square root function (which you should not hesitate to use), this is a good example of an occasion when you should be 'eyeballing' the result. For example, while you cannot easily work out in your head what the square root of 14 is, you do know that it must be somewhere between 3 and 4, since 3 is the square root of 9 and 4 is the square root of 16; if you come out with something larger or smaller, something has gone wrong somewhere!

In many of the formulae in this book, you will find that the square root sign extends over more than one number, e.g.:

$$\sqrt{45 + 19} = \sqrt{64} = 8$$

Do make sure that you complete all the calculations under the square root symbol before computing the square root.

## ROUNDING UP DECIMAL PLACES

When using decimals in fairly complicated calculations, you can often end up with a whole row of figures to the right of the decimal point. To continue your calculations with all these numbers is both cumbersome and unnecessarily accurate. Therefore, it is easier to limit the number of figures to the right of the decimal point to 2 or 3. In order to do this correctly, we do not simply chop off the excess figures, but **round them up**.

This is done by starting with the figure on the extreme right of the decimal point. If this figure is equal to 5 or larger, then the number to its immediate left is increased by 1. If the end figure is less than 5, then number to its left remains the same, e.g.:

9.14868125 becomes
9.1486813

If you wish to drop the 3, the same rule applies, so that the above decimal becomes:

9.149681

If you wish to cut down the number of decimal places to 2, the process is:

9.148681 becomes
9.14868  which becomes
9.1487   which becomes
9.149    which becomes
9.15

While this process is relatively straightforward in the above example, look at the following decimal number, which we wish to round up to two places:

7.19498

Here, dropping the last number changes the 9 to a 10, and this automatically changes the 4 to 5 which in turn changes the next 9 into a 10, such that the end result is 7.2, even though we were rounding up to 2 decimal places, thus:

7.19498 becomes
7.195    which becomes
7.2

Throughout this book, the figures have been rounded to three decimal places. If you have chosen to round up to two decimal places throughout the calculations, you will find that the end result is slightly different. Don't worry about this unless there is a massive discrepancy which will probably mean that something has gone wrong somewhere in your calculations.

# Appendix 2

# Statistical probability tables

**Table A2.1** Critical values of $\chi^2$ at various levels of probability. For your $\chi^2$ value to be significant at a particular probability level, it should be *equal to* or *larger than* the critical values associated with the df in your study. (Reproduced From Lindley DV, Scott WF (1984) New Cambridge Elementary Statistical Tables, 10th edn. Cambridge University Press, with permission.)

| | Level of significance for a two-tailed test | | | | |
|---|---|---|---|---|---|
| df | .10 | .05 | .02 | .01 | .001 |
| 1 | 2.71 | 3.84 | 5.41 | 6.64 | 10.83 |
| 2 | 4.60 | 5.99 | 7.82 | 9.21 | 13.82 |
| 3 | 6.25 | 7.82 | 9.84 | 11.34 | 16.27 |
| 4 | 7.78 | 9.49 | 11.67 | 13.28 | 18.46 |
| 5 | 9.24 | 11.07 | 13.39 | 15.09 | 20.52 |
| 6 | 10.64 | 12.59 | 15.03 | 16.81 | 22.46 |
| 7 | 12.02 | 14.07 | 16.62 | 18.48 | 24.32 |
| 8 | 13.36 | 15.51 | 18.17 | 20.09 | 26.12 |
| 9 | 14.68 | 16.92 | 19.68 | 21.67 | 27.88 |
| 10 | 15.99 | 18.31 | 21.16 | 23.21 | 29.59 |
| 11 | 17.28 | 19.68 | 22.62 | 24.72 | 31.26 |
| 12 | 18.55 | 21.03 | 24.05 | 26.22 | 32.91 |
| 13 | 19.81 | 22.36 | 25.47 | 27.69 | 34.53 |
| 14 | 21.06 | 23.68 | 26.87 | 29.14 | 36.12 |
| 15 | 22.31 | 25.00 | 28.26 | 30.58 | 37.70 |
| 16 | 23.54 | 26.30 | 29.63 | 32.00 | 39.29 |
| 17 | 24.77 | 27.59 | 31.00 | 33.41 | 40.75 |
| 18 | 25.99 | 28.87 | 32.35 | 34.80 | 42.31 |
| 19 | 27.20 | 30.14 | 33.69 | 36.19 | 43.82 |
| 20 | 28.41 | 31.41 | 35.02 | 37.57 | 45.32 |
| 21 | 29.62 | 32.67 | 36.34 | 38.93 | 46.80 |
| 22 | 30.81 | 33.92 | 37.66 | 40.29 | 48.27 |
| 23 | 32.01 | 35.17 | 38.97 | 41.64 | 49.73 |
| 24 | 33.20 | 36.42 | 40.27 | 42.98 | 51.18 |
| 25 | 34.38 | 37.65 | 41.57 | 44.31 | 52.62 |
| 26 | 35.56 | 38.88 | 42.86 | 45.64 | 54.05 |
| 27 | 36.74 | 40.11 | 44.14 | 46.97 | 55.48 |
| 28 | 37.92 | 41.34 | 45.42 | 48.28 | 56.89 |
| 29 | 39.09 | 42.56 | 46.69 | 49.59 | 58.30 |
| 30 | 40.26 | 43.77 | 47.96 | 50.89 | 59.70 |

*NB* If you have a one-tailed hypothesis, look up your value as usual and simply *halve* the associated $p$ value shown for a two-tailed hypothesis.

**Table A2.2** **Critical values of** $T$ (Wilcoxon test) at various levels of probability. (For your $T$ value to be significant at a particular probability level, it should be *equal to* or *less than* critical values associated with the $N$ in your study)

| | Level of significance for one-tailed test | | | | | Level of significance for one-tailed test | | | |
|---|---|---|---|---|---|---|---|---|---|
| | .05 | .025 | .01 | .005 | | .05 | .025 | .01 | .005 |
| | Level of significance for two-tailed test | | | | | Level of significance for two-tailed test | | | |
| $N$ | .10 | .05 | .02 | .01 | $N$ | .10 | .05 | .02 | .01 |
| 5 | 1 | - | - | - | 28 | 130 | 117 | 102 | 92 |
| 6 | 2 | 1 | - | - | 29 | 141 | 127 | 111 | 100 |
| 7 | 4 | 2 | 0 | - | 30 | 152 | 137 | 120 | 109 |
| 8 | 6 | 4 | 2 | 0 | 31 | 163 | 148 | 130 | 118 |
| 9 | 8 | 6 | 3 | 2 | 32 | 175 | 159 | 141 | 128 |
| 10 | 11 | 8 | 5 | 3 | 33 | 188 | 171 | 151 | 138 |
| 11 | 14 | 11 | 7 | 5 | 34 | 201 | 183 | 162 | 149 |
| 12 | 17 | 14 | 10 | 7 | 35 | 214 | 195 | 174 | 160 |
| 13 | 21 | 17 | 13 | 10 | 36 | 228 | 208 | 186 | 171 |
| 14 | 26 | 21 | 16 | 13 | 37 | 242 | 222 | 198 | 183 |
| 15 | 30 | 25 | 20 | 16 | 38 | 256 | 235 | 211 | 195 |
| 16 | 36 | 30 | 24 | 19 | 39 | 271 | 250 | 224 | 208 |
| 17 | 41 | 35 | 28 | 23 | 40 | 287 | 264 | 238 | 221 |
| 18 | 47 | 40 | 33 | 28 | 41 | 303 | 279 | 252 | 234 |
| 19 | 54 | 46 | 38 | 32 | 42 | 319 | 295 | 267 | 248 |
| 20 | 60 | 52 | 43 | 37 | 43 | 336 | 311 | 281 | 262 |
| 21 | 68 | 59 | 49 | 43 | 44 | 353 | 327 | 297 | 277 |
| 22 | 75 | 66 | 56 | 49 | 45 | 371 | 344 | 313 | 292 |
| 23 | 83 | 73 | 62 | 55 | 46 | 389 | 361 | 329 | 307 |
| 24 | 92 | 81 | 69 | 61 | 47 | 408 | 379 | 345 | 323 |
| 25 | 101 | 90 | 77 | 68 | 48 | 427 | 397 | 362 | 339 |
| 26 | 110 | 98 | 85 | 76 | 49 | 446 | 415 | 380 | 356 |
| 27 | 120 | 107 | 93 | 84 | 50 | 466 | 434 | 398 | 373 |

Dashes in the table indicate that no decision is possible at the stated level of significance.

**Table A2.3**   Critical values of $\chi_r^2$ (Friedman test) at various levels of probability. (For your $\chi_r^2$ value to be significant at a particular probability level, it should be *equal to* or *larger than* the critical values associated with the $C$ and $N$ in your study)
**a. Critical values for three conditions ($C = 3$)**

| N = 2 | | N = 3 | | N = 4 | | N = 5 | | N = 6 | | N = 7 | | N = 8 | | N = 9 | |
|---|---|---|---|---|---|---|---|---|---|---|---|---|---|---|---|
| $\chi_r^2$ | p | $\chi_r^2$ | p | $\chi_r^2$ | p | $\chi_r^2$ | p | $\chi_r^2$ | p | $\chi_r^2$ | p | $\chi_r^2$ | p | $\chi_r^2$ | p |
| 0 | 1.000 | .000 | 1.000 | .0 | 1.000 | .0 | 1.000 | .00 | 1.000 | .000 | 1.000 | .00 | 1.000 | .000 | 1.000 |
| 1 | .833 | .667 | .944 | .5 | .931 | .4 | .954 | .33 | .956 | .286 | .964 | .25 | .967 | .222 | .971 |
| 3 | .500 | 2.000 | .528 | 1.5 | .653 | 1.2 | .691 | 1.00 | .740 | .857 | .768 | .75 | .794 | .667 | .814 |
| 4 | .167 | 2.667 | .361 | 2.0 | .431 | 1.6 | .522 | 1.33 | .570 | 1.143 | .620 | 1.00 | .654 | .889 | .865 |
| | | 4.667 | .194 | 3.5 | .273 | 2.8 | .367 | 2.33 | .430 | 2.000 | .486 | 1.75 | .531 | 1.556 | .569 |
| | | 6.000 | .028 | 4.5 | .125 | 3.6 | .182 | 3.00 | .252 | 2.571 | .305 | 2.25 | .355 | 2.000 | .398 |
| | | | | 6.0 | .069 | 4.8 | .124 | 4.00 | .184 | 3.429 | .237 | 3.00 | .285 | 2.667 | .328 |
| | | | | 6.5 | .042 | 5.2 | .093 | 4.33 | .142 | 3.714 | .192 | 3.25 | .236 | 2.889 | .278 |
| | | | | 8.0 | .0046 | 6.4 | .039 | 5.33 | .072 | 4.571 | .112 | 4.00 | .149 | 3.556 | .187 |
| | | | | | | 7.6 | .024 | 6.33 | .052 | 5.429 | .085 | 4.75 | .120 | 4.222 | .154 |
| | | | | | | 8.4 | .0085 | 7.00 | .029 | 6.000 | .052 | 5.25 | .079 | 4.667 | .107 |
| | | | | | | 10.0 | .00077 | 8.33 | .012 | 7.143 | .027 | 6.25 | .047 | 5.556 | .069 |
| | | | | | | | | 9.00 | .0081 | 7.714 | .021 | 6.75 | .038 | 6.000 | .057 |
| | | | | | | | | 9.33 | .0055 | 8.000 | .016 | 7.00 | .030 | 6.222 | .048 |
| | | | | | | | | 10.33 | .0017 | 8.857 | .0084 | 7.75 | .018 | 6.889 | .031 |
| | | | | | | | | 12.00 | .00013 | 10.286 | .0036 | 9.00 | .0099 | 8.000 | .019 |
| | | | | | | | | | | 10.571 | .0027 | 9.25 | .0080 | 8.222 | .016 |
| | | | | | | | | | | 11.143 | .0012 | 9.75 | .0048 | 8.667 | .010 |
| | | | | | | | | | | 12.286 | .00032 | 10.75 | .0024 | 9.556 | .0060 |
| | | | | | | | | | | 14.000 | .000021 | 12.00 | .0011 | 10.667 | .0035 |
| | | | | | | | | | | | | 12.25 | .00086 | 10.889 | .0029 |
| | | | | | | | | | | | | 13.00 | .00026 | 11.556 | .0013 |
| | | | | | | | | | | | | 14.25 | .000061 | 12.667 | .00066 |
| | | | | | | | | | | | | 16.00 | .0000036 | 13.556 | .00035 |
| | | | | | | | | | | | | | | 14.000 | .00020 |
| | | | | | | | | | | | | | | 14.222 | .000097 |
| | | | | | | | | | | | | | | 14.889 | .000054 |
| | | | | | | | | | | | | | | 16.222 | .000011 |
| | | | | | | | | | | | | | | 18.000 | .0000006 |

*NB* These values are all for a two-tailed test only.

**Table A2.3** (contd) Critical values of $\chi_r^2$ (Friedman test). (For your $\chi_r^2$ value to be significant at a particular probability level, it should be *equal to* or *larger than* the critical values associated with the $C$ and $N$ in your study.)

**b. Critical values for four conditions ($C$ = 4)**

| $N = 2$ | | $N = 3$ | | $N = 4$ | | | |
|---|---|---|---|---|---|---|---|
| $\chi r^2$ | $p$ | $\chi r^2$ | $p$ | $\chi r^2$ | $p$ | $\chi r^2$ | $p$ |
| .0 | 1.000 | .0 | 1.000 | .0 | 1.000 | 5.7 | .141 |
| .6 | .958 | .6 | .958 | .3 | .992 | 6.0 | .105 |
| 1.2 | .834 | 1.0 | .910 | .6 | .928 | 6.3 | .094 |
| 1.8 | .792 | 1.8 | .727 | .9 | .900 | 6.6 | .077 |
| 2.4 | .625 | 2.2 | .608 | 1.2 | .800 | 6.9 | .068 |
| 3.0 | .542 | 2.6 | .524 | 1.5 | .754 | 7.2 | .054 |
| 3.6 | .458 | 3.4 | .446 | 1.8 | .677 | 7.5 | .052 |
| 4.2 | .375 | 3.8 | .342 | 2.1 | .649 | 7.8 | .036 |
| 4.8 | .208 | 4.2 | .300 | 2.4 | .524 | 8.1 | .033 |
| 5.4 | .167 | 5.0 | .207 | 2.7 | .508 | 8.4 | .019 |
| 6.0 | .042 | 5.4 | .175 | 3.0 | .432 | 8.7 | .014 |
| | | 5.8 | .148 | 3.3 | .389 | 9.3 | .012 |
| | | 6.6 | .075 | 3.6 | .355 | 9.6 | .0069 |
| | | 7.0 | .054 | 3.9 | .324 | 9.9 | .0062 |
| | | 7.4 | .033 | 4.5 | .242 | 10.2 | .0027 |
| | | 8.2 | .017 | 4.8 | .200 | 10.8 | .0016 |
| | | 9.0 | .0017 | 5.1 | .190 | 11.1 | .00094 |
| | | | | 5.4 | .158 | 12.0 | .000072 |

*NB* These values are all for a two-tailed test only.

**Table A2.4**   Critical values of $L$ (Page's $L$ trend test) at various levels of probability. (For your $L$ value to be significant at a particular probability level, it should be *equal to* or *larger* than the critical values associated with the $C$ and $N$ in your study.)

| N | 3 | 4 | 5 | 6 | p< |
|---|---|---|---|---|---|
| | | | **C** | | |
| | | | (*no. of conditions*) | | |
| 2 | - | - | 109 | 178 | .001 |
| | - | 60 | 106 | 173 | .01 |
| | 28 | 58 | 103 | 166 | .05 |
| 3 | - | 89 | 160 | 260 | .001 |
| | 42 | 87 | 155 | 252 | .01 |
| | 41 | 84 | 150 | 244 | .05 |
| 4 | 56 | 117 | 210 | 341 | .001 |
| | 55 | 114 | 204 | 331 | .01 |
| | 54 | 111 | 197 | 321 | .05 |
| 5 | 70 | 145 | 259 | 420 | .001 |
| | 68 | 141 | 251 | 409 | .01 |
| | 66 | 137 | 244 | 397 | .05 |
| 6 | 83 | 172 | 307 | 499 | .001 |
| | 81 | 167 | 299 | 486 | .01 |
| | 79 | 163 | 291 | 474 | .05 |
| 7 | 96 | 198 | 355 | 577 | .001 |
| | 93 | 193 | 346 | 563 | .01 |
| | 91 | 189 | 338 | 550 | .05 |
| 8 | 109 | 225 | 403 | 655 | .001 |
| | 106 | 220 | 393 | 640 | .01 |
| | 104 | 214 | 384 | 625 | .05 |
| 9 | 121 | 252 | 451 | 733 | .001 |
| | 119 | 246 | 441 | 717 | .01 |
| | 116 | 240 | 431 | 701 | .05 |
| 10 | 134 | 278 | 499 | 811 | .001 |
| | 131 | 272 | 487 | 793 | .01 |
| | 128 | 266 | 477 | 777 | .05 |
| 11 | 147 | 305 | 546 | 888 | .001 |
| | 144 | 298 | 534 | 869 | .01 |
| | 141 | 292 | 523 | 852 | .05 |
| 12 | 160 | 331 | 593 | 965 | .001 |
| | 156 | 324 | 581 | 946 | .01 |
| | 153 | 317 | 570 | 928 | .05 |

*NB*   These values are for a one-tailed test only.

**Table A2.5**  Critical values of *t* (related and unrelated *t* tests) at various levels of probability. For your *t* value to be significant at a particular probability level, it should be *equal to* or *larger than* critical values associated with the df in your study. (Reproduced from Lindley DV, Scott WF (1984) New Cambridge Elementary Statistical Tables, 10th edn. Cambridge University Press, with permission.)

| df | Level of significance for one-tailed test | | | | | |
|---|---|---|---|---|---|---|
| | .10 | .05 | .025 | .01 | .005 | .0005 |
| | Level of significance for two-tailed test | | | | | |
| | .20 | .10 | .05 | .02 | .01 | .001 |
| 1 | 3.078 | 6.314 | 12.706 | 31.821 | 63.657 | 636.619 |
| 2 | 1.886 | 2.920 | 4.303 | 6.965 | 9.925 | 31.598 |
| 3 | 1.638 | 2.353 | 3.182 | 4.541 | 5.841 | 12.941 |
| 4 | 1.533 | 2.132 | 2.776 | 3.747 | 4.604 | 8.610 |
| 5 | 1.476 | 2.015 | 2.571 | 3.365 | 4.032 | 6.859 |
| 6 | 1.440 | 1.943 | 2.447 | 3.143 | 3.707 | 5.959 |
| 7 | 1.415 | 1.895 | 2.365 | 2.998 | 3.499 | 5.405 |
| 8 | 1.397 | 1.860 | 2.306 | 2.896 | 3.355 | 5.041 |
| 9 | 1.383 | 1.833 | 2.262 | 2.821 | 3.250 | 4.781 |
| 10 | 1.372 | 1.812 | 2.228 | 2.764 | 3.169 | 4.587 |
| 11 | 1.363 | 1.796 | 2.201 | 2.718 | 3.106 | 4.437 |
| 12 | 1.356 | 1.782 | 2.179 | 2.681 | 3.055 | 4.318 |
| 13 | 1.350 | 1.771 | 2.160 | 2.650 | 3.012 | 4.221 |
| 14 | 1.345 | 1.761 | 2.145 | 2.624 | 2.977 | 4.140 |
| 15 | 1.341 | 1.753 | 2.131 | 2.602 | 2.947 | 4.073 |
| 16 | 1.337 | 1.746 | 2.120 | 2.583 | 2.921 | 4.015 |
| 17 | 1.333 | 1.740 | 2.110 | 2.567 | 2.898 | 3.965 |
| 18 | 1.330 | 1.734 | 2.101 | 2.552 | 2.878 | 3.922 |
| 19 | 1.328 | 1.729 | 2.093 | 2.539 | 2.861 | 3.883 |
| 20 | 1.325 | 1.725 | 2.086 | 2.528 | 2.845 | 3.850 |
| 21 | 1.323 | 1.721 | 2.080 | 2.518 | 2.831 | 3.819 |
| 22 | 1.321 | 1.717 | 2.074 | 2.508 | 2.819 | 3.792 |
| 23 | 1.319 | 1.714 | 2.069 | 2.500 | 2.807 | 3.767 |
| 24 | 1.318 | 1.711 | 2.064 | 2.492 | 2.797 | 3.745 |
| 25 | 1.316 | 1.708 | 2.060 | 2.485 | 2.787 | 3.725 |
| 26 | 1.315 | 1.706 | 2.056 | 2.479 | 2.779 | 3.707 |
| 27 | 1.314 | 1.703 | 2.052 | 2.473 | 2.771 | 3.690 |
| 28 | 1.313 | 1.701 | 2.048 | 2.467 | 2.763 | 3.674 |
| 29 | 1.311 | 1.699 | 2.045 | 2.462 | 2.756 | 3.659 |
| 30 | 1.310 | 1.697 | 2.042 | 2.457 | 2.750 | 3.646 |
| 40 | 1.303 | 1.684 | 2.021 | 2.423 | 2.704 | 3.551 |
| 60 | 1.296 | 1.671 | 2.000 | 2.390 | 2.660 | 3.460 |
| 120 | 1.289 | 1.658 | 1.980 | 2.358 | 2.617 | 3.373 |
| ∞ | 1.282 | 1.645 | 1.960 | 2.326 | 2.576 | 3.291 |

*NB*  When there is no exact df use the next lowest number, except for very large dfs (well over 120), when you should use the infinity row. This is marked ∞.

**Table A2.6** Critical values of $F$ (anovas) at various levels of probability. For your $F$ value to be significant at a particular probability level, it should be *equal to* or *larger than* the critical values associated with $v_1$ and $v_2$ in your study. (Reproduced from Lindley DV, Scott WF (1984) New Cambridge Elementary Statistical Tables, 10th edn. Cambridge University Press, with permission.)
**a. Critical value of $F$ at $p < .05$**

| $v_2$ | $v_1$ | | | | | | | | | | | |
|---|---|---|---|---|---|---|---|---|---|---|---|---|
| | 1 | 2 | 3 | 4 | 5 | 6 | 7 | 8 | 10 | 12 | 24 | $\infty$ |
| 1 | 161.4 | 199.5 | 215.7 | 224.6 | 230.2 | 234.0 | 236.8 | 238.9 | 241.9 | 243.9 | 249.0 | 254.3 |
| 2 | 18.5 | 19.0 | 19.2 | 19.2 | 19.3 | 19.3 | 19.4 | 19.4 | 19.4 | 19.4 | 19.5 | 19.5 |
| 3 | 10.13 | 9.55 | 9.28 | 9.12 | 9.01 | 8.94 | 8.89 | 8.85 | 8.79 | 8.74 | 8.64 | 8.53 |
| 4 | 7.71 | 6.94 | 6.59 | 6.39 | 6.26 | 6.16 | 6.09 | 6.04 | 5.96 | 5.91 | 5.77 | 5.63 |
| 5 | 6.61 | 5.79 | 5.41 | 5.19 | 5.05 | 4.95 | 4.88 | 4.82 | 4.74 | 4.68 | 4.53 | 4.36 |
| 6 | 5.99 | 5.14 | 4.76 | 4.53 | 4.39 | 4.28 | 4.21 | 4.15 | 4.06 | 4.00 | 3.84 | 3.67 |
| 7 | 5.59 | 4.74 | 4.35 | 4.12 | 3.97 | 3.87 | 3.79 | 3.73 | 3.64 | 3.57 | 3.41 | 3.23 |
| 8 | 5.32 | 4.46 | 4.07 | 3.84 | 3.69 | 3.58 | 3.50 | 3.44 | 3.35 | 3.28 | 3.12 | 2.93 |
| 9 | 5.12 | 4.26 | 3.86 | 3.63 | 3.48 | 3.37 | 3.29 | 3.23 | 3.14 | 3.07 | 2.90 | 2.71 |
| 10 | 4.96 | 4.10 | 3.71 | 3.48 | 3.33 | 3.22 | 3.14 | 3.07 | 2.98 | 2.91 | 2.74 | 2.54 |
| 11 | 4.84 | 3.98 | 3.59 | 3.36 | 3.20 | 3.09 | 3.01 | 2.95 | 2.85 | 2.79 | 2.61 | 2.40 |
| 12 | 4.75 | 3.89 | 3.49 | 3.26 | 3.11 | 3.00 | 2.91 | 2.85 | 2.75 | 2.69 | 2.51 | 2.30 |
| 13 | 4.67 | 3.81 | 3.41 | 3.18 | 3.03 | 2.92 | 2.83 | 2.77 | 2.67 | 2.60 | 2.42 | 2.21 |
| 14 | 4.60 | 3.74 | 3.34 | 3.11 | 2.96 | 2.85 | 2.76 | 2.70 | 2.60 | 2.53 | 2.35 | 2.13 |
| 15 | 4.54 | 3.68 | 3.29 | 3.06 | 2.90 | 2.79 | 2.71 | 2.64 | 2.54 | 2.48 | 2.29 | 2.07 |
| 16 | 4.49 | 3.63 | 3.24 | 3.01 | 2.85 | 2.74 | 2.66 | 2.59 | 2.49 | 2.42 | 2.24 | 2.01 |
| 17 | 4.45 | 3.59 | 3.20 | 2.96 | 2.81 | 2.70 | 2.61 | 2.55 | 2.45 | 2.38 | 2.19 | 1.96 |
| 18 | 4.41 | 3.55 | 3.16 | 2.93 | 2.77 | 2.66 | 2.58 | 2.51 | 2.41 | 2.34 | 2.15 | 1.92 |
| 19 | 4.38 | 3.52 | 3.13 | 2.90 | 2.74 | 2.63 | 2.54 | 2.48 | 2.38 | 2.31 | 2.11 | 1.88 |
| 20 | 4.35 | 3.49 | 3.10 | 2.87 | 2.71 | 2.60 | 2.51 | 2.45 | 2.35 | 2.28 | 2.08 | 1.84 |
| 21 | 4.32 | 3.47 | 3.07 | 2.84 | 2.68 | 2.57 | 2.49 | 2.42 | 2.32 | 2.25 | 2.05 | 1.81 |
| 22 | 4.30 | 3.44 | 3.05 | 2.82 | 2.66 | 2.55 | 2.46 | 2.40 | 2.30 | 2.23 | 2.03 | 1.78 |
| 23 | 4.28 | 3.42 | 3.03 | 2.80 | 2.64 | 2.53 | 2.44 | 2.37 | 2.27 | 2.20 | 2.00 | 1.76 |
| 24 | 4.26 | 3.40 | 3.01 | 2.78 | 2.62 | 2.51 | 2.42 | 2.36 | 2.25 | 2.18 | 1.98 | 1.73 |
| 25 | 4.24 | 3.39 | 2.99 | 2.76 | 2.60 | 2.49 | 2.40 | 2.34 | 2.24 | 2.16 | 1.96 | 1.71 |
| 26 | 4.23 | 3.37 | 2.98 | 2.74 | 2.59 | 2.47 | 2.39 | 2.32 | 2.22 | 2.15 | 1.95 | 1.69 |
| 27 | 4.21 | 3.35 | 2.96 | 2.73 | 2.57 | 2.46 | 2.37 | 2.31 | 2.20 | 2.13 | 1.93 | 1.67 |
| 28 | 4.20 | 3.34 | 2.95 | 2.71 | 2.56 | 2.45 | 2.36 | 2.29 | 2.19 | 2.12 | 1.91 | 1.65 |
| 29 | 4.18 | 3.33 | 2.93 | 2.70 | 2.55 | 2.43 | 2.35 | 2.28 | 2.18 | 2.10 | 1.90 | 1.64 |
| 30 | 4.17 | 3.32 | 2.92 | 2.69 | 2.53 | 2.42 | 2.33 | 2.27 | 2.16 | 2.09 | 1.89 | 1.62 |
| 32 | 4.15 | 3.29 | 2.90 | 2.67 | 2.51 | 2.40 | 2.31 | 2.24 | 2.14 | 2.07 | 1.86 | 1.59 |
| 34 | 4.13 | 3.28 | 2.88 | 2.65 | 2.49 | 2.38 | 2.29 | 2.23 | 2.12 | 2.05 | 1.84 | 1.57 |
| 36 | 4.11 | 3.26 | 2.87 | 2.63 | 2.48 | 2.36 | 2.28 | 2.21 | 2.11 | 2.03 | 1.82 | 1.55 |
| 38 | 4.10 | 3.24 | 2.85 | 2.62 | 2.46 | 2.35 | 2.26 | 2.19 | 2.09 | 2.02 | 1.81 | 1.53 |
| 40 | 4.08 | 3.23 | 2.84 | 2.61 | 2.45 | 2.34 | 2.25 | 2.18 | 2.08 | 2.00 | 1.79 | 1.51 |
| 60 | 4.00 | 3.15 | 2.76 | 2.53 | 2.37 | 2.25 | 2.17 | 2.10 | 1.99 | 1.92 | 1.70 | 1.39 |
| 120 | 3.92 | 3.07 | 2.68 | 2.45 | 2.29 | 2.18 | 2.09 | 2.02 | 1.91 | 1.83 | 1.61 | 1.25 |
| $\infty$ | 3.84 | 3.00 | 2.60 | 2.37 | 2.21 | 2.10 | 2.01 | 1.94 | 1.83 | 1.75 | 1.52 | 1.00 |

*NB* When there is no exact number for the df, use the next lowest number. For very large dfs (well over 120) you should use the row for infinity. This is indicated $\infty$.

These values are all for a two-tailed test only.

**Table A2.6** (contd) Critical values of $F$ (anovas) at various levels of probability. (For your $F$ value to be significant at a particular probability level, it should be *equal to* or *larger than* the critical values associated with $\nu_1$ and $\nu_2$ in your study.)
**b. Critical values of $F$ at $p < .025$**

| $\nu_2$ | $\nu_1$ | | | | | | | | | | | |
|---|---|---|---|---|---|---|---|---|---|---|---|---|
| | 1 | 2 | 3 | 4 | 5 | 6 | 7 | 8 | 10 | 12 | 24 | $\infty$ |
| 1 | 648 | 800 | 864 | 900 | 922 | 937 | 948 | 957 | 969 | 977 | 997 | 1018 |
| 2 | 38.5 | 39.0 | 39.2 | 39.2 | 39.3 | 39.3 | 39.4 | 39.4 | 39.4 | 39.4 | 39.5 | 39.5 |
| 3 | 17.4 | 16.0 | 15.4 | 15.1 | 14.9 | 14.7 | 14.6 | 14.5 | 14.4 | 14.3 | 14.1 | 13.9 |
| 4 | 12.22 | 10.65 | 9.98 | 9.60 | 9.36 | 9.20 | 9.07 | 8.98 | 8.84 | 8.75 | 8.51 | 8.26 |
| 5 | 10.01 | 8.43 | 7.76 | 7.39 | 7.15 | 6.98 | 6.85 | 6.76 | 6.62 | 6.52 | 6.28 | 6.02 |
| 6 | 8.81 | 7.26 | 6.60 | 6.23 | 5.99 | 5.82 | 5.70 | 5.60 | 5.46 | 5.37 | 5.12 | 4.85 |
| 7 | 8.07 | 6.54 | 5.89 | 5.52 | 5.29 | 5.12 | 4.99 | 4.90 | 4.76 | 4.67 | 4.42 | 4.14 |
| 8 | 7.57 | 6.06 | 5.42 | 5.05 | 4.82 | 4.65 | 4.53 | 4.43 | 4.30 | 4.20 | 3.95 | 3.67 |
| 9 | 7.21 | 5.71 | 5.08 | 4.72 | 4.48 | 4.32 | 4.20 | 4.10 | 3.96 | 3.87 | 3.61 | 3.33 |
| 10 | 6.94 | 5.46 | 4.83 | 4.47 | 4.24 | 4.07 | 3.95 | 3.85 | 3.72 | 3.62 | 3.37 | 3.08 |
| 11 | 6.72 | 5.26 | 4.63 | 4.28 | 4.04 | 3.88 | 3.76 | 3.66 | 3.53 | 3.43 | 3.17 | 2.88 |
| 12 | 6.55 | 5.10 | 4.47 | 4.12 | 3.89 | 3.73 | 3.61 | 3.51 | 3.37 | 3.28 | 3.02 | 2.72 |
| 13 | 6.41 | 4.97 | 4.35 | 4.00 | 3.77 | 3.60 | 3.48 | 3.39 | 3.25 | 3.15 | 2.89 | 2.60 |
| 14 | 6.30 | 4.86 | 4.24 | 3.89 | 3.66 | 3.50 | 3.38 | 3.29 | 3.15 | 3.05 | 2.79 | 2.49 |
| 15 | 6.20 | 4.76 | 4.15 | 3.80 | 3.58 | 3.41 | 3.29 | 3.20 | 3.06 | 2.96 | 2.70 | 2.40 |
| 16 | 6.12 | 4.69 | 4.08 | 3.73 | 3.50 | 3.34 | 3.22 | 3.12 | 2.99 | 2.89 | 2.63 | 2.32 |
| 17 | 6.04 | 4.62 | 4.01 | 3.66 | 3.44 | 3.28 | 3.16 | 3.06 | 2.92 | 2.82 | 2.56 | 2.25 |
| 18 | 5.98 | 4.56 | 3.95 | 3.61 | 3.38 | 3.22 | 3.10 | 3.01 | 2.87 | 2.77 | 2.50 | 2.19 |
| 19 | 5.92 | 4.51 | 3.90 | 3.56 | 3.33 | 3.17 | 3.05 | 2.96 | 2.82 | 2.72 | 2.45 | 2.13 |
| 20 | 5.87 | 4.46 | 3.86 | 3.51 | 3.29 | 3.13 | 3.01 | 2.91 | 2.77 | 2.68 | 2.41 | 2.09 |
| 21 | 5.83 | 4.42 | 3.82 | 3.48 | 3.25 | 3.09 | 2.97 | 2.87 | 2.73 | 2.64 | 2.37 | 2.04 |
| 22 | 5.79 | 4.38 | 3.78 | 3.44 | 3.22 | 3.05 | 2.93 | 2.84 | 2.70 | 2.60 | 2.33 | 2.00 |
| 23 | 5.75 | 4.35 | 3.75 | 3.41 | 3.18 | 3.02 | 2.90 | 2.81 | 2.67 | 2.57 | 2.30 | 1.97 |
| 24 | 5.72 | 4.32 | 3.72 | 3.38 | 3.15 | 2.99 | 2.87 | 2.78 | 2.64 | 2.54 | 2.27 | 1.94 |
| 25 | 5.69 | 4.29 | 3.69 | 3.35 | 3.13 | 2.97 | 2.85 | 2.75 | 2.61 | 2.51 | 2.24 | 1.91 |
| 26 | 5.66 | 4.27 | 3.67 | 3.33 | 3.10 | 2.94 | 2.82 | 2.73 | 2.59 | 2.49 | 2.22 | 1.88 |
| 27 | 5.63 | 4.24 | 3.65 | 3.31 | 3.08 | 2.92 | 2.80 | 2.71 | 2.57 | 2.47 | 2.19 | 1.85 |
| 28 | 5.61 | 4.22 | 3.63 | 3.29 | 3.06 | 2.90 | 2.78 | 2.69 | 2.55 | 2.45 | 2.17 | 1.83 |
| 29 | 5.59 | 4.20 | 3.61 | 3.27 | 3.04 | 2.88 | 2.76 | 2.67 | 2.53 | 2.43 | 2.15 | 1.81 |
| 30 | 5.57 | 4.18 | 3.59 | 3.25 | 3.03 | 2.87 | 2.75 | 2.65 | 2.51 | 2.41 | 2.14 | 1.79 |
| 32 | 5.53 | 4.15 | 3.56 | 3.22 | 3.00 | 2.84 | 2.72 | 2.62 | 2.48 | 2.38 | 2.10 | 1.75 |
| 34 | 5.50 | 4.12 | 3.53 | 3.19 | 2.97 | 2.81 | 2.69 | 2.59 | 2.45 | 2.35 | 2.08 | 1.72 |
| 36 | 5.47 | 4.09 | 3.51 | 3.17 | 2.94 | 2.79 | 2.66 | 2.57 | 2.43 | 2.33 | 2.05 | 1.69 |
| 38 | 5.45 | 4.07 | 3.48 | 3.15 | 2.92 | 2.76 | 2.64 | 2.55 | 2.41 | 2.31 | 2.03 | 1.66 |
| 40 | 5.42 | 4.05 | 3.46 | 3.13 | 2.90 | 2.74 | 2.62 | 2.53 | 2.39 | 2.29 | 2.01 | 1.64 |
| 60 | 5.29 | 3.93 | 3.34 | 3.01 | 2.79 | 2.63 | 2.51 | 2.41 | 2.27 | 2.17 | 1.88 | 1.48 |
| 120 | 5.15 | 3.80 | 3.23 | 2.89 | 2.67 | 2.52 | 2.39 | 2.30 | 2.16 | 2.05 | 1.76 | 1.31 |
| $\infty$ | 5.02 | 3.69 | 3.12 | 2.79 | 2.57 | 2.41 | 2.29 | 2.19 | 2.05 | 1.94 | 1.64 | 1.00 |

*NB* When there is no exact number for the df, use the next lowest number. For very large dfs (i.e. well over 120) you should use the row for infinity, marked $\infty$.

These values are all for a two-tailed test only.

**Table A2.6** (contd) Critical values of $F$ (anovas) at various levels of probability. (For your $F$ value to be significant at a particular probability level, it should be *equal to* or *larger* than the critical values associated with $v_1$ and $v_2$ in your study.)
**c. Critical values of $F$ at $p < .01$**

| $v_2$ | $v_1$ 1 | 2 | 3 | 4 | 5 | 6 | 7 | 8 | 10 | 12 | 24 | ∞ |
|---|---|---|---|---|---|---|---|---|---|---|---|---|
| 1 | 4052 | 5000 | 5403 | 5625 | 5764 | 5859 | 5928 | 5981 | 6056 | 6106 | 6235 | 6366 |
| 2 | 98.5 | 99.0 | 99.2 | 99.2 | 99.3 | 99.3 | 99.4 | 99.4 | 99.4 | 99.4 | 99.5 | 99.5 |
| 3 | 34.1 | 30.8 | 29.5 | 28.7 | 28.2 | 27.9 | 27.7 | 27.5 | 27.2 | 27.1 | 26.6 | 26.1 |
| 4 | 21.2 | 18.0 | 16.7 | 16.0 | 15.5 | 15.2 | 15.0 | 14.8 | 14.5 | 14.4 | 13.9 | 13.5 |
| 5 | 16.26 | 13.27 | 12.06 | 11.39 | 10.97 | 10.67 | 10.46 | 10.29 | 10.05 | 9.89 | 9.47 | 9.02 |
| 6 | 13.74 | 10.92 | 9.78 | 9.15 | 8.75 | 8.47 | 8.26 | 8.10 | 7.87 | 7.72 | 7.31 | 6.88 |
| 7 | 12.25 | 9.55 | 8.45 | 7.85 | 7.46 | 7.19 | 6.99 | 6.84 | 6.62 | 6.47 | 6.07 | 5.65 |
| 8 | 11.26 | 8.65 | 7.59 | 7.01 | 6.63 | 6.37 | 6.18 | 6.03 | 5.81 | 5.67 | 5.28 | 4.86 |
| 9 | 10.56 | 8.02 | 6.99 | 6.42 | 6.06 | 5.80 | 5.61 | 5.47 | 5.26 | 5.11 | 4.73 | 4.31 |
| 10 | 10.04 | 7.56 | 6.55 | 5.99 | 5.64 | 5.39 | 5.20 | 5.06 | 4.85 | 4.71 | 4.33 | 3.91 |
| 11 | 9.65 | 7.21 | 6.22 | 5.67 | 5.32 | 5.07 | 4.89 | 4.74 | 4.54 | 4.40 | 4.02 | 3.60 |
| 12 | 9.33 | 6.93 | 5.95 | 5.41 | 5.06 | 4.82 | 4.64 | 4.50 | 4.30 | 4.16 | 3.78 | 3.36 |
| 13 | 9.07 | 6.70 | 5.74 | 5.21 | 4.86 | 4.62 | 4.44 | 4.30 | 4.10 | 3.96 | 3.59 | 3.17 |
| 14 | 8.86 | 6.51 | 5.56 | 5.04 | 4.70 | 4.46 | 4.28 | 4.14 | 3.94 | 3.80 | 3.43 | 3.00 |
| 15 | 8.68 | 6.36 | 5.42 | 4.89 | 4.56 | 4.32 | 4.14 | 4.00 | 3.80 | 3.67 | 3.29 | 2.87 |
| 16 | 8.53 | 6.23 | 5.29 | 4.77 | 4.44 | 4.20 | 4.03 | 3.89 | 3.69 | 3.55 | 3.18 | 2.75 |
| 17 | 8.40 | 6.11 | 5.18 | 4.67 | 4.34 | 4.10 | 3.93 | 3.79 | 3.59 | 3.46 | 3.08 | 2.65 |
| 18 | 8.29 | 6.01 | 5.09 | 4.58 | 4.25 | 4.01 | 3.84 | 3.71 | 3.51 | 3.37 | 3.00 | 2.57 |
| 19 | 8.18 | 5.93 | 5.01 | 4.50 | 4.17 | 3.94 | 3.77 | 3.63 | 3.43 | 3.30 | 2.92 | 2.49 |
| 20 | 8.10 | 5.85 | 4.94 | 4.43 | 4.10 | 3.87 | 3.70 | 3.56 | 3.37 | 3.23 | 2.86 | 2.42 |
| 21 | 8.02 | 5.78 | 4.87 | 4.37 | 4.04 | 3.81 | 3.64 | 3.51 | 3.31 | 3.17 | 2.80 | 2.36 |
| 22 | 7.95 | 5.72 | 4.82 | 4.31 | 3.99 | 3.76 | 3.59 | 3.45 | 3.26 | 3.12 | 2.75 | 2.31 |
| 23 | 7.88 | 5.66 | 4.76 | 4.26 | 3.94 | 3.71 | 3.54 | 3.41 | 3.21 | 3.07 | 2.70 | 2.26 |
| 24 | 7.82 | 5.61 | 4.72 | 4.22 | 3.90 | 3.67 | 3.50 | 3.36 | 3.17 | 3.03 | 2.66 | 2.21 |
| 25 | 7.77 | 5.57 | 4.68 | 4.18 | 3.86 | 3.63 | 3.46 | 3.32 | 3.13 | 2.99 | 2.62 | 2.17 |
| 26 | 7.72 | 5.53 | 4.64 | 4.14 | 3.82 | 3.59 | 3.42 | 3.29 | 3.09 | 2.96 | 2.58 | 2.13 |
| 27 | 7.68 | 5.49 | 4.60 | 4.11 | 3.78 | 3.56 | 3.39 | 3.26 | 3.06 | 2.93 | 2.55 | 2.10 |
| 28 | 7.64 | 5.45 | 4.57 | 4.07 | 3.75 | 3.53 | 3.36 | 3.23 | 3.03 | 2.90 | 2.52 | 2.06 |
| 29 | 7.60 | 5.42 | 4.54 | 4.04 | 3.73 | 3.50 | 3.33 | 3.20 | 3.00 | 2.87 | 2.49 | 2.03 |
| 30 | 7.56 | 5.39 | 4.51 | 4.02 | 3.70 | 3.47 | 3.30 | 3.17 | 2.98 | 2.84 | 2.47 | 2.01 |
| 32 | 7.50 | 5.34 | 4.46 | 3.97 | 3.65 | 3.43 | 3.26 | 3.13 | 2.93 | 2.80 | 2.42 | 1.96 |
| 34 | 7.45 | 5.29 | 4.42 | 3.93 | 3.61 | 3.39 | 3.22 | 3.09 | 2.90 | 2.76 | 2.38 | 1.91 |
| 36 | 7.40 | 5.25 | 4.38 | 3.89 | 3.58 | 3.35 | 3.18 | 3.05 | 2.86 | 2.72 | 2.35 | 1.87 |
| 38 | 7.35 | 5.21 | 4.34 | 3.86 | 3.54 | 3.32 | 3.15 | 3.02 | 2.83 | 2.69 | 2.32 | 1.84 |
| 40 | 7.31 | 5.18 | 4.31 | 3.83 | 3.51 | 3.29 | 3.12 | 2.99 | 2.80 | 2.66 | 2.29 | 1.80 |
| 60 | 7.08 | 4.98 | 4.13 | 3.65 | 3.34 | 3.12 | 2.95 | 2.82 | 2.63 | 2.50 | 2.12 | 1.60 |
| 120 | 6.85 | 4.79 | 3.95 | 3.48 | 3.17 | 2.96 | 2.79 | 2.66 | 2.47 | 2.34 | 1.95 | 1.38 |
| ∞ | 6.63 | 4.61 | 3.78 | 3.32 | 3.02 | 2.80 | 2.64 | 2.51 | 2.32 | 2.18 | 1.79 | 1.00 |

*NB* When there is no exact number for the df, use the next lowest number. For very large dfs (i.e. well over 120) you should use the row for infinity, marked ∞.

These values are all for a two-tailed test only.

**Table A2.6** (contd) Critical values of $F$ (anovas) at various level of probability. (For your $F$ value to be significant at a particular probability level, it should be *equal to* or *larger than* the critical values associated with $v_1$ and $v_2$ in your study.)
**d. Critical values of $F$ at $p < .001$**

| $v_2$ | $v_1$ 1 | 2 | 3 | 4 | 5 | 6 | 7 | 8 | 10 | 12 | 24 | $\infty$ |
|---|---|---|---|---|---|---|---|---|---|---|---|---|
| 1 | *4053 | 5000 | 5404 | 5625 | 5764 | 5859 | 5929 | 5981 | 6056 | 6107 | 6235 | 6366* |
| 2 | 998.5 | 999.0 | 999.2 | 999.2 | 999.3 | 999.3 | 999.4 | 999.4 | 999.4 | 999.4 | 999.5 | 999.5 |
| 3 | 167.0 | 148.5 | 141.1 | 137.1 | 134.6 | 132.8 | 131.5 | 130.6 | 129.2 | 128.3 | 125.9 | 123.5 |
| 4 | 74.14 | 61.25 | 56.18 | 53.44 | 51.71 | 50.53 | 49.66 | 49.00 | 48.05 | 47.41 | 45.77 | 44.05 |
| 5 | 47.18 | 37.12 | 33.20 | 31.09 | 29.75 | 28.83 | 28.16 | 27.65 | 26.92 | 26.42 | 25.14 | 23.79 |
| 6 | 35.51 | 27.00 | 23.70 | 21.92 | 20.80 | 20.03 | 19.46 | 19.03 | 18.41 | 17.99 | 16.90 | 15.75 |
| 7 | 29.25 | 21.69 | 18.77 | 17.20 | 16.21 | 15.52 | 15.02 | 14.63 | 14.08 | 13.71 | 12.73 | 11.70 |
| 8 | 25.42 | 18.49 | 15.83 | 14.39 | 13.48 | 12.86 | 12.40 | 12.05 | 11.54 | 11.19 | 10.30 | 9.34 |
| 9 | 22.86 | 16.39 | 13.90 | 12.56 | 11.71 | 11.13 | 10.69 | 10.37 | 9.87 | 9.57 | 8.72 | 7.81 |
| 10 | 21.04 | 14.91 | 12.55 | 11.28 | 10.48 | 9.93 | 9.52 | 9.20 | 8.74 | 8.44 | 7.64 | 6.76 |
| 11 | 19.69 | 13.81 | 11.56 | 10.35 | 9.58 | 9.05 | 8.66 | 8.35 | 7.92 | 7.63 | 6.85 | 6.00 |
| 12 | 18.64 | 12.97 | 10.80 | 9.63 | 8.89 | 8.38 | 8.00 | 7.71 | 7.29 | 7.00 | 6.25 | 5.42 |
| 13 | 17.82 | 12.31 | 10.21 | 9.07 | 8.35 | 7.86 | 7.49 | 7.21 | 6.80 | 6.52 | 5.78 | 4.97 |
| 14 | 17.14 | 11.78 | 9.73 | 8.62 | 7.92 | 7.44 | 7.08 | 6.80 | 6.40 | 6.13 | 5.41 | 4.60 |
| 15 | 16.59 | 11.34 | 9.34 | 8.25 | 7.57 | 7.09 | 6.74 | 6.47 | 6.08 | 5.81 | 5.10 | 4.31 |
| 16 | 16.12 | 10.97 | 9.01 | 7.94 | 7.27 | 6.80 | 6.46 | 6.19 | 5.81 | 5.55 | 4.85 | 4.06 |
| 17 | 15.72 | 10.66 | 8.73 | 7.68 | 7.02 | 6.56 | 6.22 | 5.96 | 5.58 | 5.32 | 4.63 | 3.85 |
| 18 | 15.38 | 10.39 | 8.49 | 7.46 | 6.81 | 6.35 | 6.02 | 5.76 | 5.39 | 5.13 | 4.45 | 3.67 |
| 19 | 15.08 | 10.16 | 8.28 | 7.27 | 6.62 | 6.18 | 5.85 | 5.59 | 5.22 | 4.97 | 4.29 | 3.51 |
| 20 | 14.82 | 9.95 | 8.10 | 7.10 | 6.46 | 6.02 | 5.69 | 5.44 | 5.08 | 4.82 | 4.15 | 3.38 |
| 21 | 14.59 | 9.77 | 7.94 | 6.95 | 6.32 | 5.88 | 5.56 | 5.31 | 4.95 | 4.70 | 4.03 | 3.26 |
| 22 | 14.38 | 9.61 | 7.80 | 6.81 | 6.19 | 5.76 | 5.44 | 5.19 | 4.83 | 4.58 | 3.92 | 3.15 |
| 23 | 14.19 | 9.47 | 7.67 | 6.70 | 6.08 | 5.65 | 5.33 | 5.09 | 4.73 | 4.48 | 3.82 | 3.05 |
| 24 | 14.03 | 9.34 | 7.55 | 6.59 | 5.98 | 5.55 | 5.23 | 4.99 | 4.64 | 4.39 | 3.74 | 2.97 |
| 25 | 13.88 | 9.22 | 7.45 | 6.49 | 5.89 | 5.46 | 5.15 | 4.91 | 4.56 | 4.31 | 3.66 | 2.89 |
| 26 | 13.74 | 9.12 | 7.36 | 6.41 | 5.80 | 5.38 | 5.07 | 4.83 | 4.48 | 4.24 | 3.59 | 2.82 |
| 27 | 13.61 | 9.02 | 7.27 | 6.33 | 5.73 | 5.31 | 5.00 | 4.76 | 4.41 | 4.17 | 3.52 | 2.75 |
| 28 | 13.50 | 8.93 | 7.19 | 6.25 | 5.66 | 5.24 | 4.93 | 4.69 | 4.35 | 4.11 | 3.46 | 2.69 |
| 29 | 13.39 | 8.85 | 7.12 | 6.19 | 5.59 | 5.18 | 4.87 | 4.64 | 4.29 | 4.05 | 3.41 | 2.64 |
| 30 | 13.29 | 8.77 | 7.05 | 6.12 | 5.53 | 5.12 | 4.82 | 4.58 | 4.24 | 4.00 | 3.36 | 2.59 |
| 32 | 13.12 | 8.64 | 6.94 | 6.01 | 5.43 | 5.02 | 4.72 | 4.48 | 4.14 | 3.91 | 3.27 | 2.50 |
| 34 | 12.97 | 8.52 | 6.83 | 5.92 | 5.34 | 4.93 | 4.63 | 4.40 | 4.06 | 3.83 | 3.19 | 2.42 |
| 36 | 12.83 | 8.42 | 6.74 | 5.84 | 5.26 | 4.86 | 4.56 | 4.33 | 3.99 | 3.76 | 3.12 | 2.35 |
| 38 | 12.71 | 8.33 | 6.66 | 5.76 | 5.19 | 4.79 | 4.49 | 4.26 | 3.93 | 3.70 | 3.06 | 2.29 |
| 40 | 12.61 | 8.25 | 6.59 | 5.70 | 5.13 | 4.73 | 4.44 | 4.21 | 3.87 | 3.64 | 3.01 | 2.23 |
| 60 | 11.97 | 7.77 | 6.17 | 5.31 | 4.76 | 4.37 | 4.09 | 3.86 | 3.54 | 3.32 | 2.69 | 1.89 |
| 120 | 11.38 | 7.32 | 5.78 | 4.95 | 4.42 | 4.04 | 3.77 | 3.55 | 3.24 | 3.02 | 2.40 | 1.54 |
| $\infty$ | 10.83 | 6.91 | 5.42 | 4.62 | 4.10 | 3.74 | 3.47 | 3.27 | 2.96 | 2.74 | 2.13 | 1.00 |

*Critical values to the right of $V_2 = 1$ should all be multiplied by 100, i.e. 4053 should be 40 5300.

*NB* When there is no exact number for the df, use the next lowest number. For very large dfs (i.e. well over 120) you should use the row for infinity, marked $\infty$.

These values are all for a two-tailed test only.

**Table A2.7** Critical values of $U$ (Mann–Whitney $U$ test) at various levels of probability. For your $U$ value to be significant at a particular probability level, it should be *equal to* or *less than* the critical value associated with $n_1$ and $n_2$ in your study. (Reproduced from Runyon R, Haber A (1991) Fundamentals of Behavioral Statistics 7th edn. with permission of McGraw-Hill Inc.)

**a. Critical values of $U$ for a one-tailed test at .005; two-tailed test at .01***

| $n_2$ \ $n_1$ | 1 | 2 | 3 | 4 | 5 | 6 | 7 | 8 | 9 | 10 | 11 | 12 | 13 | 14 | 15 | 16 | 17 | 18 | 19 | 20 |
|---|---|---|---|---|---|---|---|---|---|---|---|---|---|---|---|---|---|---|---|---|
| 1 | - | - | - | - | - | - | - | - | - | - | - | - | - | - | - | - | - | - | - | - |
| 2 | - | - | - | - | - | - | - | - | - | - | - | - | - | - | - | - | - | - | 0 | 0 |
| 3 | - | - | - | - | - | - | - | 0 | 0 | 0 | 1 | 1 | 1 | 2 | 2 | 2 | 2 | 3 | 3 | 3 |
| 4 | - | - | - | - | - | 0 | 0 | 1 | 1 | 2 | 2 | 3 | 3 | 4 | 5 | 5 | 6 | 6 | 7 | 8 |
| 5 | - | - | - | - | 0 | 1 | 1 | 2 | 3 | 4 | 5 | 6 | 7 | 7 | 8 | 9 | 10 | 11 | 12 | 13 |
| 6 | - | - | - | 0 | 1 | 2 | 3 | 4 | 5 | 6 | 7 | 9 | 10 | 11 | 12 | 13 | 15 | 16 | 17 | 18 |
| 7 | - | - | - | 0 | 1 | 3 | 4 | 6 | 7 | 9 | 10 | 12 | 13 | 15 | 16 | 18 | 19 | 21 | 22 | 24 |
| 8 | - | - | - | 1 | 2 | 4 | 6 | 7 | 9 | 11 | 13 | 15 | 17 | 18 | 20 | 22 | 24 | 26 | 28 | 30 |
| 9 | - | - | 0 | 1 | 3 | 5 | 7 | 9 | 11 | 13 | 16 | 18 | 20 | 22 | 24 | 27 | 29 | 31 | 33 | 36 |
| 10 | - | - | 0 | 2 | 4 | 6 | 9 | 11 | 13 | 16 | 18 | 21 | 24 | 26 | 29 | 31 | 34 | 37 | 39 | 42 |
| 11 | - | - | 0 | 2 | 5 | 7 | 10 | 13 | 16 | 18 | 21 | 24 | 27 | 30 | 33 | 36 | 39 | 42 | 45 | 48 |
| 12 | - | - | 1 | 3 | 6 | 9 | 12 | 15 | 18 | 21 | 24 | 27 | 31 | 34 | 37 | 41 | 44 | 47 | 51 | 54 |
| 13 | - | - | 1 | 3 | 7 | 10 | 13 | 17 | 20 | 24 | 27 | 31 | 34 | 38 | 42 | 45 | 49 | 53 | 56 | 60 |
| 14 | - | - | 1 | 4 | 7 | 11 | 15 | 18 | 22 | 26 | 30 | 34 | 38 | 42 | 46 | 50 | 54 | 58 | 63 | 67 |
| 15 | - | - | 2 | 5 | 8 | 12 | 16 | 20 | 24 | 29 | 33 | 37 | 42 | 46 | 51 | 55 | 60 | 64 | 69 | 73 |
| 16 | - | - | 2 | 5 | 9 | 13 | 18 | 22 | 27 | 31 | 36 | 41 | 45 | 50 | 55 | 60 | 65 | 70 | 74 | 79 |
| 17 | - | - | 2 | 6 | 10 | 15 | 19 | 24 | 29 | 34 | 39 | 44 | 49 | 54 | 60 | 65 | 70 | 75 | 81 | 86 |
| 18 | - | - | 2 | 6 | 11 | 16 | 21 | 26 | 31 | 37 | 42 | 47 | 53 | 58 | 64 | 70 | 75 | 81 | 87 | 92 |
| 19 | - | 0 | 3 | 7 | 12 | 17 | 22 | 28 | 33 | 39 | 45 | 51 | 56 | 63 | 69 | 74 | 81 | 87 | 93 | 99 |
| 20 | - | 0 | 3 | 8 | 13 | 18 | 24 | 30 | 36 | 42 | 48 | 54 | 60 | 67 | 73 | 79 | 86 | 92 | 99 | 105 |

*Dashes in the table mean that no decision is possible for those $n$ values at the given level of significance.

**b. Critical values of $U$ for a one-tailed test at .01; two-tailed test at .02***

| $n_2$ \ $n_1$ | 1 | 2 | 3 | 4 | 5 | 6 | 7 | 8 | 9 | 10 | 11 | 12 | 13 | 14 | 15 | 16 | 17 | 18 | 19 | 20 |
|---|---|---|---|---|---|---|---|---|---|---|---|---|---|---|---|---|---|---|---|---|
| 1 | - | - | - | - | - | - | - | - | - | - | - | - | - | - | - | - | - | - | - | - |
| 2 | - | - | - | - | - | - | - | - | - | - | - | - | 0 | 0 | 0 | 0 | 0 | 0 | 1 | 1 |
| 3 | - | - | - | - | - | - | 0 | 0 | 1 | 1 | 1 | 2 | 2 | 2 | 3 | 3 | 4 | 4 | 4 | 5 |
| 4 | - | - | - | - | 0 | 1 | 1 | 2 | 3 | 3 | 4 | 5 | 5 | 6 | 7 | 7 | 8 | 9 | 9 | 10 |
| 5 | - | - | - | 0 | 1 | 2 | 3 | 4 | 5 | 6 | 7 | 8 | 9 | 10 | 11 | 12 | 13 | 14 | 15 | 16 |
| 6 | - | - | - | 1 | 2 | 3 | 4 | 6 | 7 | 8 | 9 | 11 | 12 | 13 | 15 | 16 | 18 | 19 | 20 | 22 |
| 7 | - | - | 0 | 1 | 3 | 4 | 6 | 7 | 9 | 11 | 12 | 14 | 16 | 17 | 19 | 21 | 23 | 24 | 26 | 28 |
| 8 | - | - | 0 | 2 | 4 | 6 | 7 | 9 | 11 | 13 | 15 | 17 | 20 | 22 | 24 | 26 | 28 | 30 | 32 | 34 |
| 9 | - | - | 1 | 3 | 5 | 7 | 9 | 11 | 14 | 16 | 18 | 21 | 23 | 26 | 28 | 31 | 33 | 36 | 38 | 40 |
| 10 | - | - | 1 | 3 | 6 | 8 | 11 | 13 | 16 | 19 | 22 | 24 | 27 | 30 | 33 | 36 | 38 | 41 | 44 | 47 |
| 11 | - | - | 1 | 4 | 7 | 9 | 12 | 15 | 18 | 22 | 25 | 28 | 31 | 34 | 37 | 41 | 44 | 47 | 50 | 53 |
| 12 | - | - | 2 | 5 | 8 | 11 | 14 | 17 | 21 | 24 | 28 | 31 | 35 | 38 | 42 | 46 | 49 | 53 | 56 | 60 |
| 13 | - | 0 | 2 | 5 | 9 | 12 | 16 | 20 | 23 | 27 | 31 | 35 | 39 | 43 | 47 | 51 | 55 | 59 | 63 | 67 |
| 14 | - | 0 | 2 | 6 | 10 | 13 | 17 | 22 | 26 | 30 | 34 | 38 | 43 | 47 | 51 | 56 | 60 | 65 | 69 | 73 |
| 15 | - | 0 | 3 | 7 | 11 | 15 | 19 | 24 | 28 | 33 | 37 | 42 | 47 | 51 | 56 | 61 | 66 | 70 | 75 | 80 |
| 16 | - | 0 | 3 | 7 | 12 | 16 | 21 | 26 | 31 | 36 | 41 | 46 | 51 | 56 | 61 | 66 | 71 | 76 | 82 | 87 |
| 17 | - | 0 | 4 | 8 | 13 | 18 | 23 | 28 | 33 | 38 | 44 | 49 | 55 | 60 | 66 | 71 | 77 | 82 | 88 | 93 |
| 18 | - | 0 | 4 | 9 | 14 | 19 | 24 | 30 | 36 | 41 | 47 | 53 | 59 | 65 | 70 | 76 | 82 | 88 | 94 | 100 |
| 19 | - | 1 | 4 | 9 | 15 | 20 | 26 | 32 | 38 | 44 | 50 | 56 | 63 | 69 | 75 | 82 | 88 | 94 | 101 | 107 |
| 20 | - | 1 | 5 | 10 | 16 | 22 | 28 | 34 | 40 | 47 | 53 | 60 | 67 | 73 | 80 | 87 | 93 | 100 | 107 | 114 |

*Dashes in the table mean that no decision is possible for those $n$ values at the given level of significance.

**Table A2.7** Critical values of $U$ (Mann-Whitney $U$ test) at various levels of probability. (For your $U$ value to be significant at a particular probability level, it should be *equal to* or *less than* the critical value associated with $n_1$ and $n_2$ in your study.)

**c. Critical values of $U$ for a one-tailed test at .025; two-tailed test at .05***

| | $n_1$ | | | | | | | | | | | | | | | | | | | |
|---|---|---|---|---|---|---|---|---|---|---|---|---|---|---|---|---|---|---|---|---|
| $n_2$ | 1 | 2 | 3 | 4 | 5 | 6 | 7 | 8 | 9 | 10 | 11 | 12 | 13 | 14 | 15 | 16 | 17 | 18 | 19 | 20 |
| 1 | - | - | - | - | - | - | - | - | - | - | - | - | - | - | - | - | - | - | - | - |
| 2 | - | - | - | - | - | - | - | 0 | 0 | 0 | 0 | 1 | 1 | 1 | 1 | 1 | 2 | 2 | 2 | 2 |
| 3 | - | - | - | - | 0 | 1 | 1 | 2 | 2 | 3 | 3 | 4 | 4 | 5 | 5 | 6 | 6 | 7 | 7 | 8 |
| 4 | - | - | - | 0 | 1 | 2 | 3 | 4 | 4 | 5 | 6 | 7 | 8 | 9 | 10 | 11 | 11 | 12 | 13 | 13 |
| 5 | - | - | 0 | 1 | 2 | 3 | 5 | 6 | 7 | 8 | 9 | 11 | 12 | 13 | 14 | 15 | 17 | 18 | 19 | 20 |
| 6 | - | - | 1 | 2 | 3 | 5 | 6 | 8 | 10 | 11 | 13 | 14 | 16 | 17 | 19 | 21 | 22 | 24 | 25 | 27 |
| 7 | - | - | 1 | 3 | 5 | 6 | 8 | 10 | 12 | 14 | 16 | 18 | 20 | 22 | 24 | 26 | 28 | 30 | 32 | 34 |
| 8 | - | 0 | 2 | 4 | 6 | 8 | 10 | 13 | 15 | 17 | 19 | 22 | 24 | 26 | 29 | 31 | 34 | 36 | 38 | 41 |
| 9 | - | 0 | 2 | 4 | 7 | 10 | 12 | 15 | 17 | 20 | 23 | 26 | 28 | 31 | 34 | 37 | 39 | 42 | 45 | 48 |
| 10 | - | 0 | 3 | 5 | 8 | 11 | 14 | 17 | 20 | 23 | 26 | 29 | 33 | 36 | 39 | 42 | 45 | 48 | 52 | 55 |
| 11 | - | 0 | 3 | 6 | 9 | 13 | 16 | 19 | 23 | 26 | 30 | 33 | 37 | 40 | 44 | 47 | 51 | 55 | 58 | 62 |
| 12 | - | 1 | 4 | 7 | 11 | 14 | 18 | 22 | 26 | 29 | 33 | 37 | 41 | 45 | 49 | 53 | 57 | 61 | 65 | 69 |
| 13 | - | 1 | 4 | 8 | 12 | 16 | 20 | 24 | 28 | 33 | 37 | 41 | 45 | 50 | 54 | 59 | 63 | 67 | 72 | 76 |
| 14 | - | 1 | 5 | 9 | 13 | 17 | 22 | 26 | 31 | 36 | 40 | 45 | 50 | 55 | 59 | 64 | 67 | 74 | 78 | 83 |
| 15 | - | 1 | 5 | 10 | 14 | 19 | 24 | 29 | 34 | 39 | 44 | 49 | 54 | 59 | 64 | 70 | 75 | 80 | 85 | 90 |
| 16 | - | 1 | 6 | 11 | 15 | 21 | 26 | 31 | 37 | 42 | 47 | 53 | 59 | 64 | 70 | 75 | 81 | 86 | 92 | 98 |
| 17 | - | 2 | 6 | 11 | 17 | 22 | 28 | 34 | 39 | 45 | 51 | 57 | 63 | 67 | 75 | 81 | 87 | 93 | 99 | 105 |
| 18 | - | 2 | 7 | 12 | 18 | 24 | 30 | 36 | 42 | 48 | 55 | 61 | 67 | 74 | 80 | 86 | 93 | 99 | 106 | 112 |
| 19 | - | 2 | 7 | 13 | 19 | 25 | 32 | 38 | 45 | 52 | 58 | 65 | 72 | 78 | 85 | 92 | 99 | 106 | 113 | 119 |
| 20 | - | 2 | 8 | 13 | 20 | 27 | 34 | 41 | 48 | 55 | 62 | 69 | 76 | 83 | 90 | 98 | 105 | 112 | 119 | 127 |

*Dashes in the table mean that no decision is possible for those $n$ values at the given level of significance.

**d. Critical values of $U$ for a one-tailed test at .05; two-tailed test at .10***

| | $n_1$ | | | | | | | | | | | | | | | | | | | |
|---|---|---|---|---|---|---|---|---|---|---|---|---|---|---|---|---|---|---|---|---|
| $n_2$ | 1 | 2 | 3 | 4 | 5 | 6 | 7 | 8 | 9 | 10 | 11 | 12 | 13 | 14 | 15 | 16 | 17 | 18 | 19 | 20 |
| 1 | - | - | - | - | - | - | - | - | - | - | - | - | - | - | - | - | - | - | 0 | 0 |
| 2 | - | - | - | - | 0 | 0 | 0 | 1 | 1 | 1 | 1 | 2 | 2 | 2 | 3 | 3 | 3 | 4 | 4 | 4 |
| 3 | - | - | 0 | 0 | 1 | 2 | 2 | 3 | 3 | 4 | 5 | 5 | 6 | 7 | 7 | 8 | 9 | 9 | 10 | 11 |
| 4 | - | - | 0 | 1 | 2 | 3 | 4 | 5 | 6 | 7 | 8 | 9 | 10 | 11 | 12 | 14 | 15 | 16 | 17 | 18 |
| 5 | - | 0 | 1 | 2 | 4 | 5 | 6 | 8 | 9 | 11 | 12 | 13 | 15 | 16 | 18 | 19 | 20 | 22 | 23 | 25 |
| 6 | - | 0 | 2 | 3 | 5 | 7 | 8 | 10 | 12 | 14 | 16 | 17 | 19 | 21 | 23 | 25 | 26 | 28 | 30 | 32 |
| 7 | - | 0 | 2 | 4 | 6 | 8 | 11 | 13 | 15 | 17 | 19 | 21 | 24 | 26 | 28 | 30 | 33 | 35 | 37 | 39 |
| 8 | - | 1 | 3 | 5 | 8 | 10 | 13 | 15 | 18 | 20 | 23 | 26 | 28 | 31 | 33 | 36 | 39 | 41 | 44 | 47 |
| 9 | - | 1 | 3 | 6 | 9 | 12 | 15 | 18 | 21 | 24 | 27 | 30 | 33 | 36 | 39 | 42 | 45 | 48 | 51 | 54 |
| 10 | - | 1 | 4 | 7 | 11 | 14 | 17 | 20 | 24 | 27 | 31 | 34 | 37 | 41 | 44 | 48 | 51 | 55 | 58 | 62 |
| 11 | - | 1 | 5 | 8 | 12 | 16 | 19 | 23 | 27 | 31 | 34 | 38 | 42 | 46 | 50 | 54 | 57 | 61 | 65 | 69 |
| 12 | - | 2 | 5 | 9 | 13 | 17 | 21 | 26 | 30 | 34 | 38 | 42 | 47 | 51 | 55 | 60 | 64 | 68 | 72 | 77 |
| 13 | - | 2 | 6 | 10 | 15 | 19 | 24 | 28 | 33 | 37 | 42 | 47 | 51 | 56 | 61 | 65 | 70 | 75 | 80 | 84 |
| 14 | - | 2 | 7 | 11 | 16 | 21 | 26 | 31 | 36 | 41 | 46 | 51 | 56 | 61 | 66 | 71 | 77 | 82 | 87 | 92 |
| 15 | - | 3 | 7 | 12 | 18 | 23 | 28 | 33 | 39 | 44 | 50 | 55 | 61 | 66 | 72 | 77 | 83 | 88 | 94 | 100 |
| 16 | - | 3 | 8 | 14 | 19 | 25 | 30 | 36 | 42 | 48 | 54 | 60 | 65 | 71 | 77 | 83 | 89 | 95 | 101 | 107 |
| 17 | - | 3 | 9 | 15 | 20 | 26 | 33 | 39 | 45 | 51 | 57 | 64 | 70 | 77 | 83 | 89 | 96 | 102 | 109 | 115 |
| 18 | - | 4 | 9 | 16 | 22 | 28 | 35 | 41 | 48 | 55 | 61 | 68 | 75 | 82 | 88 | 95 | 102 | 109 | 116 | 123 |
| 19 | 0 | 4 | 10 | 17 | 23 | 30 | 37 | 44 | 51 | 58 | 65 | 72 | 80 | 87 | 94 | 101 | 109 | 116 | 123 | 130 |
| 20 | 0 | 4 | 11 | 18 | 25 | 32 | 39 | 47 | 54 | 62 | 69 | 77 | 84 | 92 | 100 | 107 | 115 | 123 | 130 | 138 |

*Dashes in the table mean that no desicison is possible for those $n$ values at the given level of significance.

**Table A2.8** Critical values of *H* (Kruskal-Wallis test) at various levels of probability. (For your *H* value to be significant at a particular probability level, it should be *equal to* or *larger than* the critical values associated with the *ns* in your study.)

| $n_1$ | $n_2$ | $n_3$ | H | p | $n_1$ | $n_2$ | $n_3$ | H | p |
|---|---|---|---|---|---|---|---|---|---|
| 2 | 1 | 1 | 2.7000 | .500 | 4 | 3 | 1 | 5.8333 | .021 |
| 2 | 2 | 1 | 3.6000 | .200 |   |   |   | 5.2083 | .050 |
| 2 | 2 | 2 | 4.5714 | .067 |   |   |   | 5.0000 | .057 |
|   |   |   | 3.7143 | .200 |   |   |   | 4.0556 | .093 |
| 3 | 1 | 1 | 3.2000 | .300 |   |   |   | 3.8889 | .129 |
| 3 | 2 | 1 | 4.2857 | .100 | 4 | 3 | 2 | 6.4444 | .008 |
|   |   |   | 3.8571 | .133 |   |   |   | 6.3000 | .011 |
| 3 | 2 | 2 | 5.3572 | .029 |   |   |   | 5.4444 | .046 |
|   |   |   | 4.7143 | .048 |   |   |   | 5.4000 | .051 |
|   |   |   | 4.5000 | .067 |   |   |   | 4.5111 | .098 |
|   |   |   | 4.4643 | .105 |   |   |   | 4.4444 | .102 |
| 3 | 3 | 1 | 5.1429 | .043 | 4 | 3 | 3 | 6.7455 | .010 |
|   |   |   | 4.5714 | .100 |   |   |   | 6.7091 | .013 |
|   |   |   | 4.0000 | .129 |   |   |   | 5.7909 | .046 |
| 3 | 3 | 2 | 6.2500 | .011 |   |   |   | 5.7273 | .050 |
|   |   |   | 5.3611 | .032 |   |   |   | 4.7091 | .092 |
|   |   |   | 5.1389 | .061 |   |   |   | 4.7000 | .101 |
|   |   |   | 4.5556 | .100 | 4 | 4 | 1 | 6.6667 | .010 |
|   |   |   | 4.2500 | .121 |   |   |   | 6.1667 | .022 |
| 3 | 3 | 3 | 7.2000 | .004 |   |   |   | 4.9667 | .048 |
|   |   |   | 6.4889 | .011 |   |   |   | 4.8667 | .054 |
|   |   |   | 5.6889 | .029 |   |   |   | 4.1667 | .082 |
|   |   |   | 5.6000 | .050 |   |   |   | 4.0667 | .102 |
|   |   |   | 5.0667 | .086 | 4 | 4 | 2 | 7.0364 | .006 |
|   |   |   | 4.6222 | .100 |   |   |   | 6.8727 | .011 |
| 4 | 1 | 1 | 3.5714 | .200 |   |   |   | 5.4545 | .046 |
| 4 | 2 | 1 | 4.8214 | .057 |   |   |   | 5.2364 | .052 |
|   |   |   | 4.5000 | .076 |   |   |   | 4.5545 | .098 |
|   |   |   | 4.0179 | .114 |   |   |   | 4.4455 | .103 |
| 4 | 2 | 2 | 6.0000 | .014 | 4 | 4 | 3 | 7.1439 | .010 |
|   |   |   | 5.3333 | .033 |   |   |   | 7.1364 | .011 |
|   |   |   | 5.1250 | .052 |   |   |   | 5.5985 | .049 |
|   |   |   | 4.4583 | .100 |   |   |   | 5.5758 | .051 |
|   |   |   | 4.1667 | .105 |   |   |   | 4.5455 | .099 |
|   |   |   |   |   |   |   |   | 4.4773 | .102 |
|   |   |   |   |   | 4 | 4 | 4 | 7.6538 | .008 |
|   |   |   |   |   |   |   |   | 7.5385 | .011 |
|   |   |   |   |   |   |   |   | 5.6923 | .049 |
|   |   |   |   |   |   |   |   | 5.6538 | .054 |
|   |   |   |   |   |   |   |   | 4.6539 | .097 |
|   |   |   |   |   |   |   |   | 4.5001 | .104 |

*NB* These values are all for a two-tailed test only.

**Table A2.8** (contd) Critical values of $H$ (Kruskal-Wallis test) at various levels of probability. (For your $H$ values to be significant at a particular probability level, it should be *equal to* or *larger than* the critical values associated with the $n$s in your study.)

| Size of groups | | | | | Size of groups | | | | |
|---|---|---|---|---|---|---|---|---|---|
| $n_1$ | $n_2$ | $n_3$ | $H$ | $p$ | $n_1$ | $n_2$ | $n_3$ | $H$ | $p$ |
| 5 | 1 | 1 | 3.8571 | .143 | 5 | 4 | 3 | 7.4449 | .010 |
| 5 | 2 | 1 | 5.2500 | .036 | | | | 7.3949 | .011 |
| | | | 5.0000 | .048 | | | | 5.6564 | .049 |
| | | | 4.4500 | .071 | | | | 5.6308 | .050 |
| | | | 4.2000 | .095 | | | | 4.5487 | .099 |
| | | | 4.0500 | .119 | | | | 4.5231 | .103 |
| 5 | 2 | 2 | 6.5333 | .008 | 5 | 4 | 4 | 7.7604 | .009 |
| | | | 6.1333 | .013 | | | | 7.7440 | .011 |
| | | | 5.1600 | .034 | | | | 5.6571 | .049 |
| | | | 5.0400 | .056 | | | | 5.6176 | .050 |
| | | | 4.3733 | .090 | | | | 4.6187 | .100 |
| | | | 4.2933 | .122 | | | | 4.5527 | .102 |
| 5 | 3 | 1 | 6.4000 | .012 | 5 | 5 | 1 | 7.3091 | .009 |
| | | | 4.9600 | .048 | | | | 6.8364 | .011 |
| | | | 4.8711 | .052 | | | | 5.1273 | .046 |
| | | | 4.0178 | .095 | | | | 4.9091 | .053 |
| | | | 3.8400 | .123 | | | | 4.1091 | .086 |
| 5 | 3 | 2 | 6.9091 | .009 | | | | 4.0364 | .105 |
| | | | 6.8218 | .010 | 5 | 5 | 2 | 7.3385 | .010 |
| | | | 5.2509 | .049 | | | | 7.2692 | .010 |
| | | | 5.1055 | .052 | | | | 5.3385 | .047 |
| | | | 4.6509 | .091 | | | | 5.2462 | .051 |
| | | | 4.4945 | .101 | | | | 4.6231 | .097 |
| 5 | 3 | 3 | 7.0788 | .009 | | | | 4.5077 | .100 |
| | | | 6.9818 | .011 | 5 | 5 | 3 | 7.5780 | .010 |
| | | | 5.6485 | .049 | | | | 7.5429 | .010 |
| | | | 5.5152 | .051 | | | | 5.7055 | .046 |
| | | | 4.5333 | .097 | | | | 5.6264 | .051 |
| | | | 4.4121 | .109 | | | | 4.5451 | .100 |
| 5 | 4 | 1 | 6.9545 | .008 | | | | 4.5363 | .102 |
| | | | 6.8400 | .011 | 5 | 5 | 4 | 7.8229 | .010 |
| | | | 4.9855 | .044 | | | | 7.7914 | .010 |
| | | | 4.8600 | .056 | | | | 5.6657 | .049 |
| | | | 3.9873 | .098 | | | | 5.6429 | .050 |
| | | | 3.9600 | .102 | | | | 4.5229 | .099 |
| 5 | 4 | 2 | 7.2045 | .009 | | | | 4.5200 | .101 |
| | | | 7.1182 | .010 | 5 | 5 | 5 | 8.0000 | .009 |
| | | | 5.2727 | .049 | | | | 7.9800 | .010 |
| | | | 5.2682 | .050 | | | | 7.7800 | .049 |
| | | | 4.5409 | .098 | | | | 5.6600 | .051 |
| | | | 4.5182 | .101 | | | | 4.5600 | .100 |
| | | | | | | | | 4.5000 | .102 |

*NB* These values are all for a two-tailed test only.

**Table A2.9** Critical values of $S$ (Jonckheere trend test) at various levels of probability.
(For your $S$ value to be significant at a particular probability level, it should be *equal to* or *larger than* the critical values associated with $C$ and $n$ in your study.)

**a. Significance level $p < .05$**

| | | | | | $n$ | | | | |
|---|---|---|---|---|---|---|---|---|---|
| $C$ | 2 | 3 | 4 | 5 | 6 | 7 | 8 | 9 | 10 |
| 3 | 10 | 17 | 24 | 33 | 42 | 53 | 64 | 76 | 88 |
| 4 | 14 | 26 | 38 | 51 | 66 | 82 | 100 | 118 | 138 |
| 5 | 20 | 34 | 51 | 71 | 92 | 115 | 140 | 166 | 194 |
| 6 | 26 | 44 | 67 | 93 | 121 | 151 | 184 | 219 | 256 |

**b. Significance level $p < .01$**

| | | | | | | | | | |
|---|---|---|---|---|---|---|---|---|---|
| 3 | - | 23 | 32 | 45 | 59 | 74 | 90 | 106 | 124 |
| 4 | 20 | 34 | 50 | 71 | 92 | 115 | 140 | 167 | 195 |
| 5 | 26 | 48 | 72 | 99 | 129 | 162 | 197 | 234 | 274 |
| 6 | 34 | 62 | 94 | 130 | 170 | 213 | 260 | 309 | 361 |

*NB*   These values are all for a one-tailed test only.

**Table A2.10** Critical values of $r_s$ (Spearman test) at various levels of probability.
(For your $r_s$ value to be significant at a particular probability level, it should be *equal to* or *larger than* the critical values associated with $N$ in your study.)

| $N$ (number of subjects) | Level of significance for one-tailed test | | | |
|---|---|---|---|---|
| | .05 | .025 | .01 | .005 |
| | Level of significance for two-tailed test | | | |
| | .10 | .05 | .02 | .01 |
| 5 | .900 | 1.000 | 1.000 | - |
| 6 | .829 | .886 | .943 | 1.000 |
| 7 | .714 | .786 | .893 | .929 |
| 8 | .643 | .738 | .833 | .881 |
| 9 | .600 | .683 | .783 | .833 |
| 10 | .564 | .648 | .746 | .794 |
| 12 | .506 | .591 | .712 | .777 |
| 14 | .456 | .544 | .645 | .715 |
| 16 | .425 | .506 | .601 | .665 |
| 18 | .399 | .475 | .564 | .625 |
| 20 | .377 | .450 | .534 | .591 |
| 22 | .359 | .428 | .508 | .562 |
| 24 | .343 | .409 | .485 | .537 |
| 26 | .329 | .392 | .465 | .515 |
| 28 | .317 | .377 | .448 | .496 |
| 30 | .306 | .364 | .432 | .478 |

*NB*   When there is no exact number of subjects use the next lowest number.

**Table A2.11** Critical values of *r* (Pearson test) at various levels of probability. (For your *r* value to be significant at a particular probability level, it should be *equal to* or *larger* than the critical values associated with the *df* in your study. (Reproduced with kind permission of Longman Group Limited.)

| df = N − 2 | Level of significance for one-tailed test | | | | |
|---|---|---|---|---|---|
| | .05 | .025 | .01 | .005 | .0005 |
| | Level of significance for two-tailed test | | | | |
| | .01 | .05 | .02 | .01 | .001 |
| 1 | .9877 | .9969 | .9995 | .9999 | 1.0000 |
| 2 | .9000 | .9500 | .9800 | .9900 | .9990 |
| 3 | .8054 | .8783 | .9343 | .9587 | .9912 |
| 4 | .7293 | .8114 | .8822 | .9172 | .9741 |
| 5 | .6694 | .7545 | .8329 | .8745 | .9507 |
| 6 | .6215 | .7067 | .7887 | .8343 | .9249 |
| 7 | .5822 | .6664 | .7498 | .7977 | .8982 |
| 8 | .5494 | .6319 | .7155 | .7646 | .8721 |
| 9 | .5214 | .6021 | .6851 | .7348 | .8471 |
| 10 | .4973 | .5760 | .6581 | .7079 | .8233 |
| 11 | .4762 | .5529 | .6339 | .6835 | .8010 |
| 12 | .4575 | .5324 | .6120 | .6614 | .7800 |
| 13 | .4409 | .5139 | .5923 | .6411 | .7603 |
| 14 | .4259 | .4973 | .5742 | .6226 | .7420 |
| 15 | .4124 | .4821 | .5577 | .6055 | .7246 |
| 16 | .4000 | .4683 | .5425 | .5897 | .7084 |
| 17 | .3887 | .4555 | .5285 | .5751 | .6932 |
| 18 | .3783 | .4438 | .5155 | .5614 | .6787 |
| 19 | .3687 | .4329 | .5034 | .5487 | .6652 |
| 20 | .3598 | .4227 | .4921 | .5368 | .6524 |
| 25 | .3233 | .3809 | .4451 | .4869 | .5974 |
| 30 | .2960 | .3494 | .4093 | .4487 | .5541 |
| 35 | .2746 | .3246 | .3810 | .4182 | .5189 |
| 40 | .2573 | .3044 | .3578 | .3932 | .4896 |
| 45 | .2428 | .2875 | .3384 | .3721 | .4648 |
| 50 | .2306 | .2732 | .3218 | .3541 | .4433 |
| 60 | .2108 | .2500 | .2948 | .3248 | .4078 |
| 70 | .1954 | .2319 | .2737 | .3017 | .3799 |
| 80 | .1829 | .2172 | .2565 | .2830 | .3568 |
| 90 | .1726 | .2050 | .2422 | .2673 | .3375 |
| 100 | .1638 | .1946 | .2301 | .2540 | .3211 |

*NB* When there is no exact df use the next lowest number.

**Table A2.12** Critical values of $s$ (Kendall's coefficient of concordance) at various levels of probability. (For your $s$ value to be significant at a particular probability level, it should be *equal to* or *larger than* the critical values associated with $C$ and $N$ in your study.)

**a. Critical values of $s$ at $p = 0.05$**

| $C$ | $N = 3$ | $N = 4$ | $N = 5$ | $N = 6$ | $N = 7$ |
|---|---|---|---|---|---|
| 3 | - | - | 64.4 | 103.9 | 157.3 |
| 4 | - | 49.5 | 88.4 | 143.3 | 217.0 |
| 5 | - | 62.6 | 112.3 | 182.4 | 276.2 |
| 6 | - | 75.7 | 136.1 | 221.4 | 335.2 |
| 8 | 48.1 | 101.7 | 183.7 | 299.0 | 453.1 |
| 10 | 60.0 | 127.8 | 231.2 | 376.7 | 571.0 |
| 15 | 89.8 | 192.9 | 349.8 | 570.5 | 864.9 |
| 20 | 119.7 | 258.0 | 468.5 | 764.4 | 1158.7 |

**b. Critical values of $s$ at $p = 0.01$**

| $C$ | $N = 3$ | $N = 4$ | $N = 5$ | $N = 6$ | $N = 7$ |
|---|---|---|---|---|---|
| 3 | - | - | 75.6 | 122.8 | 185.6 |
| 4 | - | 61.4 | 109.3 | 176.2 | 265.0 |
| 5 | - | 80.5 | 142.8 | 229.4 | 343.8 |
| 6 | - | 99.5 | 176.1 | 282.4 | 422.6 |
| 8 | 66.8 | 137.4 | 242.7 | 388.3 | 579.9 |
| 10 | 85.1 | 175.3 | 309.1 | 494.0 | 737.0 |
| 15 | 131.0 | 269.8 | 475.2 | 758.2 | 1129.5 |
| 20 | 177.0 | 364.2 | 641.2 | 1022.2 | 1521.9 |

*NB*  The values are all for a one-tailed test only.

A dash in the table means that no decision can be made at this level.

# Appendix 3

# Answers to Activities

---

## Chapter 1

### Activity 1.1

1. 46
2. – 2
3. 43
4. 253
5. 65
6. 49
7. 54
8. 11
9. 104
10. 47
11. – 6
12. – 8
13. – 48
14. – 44
15. 42
16. – 48
17. 45
18. – 13
19. 7
20. – 240

## Chapter 4

### Activity 4.1

The following are examples of nominal levels of measurement. Any variation on these which still involved allocating patients to a category is acceptable.

1. You might measure improvement in incontinence by asking the patient 'Did you experience any improvement following therapy?'
   Yes/No
2. This might be measured by categorising the patients as (a) either having had a chest infection or (b) *not* having had a chest infection.
3. You assess whether or not a patient experienced an increased range of movement following manipulation by allocating him/her to either an 'Increase in movement' category or 'No increase in movement' category.
4. Patients could be classified as those who kept appointments and those who did not.
5. This might be assessed by asking patients to answer the following question: Did you find the treatment in the physiotherapy department to be:

acceptable ☐   not acceptable ☐

### Activity 4.2

Again, any variation on the answers suggested below is acceptable, as long as you are rank ordering your data according to the dimension you're interested in.

1. Improvement in incontinence might be measured by asking the patients to answer the following question:
   To what extent did your incontinence improvement following therapy?

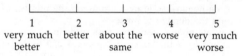

   |   |   |   |   |   |
   |---|---|---|---|---|
   | 1 | 2 | 3 | 4 | 5 |
   | very much better | better | about the same | worse | very much worse |

   Alternatively, you could rank order your subjects according to how much they improved.

2. This might be measured by assessing the patients along a scale of incidence of chest infection thus:
   The incidence of chest infection following breathing exercises was

   | 1 | 2 | 3 | 4 | 5 | 6 | 7 |
   |---|---|---|---|---|---|---|
   | very much reduced | much reduced | marginally reduced | the same | marginally increased | much increased | very much increased |

   Similarly you could rank order the patients according to their incidence of chest infections.

3. Range of movement could be assessed by either rank ordering the subjects from the greatest increase in movement to the smallest increase, or alternatively you could use a point scale thus:
   The increase in range of movement in the leg following manipulation was

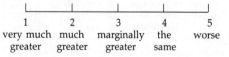

   |   |   |   |   |   |
   |---|---|---|---|---|
   | 1 | 2 | 3 | 4 | 5 |
   | very much greater | much greater | marginally greater | the same | worse |

4. Likelihood of keeping appointments could be assessed by a point scale thus:
   How likely is this patient to keep an appointment at the outpatients' clinic?

227

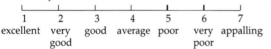

| 1 | 2 | 3 | 4 | 5 |
|---|---|---|---|---|
| very likely | quite likely | not sure | quite unlikely | very unlikely |

5. Assessing the quality of physiotherapy could be conducted along similar lines:

How would you rate the quality of the physiotherapy treatment you received?

| 1 | 2 | 3 | 4 | 5 | 6 | 7 |
|---|---|---|---|---|---|---|
| excellent | very good | good | average | poor | very poor | appalling |

## Activity 4.3

1. You could measure incontinence on an interval/ratio scale simply by monitoring the number of times a patient was incontinent or the number of ccs of urine voided accidentally.
2. Incidence of chest infection could be assessed by noting the number of times each patient suffered a chest problem following breathing exercises.
3. Range of movement could be measured in degrees.
4. The number or percentage of appointments kept and missed could be monitored for each patient.
5. You could ask the patients to rate the quality of physiotherapy by giving it marks out of 20 or 100.
6. (i) Accuracy of shooting an arrow at a target could be measured
   — on a nominal scale by counting up the number of hits and the number of misses.
   — on an ordinal scale by rank ordering each arrow's proximity to the target, giving a rank of 1 to the nearest etc.
   — on an interval/ratio scale by measuring the distance of each arrow from the target, in centimetres or inches.
   (ii) Improvement in mobility after a hip replacement operation could be measured:
   — on a nominal scale by classifying the patients according to whether they:
   a. experienced an improvement in mobility or
   b. experienced no improvement in mobility
   — on an ordinal scale using a point scale thus:
   What degree of improvement in mobility did this patient experience?

| 1 | 2 | 3 | 4 | 5 |
|---|---|---|---|---|
| great improve-ment | some improve-ment | minimal improve-ment | no improve-ment | deteriorated |

   — on an interval/ratio scale by measuring the distance walked.
   (iii) Relief of neck and arm pain following the use of a surgical collar could be measured:
   — on a nominal scale by classifying patients according to whether they experienced pain relief, or did not experience pain relief.
   — on an ordinal scale by using a point scale thus:
   How much pain relief did you experience after wearing a surgical collar?

| 1 | 2 | 3 | 4 | 5 |
|---|---|---|---|---|
| very great relief | great relief | some relief | no relief | deterioration |

   — on an interval/ratio scale by asking the patient the percentage of pain relief felt, e.g. was the pain about 50%/30%/25% less than it was prior to using the surgical collar?

7. (i) Nominal
   (ii) Ordinal (or interval if equal distances between points are assumed)
   (iii) Interval/ratio
   (iv) Interval/ratio
   (v) Interval/ratio

## Chapter 5

## Activity 5.1

1. (a) Histogram (Fig. A3.1).

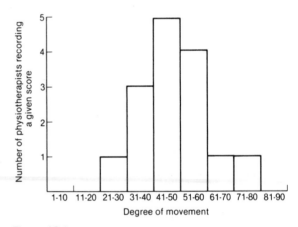

**Figure A3.1**

(b) Frequency polygon (Fig. A3.2)

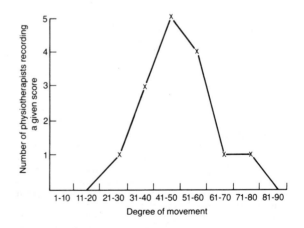

**Figure A3.2**

2. Frequency polygon with reduced number of units along horizontal axis (Fig. A3.3).

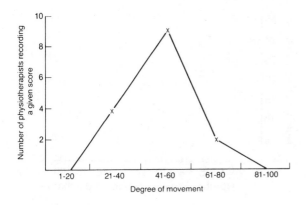

**Figure A3.3**

## Activity 5.2

1. (i) Mean : 70.333
    Median : 76
    Mode : 76
   (ii) Mean : 28.667
    Median : 27
    Mode : 17
   (iii) Mean : 50.1
    Median : 47.5
    Mode : 43

2. Set of data (i) has the largest range of scores while (ii) has the smallest.

## Activity 5.3

1. (i) Range : 24
    Deviation : 14 − 19.444 = − 5.444
         9 − 19.444 = − 10.444
         21 − 19.444 = + 1.556
         23 − 19.444 = + 3.556
         18 − 19.444 = − 1.444
         17 − 19.444 = − 2.444
         33 − 19.444 = + 13.556
         28 − 19.444 = + 8.556
         12 − 19.444 = − 7.444
    Variance : 474.221
    Standard deviation : 7.259
   (ii) Range : 33
    Deviation : 71 − 67.571 = + 3.429
         50 − 67.571 = − 17.571
         48 − 67.571 = − 19.571
         64 − 67.571 = − 3.571
         80 − 67.571 = + 12.429
         81 − 67.571 = + 13.429
         79 − 67.571 = + 11.429
    Variance : 1181.714
    Standard deviation : 12.993

2. You might assess the reliability of the goniometer by taking several readings (e.g. 10) of the same joint on, say five different occasions. For each set of 10 readings you might calculate the mean and the median to assess the homogeneity or similarity of the scores. You might also wish to calculate the range and the standard deviation to find out how disparate the readings are.

## Activity 5.4

1. 95% of patients will have heart rates of between 66 and 98 during weeks 10–20 of pregnancy.
2. 2.36% of patients will have heart rates of between 99 and 106.
3. This patient comes in 0.135% of the population in terms of heart rate.

## Chapter 6

## Activity 6.1

The two variables in each hypothesis are:

1. Age of patient (child or adolescent) and progress rate on traction
2. Sex (male or female) and responsiveness to heat treatment.
3. Sex (male or female) and incidence of chest infections.
4. Type of clinic (outpatients or sports injuries) and recovery rate for leg fractures.
5. Type of training establishment (hospital-based or university-based) and professional competence.

## Activity 6.2

The null hypotheses for these experimental hypotheses are:

1. There is no relationship between age of patient and progress rates on traction following leg fractures.
2. There is no relationship between the sex of arthritis patients and reponsiveness to heat treatment.
3. There is no relationship between sex of patient and incidence of chest infections following cardiothoracic surgery.
4. There is no relationship between the type of physiotherapy clinic and recovery rates for leg fractures.
5. There is no relationship between type of training establishment and professional competence in physiotherapists.

## Activity 6.3

1. IV = sex of patient.
   DV = tendency to complain about pain.
   IV manipulated by selecting one group of male patients and one group of female patients.
2. IV = type of walking aid.
   DV = mobility.
   IV manipulated by selecting a number of patients and deciding which walking aid each should receive.
3. IV = type of hospital.
   DV = absenteeism.
   IV manipulated by selecting one group of physiotherapists working in a psychiatric hospital and another group working in a general hospital.

4. IV = sex of patient.
   DV = degree of rapport.
   IV manipulated by selecting one group of male patients and one group of female patients.
5. IV = physiotherapy schools' entry requirements.
   DV = pass rate on CSP exam.
   IV manipulated by selecting a number of schools requiring 'A'-level physics and a number of schools not requiring 'A'-level physics.

## Activity 6.4

Other possible explanations for a more tolerant attitude amongst these physiotherapists might be:

1. Simply the fact that they were a bit older and therefore a bit wiser, and perhaps as a result a bit more tolerant.
2. Experiencing a period of illness themselves which made them more aware of the patient's perspective.
3. Reading a book on attitude change.
4. Attending another sort of course.

Plus, of course, many other possible reasons.

## Activity 6.5

Designs for hypotheses on page 55

1.

|  | Pre-test measure of DV | Condition | Post-test measure of DV |
|---|---|---|---|
| Experimental Group | Compliance | Information | Compliance |
| Control Group | Compliance | No Information | Compliance |

2.

|  | Pre-test measure of DV | Condition | Post-test measure of DV |
|---|---|---|---|
| Experimental Group | Sympathy | Experience as hospital patient | Sympathy |
| Control Group | Sympathy | No experience as hospital patient | Sympathy |

3.

|  | Condition | Measure of DV |
|---|---|---|
| Experimental Group 1 | < 5 years | Motivation |
| Experimental Group 2 | > 10 years | Motivation |

## Activity 6.6

See Fig. A3.4.

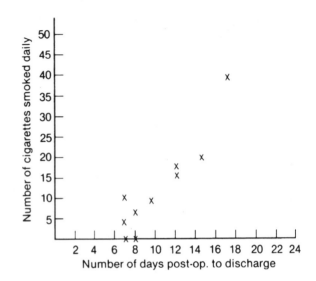

**Figure A3.4** Relationship between the number of cigarettes smoked daily and the number of days to discharge after cardiothoracic surgery.

## Activity 6.7

1. (i) A positive correlation is predicted, with high scores on age being associated with high scores on recovery time. This would be represented by a general upward slope on a scattergram and a correlation coefficient of around + 1.0.
   (ii) A negative correlation is predicted with high scores on distance being associated with low scores on attendance. This would be represented by a general downward slope on a scattergram and a correlation coefficient of around – 1.0.
   (iii) A positive correlation is predicted with low scores on 'A'-levels being associated with low final exam scores. An upward slope and a correlation coefficient of around + 1.0 would be anticipated.
   (iv) A negative correlation is predicted with high scores on fibre intake being associated with low scores on incidence of diverticulitis. A general downward slope and a correlation coefficient of around – 1.0 would be predicted.
2. From strongest to weakest, the coefficients are:
   – 0.73  + 0.61  – 0.42  + 0.21  – 0.17  + 0.09

## Chapter 8

### Activity 8.1

Some of the constant and random errors involved in these experiments are outlined in Tables A3.1 and A3.2. You may have thought of many more.

**Table A3.1** Hypothesis: Men are more likely to suffer respiratory complications following cardiothoracic surgery

| Constant error | Solution | Random error | Solution |
|---|---|---|---|
| 1. Age of patient | Ensure both groups are of comparable age | 1. Personality | |
| 2. Nature of illness | Ensure both groups are being treated for the same complaint | 2. Attitude | |
| 3. Previous health | Establish comparability of previous health in both groups | 3. Supportive family | Random selection of patients in each group |
| 4. Previous relevant illnesses | Ensure both groups have had similar number/ types of relevant illness | 4. Biochemical make-up | |
| 5. Smoker/ Non-smoker | Ensure that no S in either group smokes | 5. Inherent and undetected lung defects | |
| 6. Vital capacity | Ensure that both groups have comparable vital capacity | | |

**Table A3.2** Hypothesis: Outpatient clinics achieve better recovery rates for leg fractures than specific sports injuries clinics

| Constant error | Solution | Random error | Solution |
|---|---|---|---|
| 1. Age of patient | Ensure both groups of patients are of comparable age | 1. Motivation of patient and therapist | |
| 2. Nature of fracture | Ensure the type of fracture is the same in each case | 2. Personality of patient and therapist | Randomly select patients from each situation to take part in the experiment |
| 3. Fitness of patient | Ensure comparability of previous fitness in both groups | 3. Attitude of patient and therapist | |
| 4. Sex of patient | Ensure both groups comprise either all males, all females, or an equal number of each sex | 4. Biochemical make-up | |

**Table A3.2** *(cont'd)*

| Constant error | Solution | Random error | Solution |
|---|---|---|---|
| 5. Amount of time spent in treatment | Ensure that the amount of treatment is standardised in each case | 5. Inherent and undetected bone defects | |
| 6. Quality of treatment | Ensure that the type and quality of treatment is standardised in each case | | |

### Activity 8.2

From greatest support to least:
$p = 0.01\%$   $p = 3\%$   $p = 5\%$   $p = 7\%$   $p = 15\%$
$p = 19\%$
Converted to a decimal:
$p = 0.0001$   $p = 0.03$   $p = 0.05$   $p = 0.07$
$p = 0.15$   $p = 0.19$

### Activity 8.3

See Table A3.3.

| | % probability that the results are due to chance |
|---|---|
| $p = 0.01$ | 1% |
| $p = 0.07$ | 7% |
| $p = 0.03$ | 3% |
| $p = 0.05$ | 5% |
| $p = 0.50$ | 50% |

## Chapter 9

### Activity 9.1

1. Chi-squared test (data is nominal).
2. Wilcoxon or related $t$ test.
3. Spearman (data is ordinal for grade of physiotherapist).
4. Mann–Whitney $U$ test (data is ordinal).
5. Friedman or one-way anova for related samples.
6. Kruskal–Wallis (data is ordinal).

### Activity 9.2

1. one-tailed (*more* effective).
2. two-tailed (*differentially* effective).
3. one-tailed (*fewer* complaints).
4. two-tailed (*difference* in strength).
5. one-tailed (*diminishes* vital capacity).
**Converting the one-tailed hypotheses to two-tailed.**
1. There is a difference in the effectiveness of praise as a motivator when used in a group or a one-to-one situation.
2. There is a difference in the number of complaints made by patients who attend either for rigorous exercise regimes or heat treatment in back schools.
3. The application of lumbar traction alters vital capacity.
**Converting the two-tailed hypotheses to one-tailed.**

1. Paraffin wax is more (less) effective than hot soaks as a preparation for mobilising exercises in post-fracture patients.
2. Strength of muscle contraction in a selected muscle group is reduced (increased) more by 2 minutes infrared radiation than by 2 minutes specific warm-up.

## Chapter 13

## Activity 13.1

1.  (i) $p < 0.025$    significant
    (ii) $p < 0.005$    significant
    (iii) $p = 0.02$    significant
    (iv) $p$ is *greater than* 0.05, and is therefore not significant
    (v) $p < 0.001$    significant
    (vi) $p < 0.05$    significant

2. $\chi^2 = 9.6; p < 0.01$
    Using the McNemar test ($\chi^2 = 9.6$) the results were significant ($p < 0.01$ two-tailed). These results suggest that providing information about the reasons for changing on-call duty hours significantly alters physiotherapists' views in favour of the change.

## Activity 13.2

1. See Table A3.4.

**Table A3.4**

| Subject | Condition A | Condition B | d | Rank |
|---------|-------------|-------------|------|------|
| 1 | 10 | 9 | + 1 | 3.5 |
| 2 | 8 | 9 | − 1 | 3.5 |
| 3 | 9 | 7 | + 2 | 7 |
| 4 | 6 | 7 | − 1 | 3.5 |
| 5 | 5 | 4 | + 1 | 3.5 |
| 6 | 8 | 3 | + 5 | 11 |
| 7 | 7 | 6 | + 1 | 3.5 |
| 8 | 9 | 9 | 0 | omit |
| 9 | 9 | 6 | + 3 | 8 |
| 10 | 5 | 6 | − 1 | 3.5 |
| 11 | 7 | 3 | + 4 | 9.5 |
| 12 | 8 | 4 | + 4 | 9.5 |

2.  (i) $p < 0.05$    significant
    (ii) $p < 0.01$    significant
    (iii) $p < 0.025$    significant
    (iv) $p < 0.01$    significant
    (v) $p < 0.1$    not significant
    (vi) $p < 0.05$    significant
    (vii) $p = 0.01$    significant
    (viii) $p < 0.01$    significant

3. $T = 0$
    $N = 9$
    $p < 0.005$, one-tailed
    Using a Wilcoxon on the data ($T = 0, N = 9$) the results were found to be significant at $p < 0.005$ (one-tailed). These results support the hypothesis that traction is

significantly more effective than surgical collars in the treatment of cervical spondylosis.

## Activity 13.3

1.  (i) $p = 0.033$    significant
    (ii) $p < 0.02$    significant
    (iii) $p < 0.072$    not significant
    (iv) $p < 0.001$    significant
    (v) $p < 0.008$    significant
    (If you got any of these wrong, or are confused about the answers, do check that you were using the correct table.
2. $\chi r^2 = 2.658, p < 0.305$; not significant
    Using a Friedman test to analyse the data, the results were not significant ($\chi r^2 = 2.658, p < 0.305$). This suggests that there is no significant difference in the tone of the quadriceps muscle between Asian, Caucasian and African-Caribbean children. The null hypothesis can therefore be accepted.

## Activity 13.4

1.  (i) $p < 0.01$    significant
    (ii) $p = 0.05$    significant
    (iii) $p < 0.05$    significant
    (iv) $p < 0.001$    significant
    (v) $p$ is greater than 0.05 and is therefore not significant
2. $L = 105$    $p < 0.05$
    Using the Page's $L$ trend test to analyse the data, the results were significant ($L = 105, p < 0.05$). These results support the experimental hypothesis that hydrotherapy is more effective than exercise, which in turn is more effective than massage in the mobilistiaon of lower limbs paralysed following a stroke.

## Chapter 14

## Activity 14.1

1.  (i) $p < 0.025$    significant
    (ii) $p < 0.1$    not significant
    (iii) $p < 0.01$    significant
    (iv) $p < 0.01$    significant
    (v) $p < 0.02$    significant
2. $t = 2.362$; df $= 11$; $p < 0.025$
    Using a related $t$ test to analyse the data, the results were found to be significant at $p < 0.025$ ($t = 2.362$, df $= 11$). This suggests that student physiotherapists with 'A'-level physics do better in their 1st year theory exam marks than students without 'A'-level physics. The null hypothesis can therefore be rejected in favour of the experimental hypothesis.

## Activity 14.2

1.  (i) $p < 0.05$    significant
    (ii) $p < 0.01$    significant
    (iii) $p$ is greater than 0.05 and is therefore not significant
    (iv) $p < 0.025$    significant
    (v) $p < 0.05$    significant
    (iv) $p < 0.025$    significant

2. See Table A3.5.

**Table A3.5**

| Source of variation in scores | SS | df | MS | F ratios |
|---|---|---|---|---|
| Variation in scores between conditions | 31.445 | 2 | 15.723 | 3.529 |
| Variation in scores between subjects | 76.278 | 5 | 15.256 | 3.424 |
| Variation in scores due to random error | 44.555 | 10 | 4.456 | |
| Total | 152.278 | 17 | | |

$F$ ratio $= 3.529$; $df_{bet} = 2$; $df_{error} = 10$; $p$ is not significant.
$F$ ratio$_{subj} = 3.424$; $df_{subj} = 5$; $df_{error} = 10$
$p < 0.05$; significant

These results suggest that there is no significant effect from the different types of therapy used, but that the sets of matched subjects *were* significantly different from one another, and were therefore an atypical sample. These results can be expressed in the following way:

Using a one-way anova for related samples, no significant differences were found between the three treatment conditions ($F = 3.529$, $df_{bet} = 2$, $df_{error} = 10$). This suggests that the type of therapy used on hip replacement patients has no significant effect on mobility after 1 week. However, significant differences were found between the sets of matched subjects, ($F = 3.424$, $df_{subj} = 5$, $df_{error} = 10$, $p < 0.05$). This indicates that the subject sample was an atypical group and may represent a flaw in the sampling procedure. The null hypothesis must therefore be accepted.

## Activity 14.3

Comparisons:
a. *Condition 1* (seminar) × *Condition 2* (tutorial)
($F^1 = (C - 1)$ 3.29 $= 9.87$)
$F = 2.8$ $p > 0.05$ not significant
This suggests that the tutorial method is not significantly more effective than seminars in promoting understanding among a group of physiotherapy students.
b. *Condition 1* (seminar) × *Condition 3* (lecture)
($F^1 = (C - 1)$ 3.29 $= 9.87$)
$F = 0.194$; not significant
This suggests that there is no difference in the effectiveness of seminar or lecture methods in developing understanding among physiotherapy students.
c. *Condition 1* (seminar) × *Condition 4* (reading)
($F^1 = (C - 1)$ 3.29 $= 9.87$)
$F = 6.078$ $p > 0.05$ not significant
This suggests that seminars are no more effective than reading for developing understanding in a group of physiotherapy students.
d. *Condition 2* (tutorial) × *Condition 3* (lecture)
($F^1 = (C - 1)$ 3.29 $= 9.87$)
$F = 4.465$ $p > 0.05$ not significant
These results indicate that the tutorial is no more effective than lectures in developing student physiotherapists' understanding.

e. *Condition 2* (tutorial) × *Condition 4* (reading)
($F^1 = (C - 1)$ 5.42 $= 16.26$)
$F = 17.124$ $p < 0.01$, significant
These results suggest that tutorials are significantly more effective than reading for developing understanding in a group of physiotherapy students.
f. *Condition 3* (lecture) × *Condition 4* (reading)
($F^1 = (C - 1)$ 3.29 $= 9.87$)
$F = 4.101$ $p > 0.05$ not significant
These results suggest that lectures are no more effective than reading in promoting physiotherapy students' understanding.

## Chapter 15

## Activity 15.1

1. (i) $p < 0.025$ significant
(ii) $p < 0.02$ significant
(iii) $p < 0.05$ significant
(iv) $p$ is greater than 0.10 and is therefore not significant
(v) $p < 0.005$ significant
2. $\chi^2$ 8.377 df $= 1$, $p < 0.005$
Using a $\chi^2$ to analyse the data ($\chi^2 = 8.377$, df $= 1$) the results were significant ($p < 0.005$, one-tailed). This means that the null hypothesis can be rejected and that teachers of physiotherapy are more likely to study for Open University degree courses than clinically-based physiotherapists.

## Activity 15.2

1. (i) $p < 0.05$ significant
(ii) $p = 0.05$ significant
(iii) $p < 0.01$ significant
(iv) $p < 0.005$ significant
(v) $p < 0.05$ significant
(vi) $p$ is larger than 0.10 and is therefore not significant
2. $U = 45$, $p < 0.01$, one-tailed test
Using a Mann–Whitney $U$ test on the data ($U = 45$, $N_1 = 14$, $N_2 = 14$) the results were found to be significant at $p < 0.01$ for a one-tailed hypothesis. This suggests that the experimental hypothesis has been supported and that paraffin wax is more effective than a hot soak as a preparation for mobilising exercises on post-fracture patients.

## Activity 15.3

1. (i) $p < 0.046$ significant
(ii) $p = 0.049$ significant
(iii) $p < 0.05$ significant
(iv) $p < 0.011$ significant
(v) $p < 0.01$ significant
(vi) $p$ is larger than 0.05 and is therefore not significant
2. $H = 6.26$, $N_1 = 5$, $N_2 = 5$, $N_3 = 5$ $p < 0.049$
Using a Kruskal–Wallis test on the data ($H = 6.26$, $N_1 = 5$, $N_2 = 5$, $N_3 = 5$), the results were found to be significant $p < 0.049$ for a two-tailed test). This suggests that the three methods of giving postnatal exercise instructions are differentially effective. This means the null hypothesis can be rejected and the experimental hypothesis supported.

## Activity 15.4

1. (i) $p < 0.01$    significant
   (ii) $p$ is greater than 0.05 and so the results are not significant
   (iii) $p < 0.05$    significant
   (iv) $p < 0.01$    significant
   (v) $p < 0.05$    significant
   (vi) $p$ is greater than 0.05 and therefore the results are not significant
2. $A = 128$, $B = 192$, $S = 64$, $C = 3$, $n = 8$, $p < 0.05$
   Using a Jonckheere trend test to analyse the results ($S = 64$, $C = 3$, $n = 8$) the results were found to be significant ($p < 0.05$, one-tailed). This suggests that there is a significant trend in the probability of keeping outpatients' appointments, according to social class, with social class 3 being the most likely to keep them, followed by social class 2, and finally class 4. The null hypothesis can be rejected.

## Activity 15.5

1. (i) $p$ is greater than 10% and so the results are not significant.
   (ii) $p < 0.05$    significant
   (iii) $p < 0.05$    significant
   (iv) $p$ is greater than 5%, and so the results not significant
   (v) $p < 0.02$    significant
2. $\chi^2 = 5.095$, df $= 2$, $p$ is greater than 5% and so is not significant.
   Using an extended $\chi^2$ on the data, ($\chi^2 = 5.095$, df $= 2$) the results were found to be not significant ($p$ is greater than 5%). Therefore the null hypothesis is accepted; there is no significant relationship between keeping an outpatients' appointment and ease of journey, using public transport.

## Chapter 16

## Activity 16.1

1. (i) $p < 0.05$    significant
   (ii) $p < 0.02$    significant
   (iii) $p = 0.01$    significant
   (iv) $p$ is larger than 5% and so the results are not significant
   (v) $p < 0.01$    significant
2. $t = 2.43$; df $= 25$; $p < 0.025$
   Using an unrelated $t$ test on the data ($t = 2.43$, df $= 25$), the results were significant ($p < 0.025$ for a one-tailed test). The null hypothesis can be rejected. This suggests that absenteeism is significantly greater among basic grade physiotherapists than among senior IIs.

## Activity 16.2

1. (i) $p < 0.01$    significant
   (ii) $p < 0.001$    significant
   (iii) $p < 0.05$    significant
   (vi) $p < 0.01$    significant
2. $F = 2.171$, $p$ is greater than 5% and is therefore not significant.

### Table A3.6

| Source of variation | SS | df | MS | F ratio |
|---|---|---|---|---|
| Variation due to treatment, i.e. *between conditions* | 180.952 | 2 | 90.476 | 2.171 |
| Variation due to *random error* | 750 | 18 | 41.667 | |
| Total | 930.952 | 20 | | |

Using a one-way anova (see Table A3.6) for unrelated subject designs on the data ($F = 2.171$, df$_{bet} = 2$, df$_{error} = 18$) the results were found to be not significant ($p$ is greater than 5%). This means that the null hypothesis must be accepted and that there is no relationship between the age of cystic fibrosis patients and the efficacy of clapping.

## Activity 16.3

1. a. Comparison of 1975 and 1980
      $F = 4.982$
      $p$ is not significant
      i.e. 'A'-level results were not significantly higher in 1980 than in 1975.
   b. Comparison of 1975 and 1985
      $F = 35.124$
      $p < 0.001$
      i.e. 'A'-level results were significantly higher in 1985 than in 1975.
   c. Comparison of 1980 and 1985
      $F = 13.649$
      $p < 0.01$
      i.e. 'A'-level results were significantly higher in 1985 than in 1980.

## Chapter 17

## Activity 17.1

1. $H_1$   There is a relationship between the age of the patient and vital capacity.
   a. *Correlational design*
      You would select one group of subjects who represented a whole range of ages (e.g. 15–65). You would then measure their vital capacities to see if there was any correlation between age and vital capacity.
   b. *Experimental design*
      You have two possible options here.
      Firstly, you might select two groups of subjects one being at the young/ish end of the age range and the other being at the older end.
         Group 1    15–30 years (for example)
         Group 2    50–65 years (for example)
      You would measure their vital capacities to see if there was any difference between the groups.
      Alternatively, you might select a third group who represented a mid age range thus:
         Group 1    15–25 years (for example)
         Group 2    35–45 years (for example)
         Group 3    55–65 years (for example)
      Again you would compare their vital capacities for differences between the groups.

## Activity 17.2

1. $p < 0.01$
   $p$ = not significant
   $p$ = 0.02
   $p$ = not significant
   $p < 0.005$
2. Results of the calculation of the Spearman rho:
   $r_s$ = $-0.827$
   $p$ = $< 0.01$ (two-tailed)
   Using a Spearman test on the data, ($r_s$ = $-0.827, N$ = 10) the results were found to be significant ($p < 0.01$ for a two-tailed test). This suggests that there is a significant negative correlation between the length of lunch-break and professional competence. The null hypothesis can, therefore, be rejected.

## Activity 17.3

1. (i) $p < 0.05$
   (ii) $p$ = not significant
   (iii) $p < 0.005$
   (iv) $p$ = 0.02
   (v) $p < 0.001$
2. Results of the calculation of the Pearson product moment correlation:
   $r$ = $+0.899$
   $p < 0.005$ (one-tailed)
   Using a Pearson product moment correlation test on the data ($r$ = $+0.899$, df = 6), the results were found to be significant ($p < 0.005$, for a one-tailed test). This means that there is a significant positive correlation between students' marks on their 1st year exam and their averaged continuous assessment mark through the year. The null hypothesis can therefore be rejected.

## Activity 17.4

1. (i) $p < 0.05$
   (ii) $p$ is greater than 5% and is therefore not significant.
   (iii) $p < 0.01$
   (iv) $p < 0.01$
   (v) $p$ is greater than 5% and is therefore not significant.
2. Results of the calculation of the Kendall coefficient of concordance
   $s$ = 77, $W$ = 0.616
   $p < 0.05$
   Using the Kendall coefficient of concordance on the data ($s$ = 77, $W$ = 6.61, $n$ = 5, $N$ = 4) the results were found to be significant ($P < 0.05$ for a one-tailed test). This suggests that there is significant agreement on knee movement when measured by a goniometer. The null hypothesis can be rejected.

## Activity 17.5

1. a = 0.939, b = 0.47
   a. This patient would be in labour for 11.1749 hours.
   b. This patient would be in labour for 8.459 hours.
   c. This patient would be in labour for 14.569 hours.

## Chapter 18

## Activity 18.1

1. The proportion of non-attenders in the outpatient clinic will be somewhere between 0.3–0.46 (for 95% confidence level).
2. The average amount of physiotherapy time learning disabled children will require will be between 2.25–4.15 hours, per child, per week (99% confidence level).
3. The average life expectancy of your ulatrasound machine is estimated, with 90% confidence to fall within the confidence interval of 4.07–4.53 years.

# Glossary

**abstract** (Also called a summary) a résumé usually found at the beginning of journal articles, which summarises the key features of the study.

**analysis of variance** (anova) a statistical technique which allows the simultaneous comparison of three or more sets of data derived from experimental designs. There are a number of variants on this technique which allow the researcher to analyse data from different-, same- and matched-subject designs, or a mixture of both. While there are non-parametric analyses of variance tests, the term anova is commonly taken to mean the parametric variety, while the non-parametric tests are referred to by specific names (e.g. Kruskal–Wallis test).

**apparatus** any equipment used in a research project.

**bar graph** a graph used to show the frequency of a given event by the height of vertically arranged bars or columns. These bars have spaces between them.

**baseline** a stage in a research project when the subjects receive no treatment or intervention.

**bias** any distortion in results due to flaws in the design of the study. (See also *experimenter bias*.)

**central tendency** a description of a set of results which typically makes use of the average score, the most commonly occurring score and the mid-score of that set of data.

**characteristic** this is some feature of a population for which the researcher wishes to make an estimate from a sample of that population.

**chi-squared test ($\chi^2$)** a non-parametric statistical test used to analyse two sets of nominal data from different subject designs which employ two groups of subjects only. (See also *extended $\chi^2$ test*.)

**clinical significance** the degree to which a set of results have some clinical meaning or relevance.

Sometimes results can be statistically significant but clinically meaningless.

**closed-response question** any question which is framed in such a way that only a limited number of answers are possible.

**confidence interval** a range in a set of scores derived from a sample in which the population characteristic is confidently expected to fall.

**confidence level** the degree of confidence which can be placed in an estimate of a population characteristic. It is expressed as a percentage and the most commonly used levels are 90%, 95% and 99%.

**confidence limits** the upper and lower figures of the confidence interval

**constant errors** any sources of bias and error in a research project which will influence the results in a constant and predictable way. They must be controlled or eliminated: if they are not then the conclusions may be wrong, misleading and possibly dangerous.

**control group** a group of subjects in an experimental design which does not receive any treatment or intervention. This group can then be compared with the experimental group which does receive some intervention, in order to establish the effects of the independent variable.

**correlation coefficient** a numerical value somewhere between $-1.0$ and $+1.0$ which indicates the degree and nature of the association between sets of data derived from a correlational design.

**correlational designs** designs which test an experimental hypothesis by collecting data on both the variables in the hypothesis to see if the data is related in some way. The two relationships which are of interest are *positive correlations* and *negative correlations* (see entries under these headings).

237

**counterbalancing** a technique used in research design to overcome the bias caused by order effects. It involves ensuring that the order of testing a group of subjects is alternated so that any results will not be influenced by the sequence of testing.

**data** the facts and figures collected during a research project.

**degrees of freedom** a complex concept involved in some statistical tests which refers to the extent to which data have the capacity to vary once certain limits have been imposed. It is abbreviated to df and is very easy to calculate.

**dependent variable** the variable in an experimental hypothesis which changes as a result of manipulating the independent variable. The changes in the dependent variable constitute the data in a study and can be thought of as the effects of the manipulation of the independent variable.

**descriptive statistics** methods of describing a set of results in terms of their most interesting characteristics.

**different-subject design** experimental designs which use two or more separate or different groups of subjects each of which is tested once. The groups are then compared for any differences between them. Sometimes known as a between- or unrelated-subjects design.

**discussion** a section of a research report which discusses the findings of that research.

**double-blind technique** an aspect of research design whose aim is to minimise the biasing effect that subjects and experimenters may have on the results by knowing what the aims of the study are. The double-blind procedure involves keeping the subjects ignorant of the project's aims until after the data has been collected, as well as using someone other than the main researcher to collect the data. This person will also be unaware of the purpose of the research project.

**estimation** a form of scientific 'best guessing' where estimates of a population characteristic are made on the basis of knowledge of the sample characteristic. It is a useful tool in planning.

**ethics** a set of guidelines imposed on a study to ensure that the project will not compromise or upset the subjects in any way.

**experimental condition** a group of subjects in an experimental design which receives some form of intervention or level of the independent variable. This group may be compared with other experimental groups who receive a different form of intervention or with a control group who receive no intervention at all.

**experimental design** a method of testing hypotheses which involves manipulating the independent variable(s) in the experimental hypothesis and monitoring what impact this has on the dependent variable. By doing this cause and effect can be established.

**experimental hypothesis** a prediction of a consistent and reliable relationship between two or more variables. The experimental hypothesis is the starting point of any piece of experimental research and is often referred to in the literature as $H_1$.

**experimenter bias effects** a source of bias to the results which results from the experimenter (usually unwittingly) influencing subjects' responses so that they fulfil the experimenter's aims. It can be counteracted to some extent by using a naive data collector (see single-blind procedures).

**extended chi-squared ($\chi^2$) test** a non-parametric statistical test for use with nominal data and different subject designs. It is used with more than two nominal categories and/or more than two groups of subjects.

**fatigue effects** an aspect of order problems where subjects do worse on the second or subsequent testing because of fatigue. This can mask the real effects of the independent variable.

**frequency distribution graph** a graph which presents the frequency with which any given event occurs. These graphs can be bar graphs, histograms and frequency polygons (see separate entries).

**frequency polygon** a frequency distribution graph which is characterised by the single continuous line drawn between the points on the graph.

**Friedman test** a non-parametric analysis of variance for use with same- or matched-subject design, using more than two testing conditions. The data can be ordinal or interval/ratio, but this test is most likely to be used with ordinal data.

**histogram** a frequency distribution graph characterised by the use of adjacent vertical columns.

**incidental sample** a method of selecting subjects for study which involves using the most easily available people.

**independent variable** that variable in the experimental hypothesis which is manipulated so that the impact of this on the dependent variable can be observed. It can be thought of as the cause of something happening.

**inferential statistics** a statistical technique whereby results derived from a sample of subjects are also inferred to apply to the population from which they come.

**interobserver reliability** the degree to which two or more people agree in their observations of an event.

**interval level of measurement** usually linked with the ratio level of measurement, this is a level of data which: (a) allows parametric statistical tests to be performed; (b) assumes equal intervals in measurement between the data; (c) has no absolute zero (i.e. a score of 0 does not mean the absence of that characteristic).

**interview** a conversation between the researcher and the subject which aims to elicit information relevant to the research topic. This interview may follow prescribed topics (structured interview) or may be entirely open (unstructured interview).

**introduction** (to a research report) the section of a research report which reviews the relevant literature, and provides a rationale and the aims of the study in question.

**Jonckheere trend test** a non-parametric statistical analysis which is used with three or more separate groups of subjects (a different-subject design), ordinal or interval/ratio data, and where the results are expected to be in a specified trend.

**Kendall's coefficient of concordance** a non-parametric statistical test used with correlational designs and ordinal data which assesses the extent of agreement between three or more sets of data.

**Kruskal–Wallis test** a non-parametric analysis of variance test used with three or more separate groups of subjects (a different-subject design) and ordinal or interval/ratio data.

**levels of measurement** the data collected from a piece of research fall into one of four levels of measurement, which differ in their sophistication and the type of calculation that can be performed on them. These levels are (in order of sophistication from least to most):

Nominal (least)
Ordinal
Interval
Ratio (most)

**linear regression** a statistical technique used with sets of data known to be correlated, such that values on one variable can be calculated from knowledge of the values on the other.

**literature review** a survey of all the research relevant to the topic in question, which allows the researcher to establish what has already been carried out.

**Mann–Whitney *U*-test** a non-parametric statistical test used with two separate groups of subjects (a different-subject design) and ordinal or interval/ratio data.

**matched-subject designs** types of experimental designs which involve matching subjects on all those factors which may affect the results. While these designs have the advantage of not being affected by individual differences and order effects, they are very difficult to carry out properly.

**materials** any non-mechanical items used in a piece of research, e.g. questionnaires, blood pressure sheets etc.

**McNemar test** a non-parametric statistical test used with same- or matched-subject designs, two testing conditions and nominal data. It assesses the significance of any changes noted over the two testings.

**mean** the average score in a set of data, calculated by adding all the scores up and dividing this total by the number of scores in the set of data.

**median** the middle score in a set of data, such that there are as many scores above it as below.

**method** the section of a research report which describes in detail what was done, how and with whom, in a piece of research. It should be sufficiently detailed that anyone who reads this section should be able to replicate the study exactly.

**mode** the most frequently occurring score in a set of data.

**negative correlation** the relationship between two sets of data derived from a correlational design, whereby high scores on one set of data are associated with low scores on the other.

**negative skew** a frequency distribution distorted to one side because too many subjects recorded high scores (see Fig. 5.11).

**nominal level of measurement** a very basic level of measurement (sometimes referred to as categorical data) which simply allocates subjects or their responses to named categories. It is characterised by the following:
(a) Only non-parametric statistical analyses can be performed on this data.
(b) The categories are mutually exclusive.
(c) There is no commonly understood value attached to the category labels.

**non-parametric tests** these are techniques of data analysis which are less sensitive and rather cruder than parametric tests. They can be used, in principle, with all levels of measurement, but are most commonly associated with the nominal and ordinal levels.

**normal distribution** a symmetrical bell-shaped curve which has certain properties which are critical to statistical inference.

**null hypothesis** the prediction which counters the claim made by the experimental hypothesis in a study. The null hypothesis predicts there is no relationship between the variables in the experimental hypothesis. It is often referred to in the literature as $H_0$.

**observation** a technique of conducting research which involves the researcher simply observing what goes on in naturalistic settings.

**one-tailed hypotheses or tests** these refer to hypotheses where a prediction is made that the results of the study will be in a specific direction.

**open-ended questions** questions which allow the respondent to reply in a free and unstructured way to any given question.

**order effects** a source of bias usually found in same-subject designs where the order in which the subjects were tested rather than the independent variable produces the results. This can be overcome by counterbalancing the order of testing.

**ordinal level of measurement** a type of data which allows the researcher to rank order subjects along the dimension of interest (e.g. least improvement–most improvement). An important feature of this scale is that while it allows the researcher to impose a numerical score on the subject's response, the differences between the points on the scale are not equal.

**Page's *L* trend test** a non-parametric test used with same- or matched-subject designs which yields three or more sets of ordinal or interval/ratio data. A particular characteristic is that a trend in the results is specifically predicted.

**parametric tests** techniques of statistical analysis which are said to be robust and sensitive. They require certain conditions or parameters to be fulfilled before they can be applied, the most important of which is that the data must be interval/ratio.

**Pearson test** a parametric test for use with correlational designs and interval/ratio data.

**pilot study** a preliminary run of the main study to highlight any problems which can then be corrected.

**placebo effect** an interesting phenomenon whereby subjects show a significant degree of improvement even though their treatment is known to have no use.

**point estimation** a statistical 'best guess' which provides a single figure estimate (usually an average or percentage figure) of a population characteristic based on information about the sample's characteristic.

**population** a group of people all of whom have a characteristic in common which is of interest to the researcher, e.g. talipes. The sample for study in the research is drawn from this parent population.

**population characteristic** see *characteristic*.

**positive correlation** the degree of relationship between the data from two or more variables derived from a correlational design, such that high scores on one variable are associated with high scores from the other(s), and similarly low scores are associated with low scores.

**positive skew** a frequency distribution where the data are distorted towards the lower scores, for example, where students perform badly on an exam which is too difficult (see Fig. 5.10).

**post–test** a measurement of the dependent variable which takes place after the intervention has occurred.

**practice effects** a variety of order effects whereby subjects perform better on second and subsequent testings and this improved performance masks the effects of the independent variable.

**pre-test** a measurement of the dependent variable which takes place before any intervention has occurred.

**probability** the likelihood that random error is producing the results in a study. It is expressed as a percentage or decimal and is usually abbreviated to '$p$'.

**qualitative research** techniques of research investigation which collect non-numerical information from subjects.

**quantitative research** techniques of research which collect numerical information from subjects.

**questionnaires** a method of collecting information whereby subjects answer a set of questions usually predefined by the researcher.

**quota sample** a process of selecting a sample to participate in a research study, such that pre-set quotas of subjects will be selected to represent categories deemed to be important.

**random errors** any sources of bias or error in a piece of research which will affect the results in a random and unpredictable way. They include a variety of individual differences and cannot be eliminated completely.

**random number tables** tables of randomly generated numbers which can be used to select a random sample of subjects for study.

**random selection/sample** a method of selecting subjects to take part in a study, such that every member of the parent population has an equal chance of being chosen.

**range** the difference between the lowest score and the highest score in a set of data.

**ratio level of measurement** the 'highest' level of data which is characterised by equal intervals between the data points and an absolute zero which represents an absence of the quality in question.

**references** a section in a research report which lists all the research articles referred to in the body of the report.

**related *t* test** a parametric statistical test for use with same- or matched-subject designs and two sets of interval/ratio data.

**representative sample** a sample which is typical or accurately reflects the population from which it comes.

**research proposal** an outline of an anticipated piece of research covering background literature, aims, objectives, methodology, proposed analysis, and a cost/benefit analysis. A research proposal is often required by ethical committees or when funding is applied for.

**same-subject designs** a variant of experimental design which involves testing the same group of subjects on two or more occasions. They are typically used in before/after designs.

**sample** a group of subjects selected from a parent population, who are used in a piece of research.

**scattergram** a technique of plotting data derived from correlational studies in a graph. A general upward slope to the graph indicates a positive correlation, while a general downward slope indicates a negative correlation.

**Scheffé multiple range test** a statistical technique used in conjunction with parametric anovas which have yielded significant results. The Scheffe test allows the researcher to make an objective scrutiny of the data in order to establish which parts were responsible for the significant anova results.

**significance level** A cut-off point, usually of 5% or less, such that if the results from a piece of research have a probability of 5% or less of being due to random error, then they are said to be significant.

The null (no relationship) hypothesis can then be rejected in favour of the experimental hypothesis.

**Spearman test** a non-parametric test for use with correlational designs and ordinal or interval/ratio data.

**standard deviation** a measure of the average amount that a set of scores varies or deviates from the mean.

**stratified random sample** a method of selecting a sample from a population, so that subgroups of that population are represented in the sample.

**subjects** the individual people who take part in a study.

**surveys** a method of collecting data which involves the researcher measuring relevant sample variables (often using a questionnaire) without any form of manipulation or systematic intervention.

**systematic sample** a method of selecting a sample for study by choosing every fourth, fifth or whatever, member of the parent population.

**two-tailed hypothesis or test** an experimental hypothesis which, simply predicts that the variables in the hypothesis are related, but does not specify the precise nature of that relationship.

**Type I error** a conclusion that there is a relationship between the variables in the hypothesis, when in fact there is not.

**Type II error** a conclusion that there is no relationship between the variables in the hypothesis when, in fact, there is.

**Unrelated *t* test** a parametric statistical test used with two different groups of subjects and interval/ratio data.

**variable** any event or characteristic which has the capacity to vary (e.g. weight, age etc.).

**variance** the degree to which a set of scores vary or are dispersed

**Wilcoxon test** a non-parametric statistical test used with same- or matched-subject designs, and two sets of ordinal or interval/ratio data.

# References

Cartwright A 1983 Health surveys in practice and potential. King Edward's Hospital Fund for London, London

Chalmers A F 1983 What is this thing called science? Open University Press, Milton Keynes

Darbyshire P 1986 When the face doesn't fit! Nursing Times 82 (39): 28–30

Ferguson G A 1976 Statistical analysis in psychology and education. McGraw-Hill Kogakusha, Tokyo

Gardener G 1978 Social surveys for social planners. Open University Press, Milton Keynes

Green J, D'Oliveira M 1982 Learning to use statistical tests in psychology. Open University Press, Milton Keynes

Hicks C M 1993 Effects of psychological prejudices on communication and social interaction. British Journal of Midwifery 1 (1): 10–16

Hunt M 1987 The process of translating research findings into nursing practice. Journal of Advanced Nursing 12: 101–110

McNemar Q 1962 Psychological statistics. Wiley, New York

Oppenheim A N 1966 Questionnaire design and attitude measurement. Heinemann Education, London

Peters D P, Ceci S 1982 Peer-review practices of psychological journals – the fate of accepted, published articles submitted again. Behavioural and Brain Sciences 5 (2): 187–195

Polgar S, Thomas S A 1992 Introduction to research in the health sciences. Churchill Livingstone, Edinburgh

Robson C 1974 Experiment, design and statistics in psychology. Penguin, Harmondsworth

Sanders D H, Eng R J, & Murph A F 1985 Statistics: a fresh approach. McGraw Hill, New York

Siegel S 1956 Nonparametric statistics for the behavioural sciences. McGraw Hill Kogakusha, Tokyo

# Index